VIROLOGY RESEARCH PROGRESS

VIRAL INFECTIONS

CAUSES, TREATMENT OPTIONS AND POTENTIAL COMPLICATIONS

VIROLOGY RESEARCH PROGRESS

Additional books in this series can be found on Nova's website under the Series tab.

Additional e-books in this series can be found on Nova's website under the e-book tab.

VIROLOGY RESEARCH PROGRESS

VIRAL INFECTIONS

CAUSES, TREATMENT OPTIONS AND POTENTIAL COMPLICATIONS

DEBORAH SHINN
EDITOR

New York

For permission to use material from this book please contact us:
Telephone 631-231-7269; Fax 631-231-8175
Web Site: http://www.novapublishers.com

Library of Congress Cataloging-in-Publication Data

ISBN: 978-1-63117-221-2
Library of Congress Control Number: 2014931127

Published by Nova Science Publishers, Inc. † New York

CONTENTS

PREFACE

Viral infection is a disease caused by microorganisms, which invade a living cell and use its mechanisms to reproduce. Viruses need to colonize a host organism in order to fulfill its vital functions because it lacks the biochemical organizations that replication requires. This book discusses several topics that include viral infections in obstetrics and gynecology; the management of HIV infection by Chinese medicine; antiviral activity of lactoferrin; and antiviral effects of phytochemicals of the Mediterranean medicinal plants.

Chapter 1 – Viral infection is a disease caused by infectious microorganisms, viruses, which invade a living cell and use its mechanisms to reproduce. The virus is, in fact, a microorganism whose size ranges from 10 nanometers (0.000000001 meters) to a few microns (0.0000001 meters), and then an average of 100 times smaller than a common cell. It has such a structure as having to forcibly live as a parasite. In fact, in order to fulfil its vital functions, it needs to colonize a host organism, because it lacks the biochemical organizations that the replication requests. Viruses, therefore, attack the cells of living organisms, they invade and colonize them. Once entered into a cell, they release their genetic heritage consisting of deoxy-ribonucleic acid (DNA) or ribonucleic acid (RNA), which takes control of the host cell and forces it to replicate the virus. Normally, as a result of this process, the cell, no longer able to perform its natural functions, dies (apoptosis) but first it releases the replicated viruses that go to infect new cells. In this way, the infection triggers and develops. However, there are kinds of viruses that instead of killing the host cell alter its characteristics and functions. Thus, it may happen that the guest can no longer control the natural cell division and becomes a cancer cell. It can also happen that the virus after the infection leaves the genetic heritage in a silent form within the cell. And if after some time, for any event, the balance reached perturbs the virus awakens. Thus it begins again to replicate and to trigger a relapse of the disease. The infection occurs when the virus is able to penetrate into the body nevertheless its natural defensive barriers. Once in the body, it can proliferate in the point where the entrance has occurred or through the bloodstream and/or the lymphatic vessels it can reach a target organ and attach itself to the cells of this. Obviously, an important role is also played by the way in which the transmission takes place. The modalities are varied. The most common are: 1) ingestion and so by the oral-fecal route; 2) inhalation and so by the respiratory route; 3) insect bites and so by the trans-dermal route; 4) through the microscopic lesions of the mucous membranes of the male and female genitals; 5) direct contact with blood and then by the injecting route (utilization of used syringes or toilet articles); and 6) by vertical transmission from mother to fetus through the placenta. The evolution of viral infection depends on various parameters and precisely: 1) the characteristics of the virus, i.e., the ease with which it passes from one host to another, how easily it can overcome the defences opposed by the host, how much it is able to withstand them, how much damage it is able to create; 2) the characteristics of the system that defences the host, i.e., in the human body such function is performed as the first instance by a series of natural and physical barriers (skin, mucous membranes, secretions, gastric juices, etc.), and as the second instance by the immune system: this has the task to organize the internal defence and to destroy the outsiders retained as potentially dangerous and thus also the viruses. There are substances called "antigens" localized on the surface of the virus or in its internal part that alert the immune system of the threat. The army that the immune system alerts and detaches is instead made by the white cells of the blood; and 3) the state of the environment in which the host lives, i.e., there are some factors that clearly facilitate the spread and progression of the infection: examples are the climatic conditions, etc. Once the infection has occurred, the response of the immune system is triggered which can lead to three different conditions: 1) the white cells of the blood, particularly the lymphocytes, recognize the enemy, attack it, and if possible destroy it along with the infected cells; 2) the virus instead is able to overcome the body's defences and the infection spreads; and 3) a state of equilibrium between the virus and the body that causes a chronic infection is reached. If the body can overcome the infection and heal, the lymphocytes retain memory of the intruder.

Therefore, if the same pathogen reappears in the future, they are able, on the basis of the past experience, to organize countermeasures quickly and efficiently and to eliminate the new threat. This mechanism is referred to as immunity. It is important to note that it is the basis of the operation of the vaccines. These, in fact, are made from inactivated viruses or parts of them and therefore they cannot, if inoculated, unleash a true infection, but they are equally useful to the immune system to recognize the pathogen and to develop antibodies that will then allow to immediately locate and eradicate it at his next attack. Each virus generally infects a particular cell type, such as those of the cold penetrate the cells of the respiratory tract, the rabies and encephalitis viruses infect the cells of the central nervous system (CNS). The viruses that affect the female reproductive organs and then external but also internal ones such as uterus and ovaries are Herpes Simplex Virus (HSV), Human Papilloma Virus (HPV), Human Immunodeficiency Virus (HIV), Hepatitis B Virus (HBV), and Hepatitis C Virus (HCV). HSV causes genital blisters, pain, and urinating difficulty.

HPV are almost completely asymptomatic and are accompanied by only small lesions of the genitals, but that may develop into cancerous lesions. HIV deserves a special mention, since it is the virus that causes the acquired immune deficiency syndrome (AIDS) that severely compromises the efficiency of the immune system and leaves the body at the mercy of any aggression. HBV and HCV are viruses that target the liver as an organ, but they are transmitted through unprotected sex intercourse and cause viral hepatitis B and C. Viral infections of the genital tract are particularly dangerous during pregnancy, because they can cause miscarriage and fetal malformations. Some types of viruses, as already mentioned, do not kill the host cell but alter its DNA. All this means that in the future it can degenerate and lead to cancer. The main types of viruses to which this capacity is recognized are: 1) HPV: it can lead to cancers of the cervix uteri; 2) HBV and HCV: they can induce the development of liver cancer; 3) Human Herpesvirus (HHV) 8: it causes the development of Kaposi's sarcoma in AIDS patients; and 4) Epstein-Barr Virus (EBV): the virus of the infectious mononucleosis can cause Burkitt's lymphoma, that is a neoplasm of B lymphocytes. The drugs used to fight viral infections are just called "antivirals". They work by blocking the process of replication of the virus responsible for the infection. But, since the viruses to replicate exploit the metabolic structures of the cell that they have infected, the range of action of these drugs is especially low because the structures against which they can be addressed are numerically limited. Moreover, they have a high toxicity also for the cells of the body in addition to the viral agent. All this means that the antiviral drugs are very difficult to produce and to use. And to make the situation even more difficult there is also the capability of a virus to develop resistance to them with ease.

Antiviral drugs reduce the duration of symptoms and among the most used are: 1) Acyclovir (ACV), for Herpes Zoster and genital Herpes; 2) Cidofovir, against infection by Cytomegalovirus (CMV); 3) Alpha-Interferon (IFN), against hepatitis B and C; 4) Amantadine, for type A influenza; and 5) Zanamivir, for type A and B influenza. The best cure to viral infections therefore remains prevention which is based on the vaccine when it exists. But also this weapon which mechanism has been previously described is difficult to use given the speed of certain viruses to mutate. A typical example is provided by the Influenza Virus that mutates so quickly that every year a new epidemic comes with a totally new strain, and forces to prepare a new type of vaccine to combat it. It is absolutely useless to take antibiotics for diseases caused by viruses. Antibiotics have effect on bacteria. And they should be used only on special occasions and on doctor's prescription if he believes that a secondary bacterial infection is superimposed to the viral one.

Chapter 2 – Human immunodeficiency virus (HIV) is a retrovirus that causes the immunodeficiency illness. HIV infection is an important infectious disease that can be seen around the world. This disease is still a problematic public health threat since there is still no successful therapeutic option for HIV. The management of HIV by alternative medicine is an interesting topic. Here, the authors will briefly review and discuss on the role of Chinese medicine for management of HIV infection.

Chapter 3 – Lactoferrin (Lf) is a multifunctional iron-binding glycoprotein present in most biological fluids of mammals, being abundant in milk and colostrum. It was shown that Lf is a key player in the innate immune defense, as it is rapidly released from the neutrophils during an inflammatory response. Besides the immunomodulatory activity, Lf plays a plethora of biological functions, such as anti-tumoral, bactericidal and antiviral. Most of these activities are associated with the N-terminal region of the protein.

As for other functions, the antiviral mechanism of Lf is a multifaceted property and not yet fully defined. Lf was demonstrated to exert *in vitro* and *in vivo* anti-viral activity against a broad range of RNA and DNA viruses such as influenza viruses, human immunodeficiency virus (HIV), rotaviruses, Japanese encephalitis virus (JEV), hepatitis B and C viruses (HBV and HCV) or poliovirus. The antiviral mechanisms of action of Lf were suggested to involve prevention of viral infection of the target cell by direct binding to virus particle or by competition for /or blocking the common receptors/co-receptors at the cell membrane. Since Lf binds to most cells and Lf receptors with either low or high affinity for the protein have been described, intracellular antiviral activities of Lf involving apoptosis or inflammatory pathways have been proposed. Intriguingly, several peptides derived from Lf were shown to preserve the beneficial antiviral activity of the parental protein. Moreover, synergistic effects of antiviral drugs in combination with Lf or Lf -derived peptides were reported. However, only a few antiviral studies using Lf have reached the level of clinical trials.

Despite continuous improvement of current therapies, many viruses develop resistance during treatment, therefore the search for alternative antiviral strategies remains a very hot topic. Owing to its remarkable antiviral properties and lack of cellular toxicity Lf has recently received increasing attention from virologists and clinicians, much effort being devoted in subscribing this interesting protein to a therapeutic platform.

The present work is a critical overview of the mechanisms proposed to explain the antiviral activity of Lf and Lf-derived peptides, and their use as a possible novel strategy in antiviral therapeutics.

Chapter 4 – Viral infection is an important health problem worldwide due to the rapid development of resistant mutants against current therapeutic agents. There are only a few antiviral drugs available for the treatment of viral diseases and they have generally inadequate efficacy and a number of serious adverse effects. Medicinal plants may be an alternative strategy for treatment of viral diseases. Although many herbs have a very good folkloric reputation, their antiviral properties have not yet been investigated. Medicinal plants from the Mediterranean region have been used in medicine since ancient times and are well known for their successful therapeutic activity. Many phytochemicals including glycosides, flavonoids, terpenoids, polyphenolics, coumarins, saponins, furil compounds, alkaloids, different sugars, proteins and peptides isolated from these plants demonstrated antiviral properties.

The purpose of this review is to provide the verified data on the antiviral activities of the herb extracts and pure compounds isolated from the medicinal plants of the Mediterranean flora and to discuss the various mechanisms of their actions.

In: Viral Infections
Editor: Deborah Shinn
ISBN: 978-1-63117-221-2

Chapter 1

VIRAL INFECTIONS IN OBSTETRICS AND GYNECOLOGY

Ciro Comparetto[1,*] and Franco Borruto[2]
[1]Division of Obstetrics and Gynecology,
City Hospital, Prato, Italy
[2]Professor of Obstetrics and Gynecology,
Princess Grace Hospital, Principality of Monaco

ABSTRACT

Viral infection is a disease caused by infectious microorganisms, viruses, which invade a living cell and use its mechanisms to reproduce. The virus is, in fact, a microorganism whose size ranges from 10 nanometers (0.000000001 meters) to a few microns (0.0000001 meters), and then an average of 100 times smaller than a common cell. It has such a structure as having to forcibly live as a parasite. In fact, in order to fulfil its vital functions, it needs to colonize a host organism, because it lacks the biochemical organizations that the replication requests. Viruses, therefore, attack the cells of living organisms, they invade and colonize them. Once entered into a cell, they release their genetic heritage consisting of deoxy-ribonucleic acid (DNA) or ribonucleic acid (RNA), which takes control of the host cell and forces it to replicate the virus. Normally, as a result of this process, the cell, no longer able to perform its natural functions, dies (apoptosis) but first it releases the replicated

* Corresponding author: Ciro Comparetto. E-mail: cicomp@tin.it.

viruses that go to infect new cells. In this way, the infection triggers and develops. However, there are kinds of viruses that instead of killing the host cell alter its characteristics and functions. Thus, it may happen that the guest can no longer control the natural cell division and becomes a cancer cell. It can also happen that the virus after the infection leaves the genetic heritage in a silent form within the cell. And if after some time, for any event, the balance reached perturbs the virus awakens. Thus it begins again to replicate and to trigger a relapse of the disease. The infection occurs when the virus is able to penetrate into the body nevertheless its natural defensive barriers. Once in the body, it can proliferate in the point where the entrance has occurred or through the bloodstream and/or the lymphatic vessels it can reach a target organ and attach itself to the cells of this. Obviously, an important role is also played by the way in which the transmission takes place. The modalities are varied. The most common are: 1) ingestion and so by the oral-fecal route; 2) inhalation and so by the respiratory route; 3) insect bites and so by the trans-dermal route; 4) through the microscopic lesions of the mucous membranes of the male and female genitals; 5) direct contact with blood and then by the injecting route (utilization of used syringes or toilet articles); and 6) by vertical transmission from mother to fetus through the placenta. The evolution of viral infection depends on various parameters and precisely: 1) the characteristics of the virus, i.e., the ease with which it passes from one host to another, how easily it can overcome the defences opposed by the host, how much itis able to withstand them, how much damage it is able to create; 2) the characteristics of the system that defences the host, i.e., in the human body such function is performed as the first instance by a series of natural and physical barriers (skin, mucous membranes, secretions, gastric juices, etc.), and as the second instance by the immune system: this has the task to organize the internal defence and to destroy the outsiders retained as potentially dangerous and thus also the viruses. There are substances called "antigens" localized on the surface of the virus or in its internal part that alert the immune system of the threat. The army that the immune system alerts and detaches is instead made by the white cells of the blood; and 3) the state of the environment in which the host lives, i.e., there are some factors that clearly facilitate the spread and progression of the infection: examples are the climatic conditions, etc. Once the infection has occurred, the response of the immune system is triggered which can lead to three different conditions: 1) the white cells of the blood, particularly the lymphocytes, recognize the enemy, attack it, and if possible destroy it along with the infected cells; 2) the virus instead is able to overcome the body's defences and the infection spreads; and 3) a state of equilibrium between the virus and the body that causes a chronic infection is reached. If the body can overcome the infection and heal, the lymphocytes retain memory of the intruder.

Therefore, if the same pathogen reappears in the future, they are able, on the basis of the past experience, to organize countermeasures quickly and efficiently and to eliminate the new threat. This mechanism is referred to as immunity. It is important to note that it is the basis of the operation of the vaccines. These, in fact, are made from inactivated viruses or parts of them and therefore they cannot, if inoculated, unleash a true infection, but they are equally useful to the immune system to recognize the pathogen and to develop antibodies that will then allow to immediately locate and eradicate it at his next attack. Each virus generally infects a particular cell type, such as those of the cold penetrate the cells of the respiratory tract, the rabies and encephalitis viruses infect the cells of the central nervous system (CNS). The viruses that affect the female reproductive organs and then external but also internal ones such as uterus and ovaries are Herpes Simplex Virus (HSV), Human Papilloma Virus (HPV), Human Immunodeficiency Virus (HIV), Hepatitis B Virus (HBV), and Hepatitis C Virus (HCV). HSV causes genital blisters, pain, and urinating difficulty.

HPV are almost completely asymptomatic and are accompanied by only small lesions of the genitals, but that may develop into cancerous lesions. HIV deserves a special mention, since it is the virus that causes the acquired immune deficiency syndrome (AIDS) that severely compromises the efficiency of the immune system and leaves the body at the mercy of any aggression. HBV and HCV are viruses that target the liver as an organ, but they are transmitted through unprotected sex intercourse and cause viral hepatitis B and C. Viral infections of the genital tract are particularly dangerous during pregnancy, because they can cause miscarriage and fetal malformations. Some types of viruses, as already mentioned, do not kill the host cell but alter its DNA. All this means that in the future it can degenerate and lead to cancer. The main types of viruses to which this capacity is recognized are: 1) HPV: it can lead to cancers of the cervix uteri; 2) HBV and HCV: they can induce the development of liver cancer; 3) Human Herpesvirus (HHV) 8: it causes the development of Kaposi's sarcoma in AIDS patients; and 4) Epstein-Barr Virus (EBV): the virus of the infectious mononucleosis can cause Burkitt's lymphoma, that is a neoplasm of B lymphocytes. The drugs used to fight viral infections are just called "antivirals". They work by blocking the process of replication of the virus responsible for the infection. But, since the viruses to replicate exploit the metabolic structures of the cell that they have infected, the range of action of these drugs is especially low because the structures against which they can be addressed are numerically limited. Moreover, they have a high toxicity also for the cells of the body in addition to the viral agent. All this means that the antiviral drugs are very difficult to produce and to use. And to make the situation even more difficult there is also the capability of a virus to develop resistance to them with ease.

Antiviral drugs reduce the duration of symptoms and among the most used are: 1) Acyclovir (ACV), for Herpes Zoster and genital Herpes; 2) Cidofovir, against infection by Cytomegalovirus (CMV); 3) Alpha-Interferon (IFN), against hepatitis B and C; 4) Amantadine, for type A influenza; and 5) Zanamivir, for type A and B influenza. The best cure to viral infections therefore remains prevention which is based on the vaccine when it exists. But also this weapon which mechanism has been previously described is difficult to use given the speed of certain viruses to mutate. A typical example is provided by the Influenza Virus that mutates so quickly that every year a new epidemic comes with a totally new strain, and forces to prepare a new type of vaccine to combat it. It is absolutely useless to take antibiotics for diseases caused by viruses. Antibiotics have effect on bacteria. And they should be used only on special occasions and on doctor's prescription if he believes that a secondary bacterial infection is superimposed to the viral one.

INTRODUCTION

The majority of infectious diseases in the gynecological patient arise at the mucosal surfaces. Mucosal surface pathogens must compete with organisms which are members of the normal flora and with local immunity. The host possesses a variety of defence mechanisms which operate in concert to prevent infection or alter the course of an infective process. In the surgical patient, infection usually arises as a result of disruption of anatomical barriers and implantation of organisms from the host's own flora in deeper tissues. Inflammatory and phagocytic reactions provide protection in this setting, but their effectiveness may be perturbed by such features of the surgical procedure as leaving devitalized tissue or excessive amounts of suture in the operative site, or by inadequate hemostasis. The pregnant patient appears to have increased phagocytic activity. She may have slight alterations in humoral immunity and evidence for altered cell-mediated immunity is provided [1]. The mucosal surface of the female genital tract is a complex biosystem, which provides a barrier against the outside world and participates in both innate and acquired immune defense systems. This mucosal compartment has adapted to a dynamic, non-sterile environment challenged by a variety of antigenic/inflammatory stimuli associated with sexual intercourse and endogenous vaginal microbiota. Rapid innate immune defences against microbial infection usually involve the recognition of invading pathogens by specific pattern-recognition receptors recently attributed to the family of toll-like receptors (TLR).

TLR recognize conserved pathogen-associated molecular patterns (PAMP) synthesized by microorganisms including viruses as well as endogenous ligands associated with cell damage. Members of the TLR family, which includes 10 human TLR identified to date, recognize distinct PAMP produced by various viral pathogens [2]. Innate immune responses against microorganisms at the maternal-fetal interface may have a significant impact on the success of pregnancy because intrauterine infections have been shown to be strongly associated with certain complications of pregnancy. At the maternal-fetal interface, TLR are expressed not only in the immune cells but also in nonimmune cells such as trophoblasts and decidual cells. Moreover, their expression patterns vary according to the stage of pregnancy. Increased understanding of these molecules may provide insight into site-specific immunoregulatory mechanisms in the female reproductive tract [3].

Human reproduction provides unique opportunities for the transmission of infectious agents. Furthermore, the mother and her offspring have distinct susceptibilities to infection at each stage of reproduction, from conception and gestation to parturition and the neonatal period. The impact of pathogens on reproduction can be mitigated or exacerbated depending on timing of acquisition during pregnancy.

Similarly, factors such as maternal immune response, nutritional status, or concurrent infection may modify the effect of an infectious agent [4]. Viruses and fetuses face similar immunologic challenges. Each must evade immune detection and destruction. The virus must avoid host recognition of intracellular infection; the fetus allogenic recognition. Each has manipulated the process of antigen presentation to allow survival in an immunologic environment otherwise predictably hostile.

Special classical and non-classical major histocompatibility complex (MHC) class I products are spared from down-regulation in the placenta and from viral immunoevasive strategies. Viruses rely upon some of the same strategies to avoid immune detection as do trophoblast cells. In the future, viral infections may prove a useful tool for studies of immunology at the maternal-fetal interface [5].

A major portion of the human genome appears to be of retroviral origin. These endogenous retroviral elements are expressed in a variety of normal tissues and during disease states, such as autoimmune and malignant conditions.

Recently, potential roles have been described for endogenous retroviral envelope proteins in normal differentiation of human villous cytotrophoblast into syncytiotrophoblast.

The current state of knowledge concerning the expression of the env regions of three endogenous retroviral elements (ERV-3, HERV-W, and HERV-FRD) has brought to the construction of a testable model of villous cytotrophoblast differentiation, in which a complementary expression of endogenous retroviral envelope proteins initiates human chorionic gonadotropin (hCG) production, decreased cell proliferation, and intercellular fusion [6].

Placental immune response and its tropism for specific viruses and pathogens affect the outcome of the pregnant woman's susceptibility to and severity of certain infectious diseases. The generalization of pregnancy as a condition of immune suppression or increased risk is misleading and prevents the determination of adequate guidelines for treating pregnant women during pandemics. There is a need to evaluate the interaction of each specific pathogen with the fetal/placental unit and its responses to design the adequate prophylaxis or therapy. The complexity of the immunology of pregnancy and the focus, for many years, on the concept of immunology of pregnancy as an organ transplantation have complicated the field and delayed the development of new guidelines with clinical implications that could help to answer these and other relevant questions. The challenge is to evaluate many of the "classical concepts" to define new approaches for a better understanding of the immunology of pregnancy that will benefit mothers and fetuses in different clinical scenarios [7]. Sex hormones influence susceptibility and disease predisposition for many genital tract infections. Sex steroids affect mucosal immunity, with particular reference to Human Immunodeficiency Virus (HIV) and genital herpes, and there are stage-specific effects of hormonal contraception on Human Papillomavirus (HPV) infection. Estrogen's role is important in the early stages of several infections as it stimulates antibody- and cell-mediated immune responses. There is increased expression of some cytokines in peripheral blood and vaginal fluids during the follicular phase of the menstrual cycle and with use of hormonal contraception. Whether estrogen exerts a protective or deleterious influence depends on the infecting organism and stage of infection or disease. Estrogen apparently reduces susceptibility to primary HPV infection but in the event of persistent HPV infection, sex steroid hormones (estrogen and/or progesterone) are associated with progression to cervical cancer. It is important that these stage-specific effects are better described because most vaccines will try to prevent either infection or disease. Clinicians with patients at high risk of sexually transmitted infections (STI), especially HIV, require better information on the risks associated with different hormonal contraceptive regimes [8].

Genital infections in impoverished countries take a heavy toll both in the etiology of childlessness and in pregnancy-related morbidity, both for the carrier (mother) and the passenger (fetus/newborn). Tubal damage is by far the most common single etiology in cases of childlessness. Among the three factors principally contributing to childlessness, infertility, pregnancy wastage, and child loss, tubal infertility is the predominant one. Genitally acquired infections during pregnancy contribute to pregnancy wastage in the second and third trimesters of pregnancy.

There is virtually no data to support that Hepatitis B Virus (HBV), Herpes Simplex Virus (HSV), and HPV significantly contribute to transmitted intra-uterine disease leading to pregnancy wastage. In the third category of childlessness, child loss, HSV and HIV play a well-known role. Maternal and neonatal morbidity is adversely affected by genital infections acquired during pregnancy. While hepatitis in some places is an important contributor to maternal mortality and morbidity, other viral diseases like HSV and HPV do not appear important in pregnancy-related maternal morbidity. HSV is less frequent but extremely serious when it appears [9]. Vaginal symptoms are common in the general population and are one of the most frequent reasons for patient visits to obstetrician-gynecologists. Vaginitis may have important consequences in terms of discomfort and pain, days lost from school or work, and sexual functioning and self image. Vaginitis is associated with sexually transmitted diseases (STD) and other infections of the female genital tract, including HIV, as well as adverse reproductive outcomes in pregnant and nonpregnant women. Treatment usually is directed to the specific cause of vaginal symptoms [10]. Urinary tract infections (UTI) remain some of the most common infections observed in community- and hospital-based practices. A growing proportion of these infections are caused by pathogens often associated with STD, including those of nonbacterial and viral etiologies. Consequently, multiresistant strains have become more prevalent, and the clinician must respond with a rational approach to therapy. The drugs may be effective in single- or multiple-dose regimens, depending on the condition being treated, and these should be considered important drugs in the treatment of uncomplicated and complicated adult UTI [11].

The need to screen for STD during pregnancy depends on the prevalence of the condition, its pathogenesis and the cost-benefit analysis for a population or risk group. For a few genital infections with severe impact on the outcome of the pregnancy a “screen and treat” policy is almost always cost-effective. Genital infections often remain unnoticed during pregnancy, as their signs and symptoms may be seen as part of the normal discomfort of pregnancy.

Also, it is sometimes not clear whether there are multiple partners or whether the partners have been treated, making re-infection after treatment highly likely. Partner tracing may be difficult, but the "screen and treat" policy is usually the best solution [12]. Viral infections are a common complication of pregnancy and in some cases can have profound effects for the unborn fetus. The Human Herpesvirus (HHV) family is composed of large, enveloped deoxy-ribonucleic acid (DNA) viruses that have close structural similarity. The family includes the HSV types 1 and 2, Varicella Zoster Virus (VZV), Epstein Barr Virus (EBV), Cytomegalovirus (CMV), and HHV types 6, 7, and 8. These viruses all share the ability to establish latency and reactivate at a later time. Structural fetal abnormalities can result from intrauterine infection and transmission of the infection during the pregnancy or at the time of delivery can result in important neonatal disease. Human Parvovirus B19 is a DNA virus with strong tropism for erythroid precursors and infection during pregnancy can result in fetal hydrops and stillbirth. The causative agents of hepatitis are hepatotropic viruses termed Hepatitis A, B, C, D (Deltavirus), and E. All except HBV are ribonucleic acid (RNA) viruses. Vertical transmission of maternal infection with hepatitis B and C can result in significant long term sequelae [13]. Viruses like Rubella Virus, CMV, and VZV can be transmitted from a pregnant woman to her fetus and can affect fetal development. Several factors determine the likelihood of fetal infection and the risk of consequences for the fetus, such as the timing of transmission during gestation or the immunologic status of the mother. No single diagnostic modality can be applied to all infections. Knowledge of the diagnostic methods available is essential for accurate counseling and treatment of affected pregnant women [14]. Maternal infections with Hepatitis C Virus (HCV), CMV, and HIV and their management problems continue to raise concern in obstetrics. We know that congenital human CMV infection can lead to major neurological disease with sensorineuronal loss. The current lack of trusted prognostic elements to predict impact on the infected fetus makes any prenatal diagnosis questionable. For the last 20 years, HIV mother-to-child transmission (MTCT) has decreased from 25% to less than 3%. The new problem is how to answer the more and more frequent request for pregnancy from an infected woman. The treatment must be adapted to the pregnancy in order to reduce the risks for the mother and the infant [15]. Collectively, toxoplasmosis, other infections (Coxsackievirus, Chickenpox, Parvovirus B19, Chlamydia, HIV, Human T-Lymphotropic Virus [HTLV], and Syphilis), Rubella Virus, CMV, and HSV (TORCH) infections create more neonatal morbidity than early-onset group B streptococcal sepsis.

Fortunately, the incidence of maternal infection by CMV or toxoplasmosis is low (2-10 per 1,000 births). There have been tremendous advances in direct antigen testing and in the sensitivity and specificity of immunoglobulin G (IgG) and IgM testing. Consistently, research laboratories show more accurate results than in the past. Unfortunately, commercial laboratories are using older, single-kit testing. The relatively poor degree of reliability can lead to unnecessary obstetric intervention or elective termination. Any positive pathogen-specific IgM on maternal serum should have additional confirmatory testing in a reputable research laboratory before any intervention. Direct antigen testing or multiple testing would seem to be appropriate for confirmation. This may include amniocentesis of fetal blood sampling. The research on the newer tests is based of the evaluation of blood from seriously immunocompromised subjects. Extrapolations of test accuracy to similar tests on healthy, pregnant women and their fetuses are likely to be in error. The application of these accurate tests to the obstetric population is a critical research need [16].

Infectious agents are associated with a wide range of obstetric complications and pathological processes affecting the placenta, membranes, and fetus. In some cases, there will be associated maternal symptoms and signs indicating an infectious etiology, but in the majority such infection is subclinical, and specific diagnosis or confirmation is achieved following pathological examination of the delivered placenta and/or fetus. There are two major groups of microorganism-related mechanisms associated with significant perinatal morbidity and mortality. First, ascending genital-tract infection, which ranges from localized choriodecidual inflammation to frank chorioamnionitis with fetal sepsis. This is a major cause of mid-trimester miscarriage and severe preterm delivery, and more recent data suggest that it may also have potentially important effects via cytokine release mediating neonatal cerebral injury. Second, hematogenous spread of maternal systemic infection which may result in isolated placental effects or transmission to the fetus with associated developmental abnormalities and neonatal complications. In many cases, distinctive histopathological findings are described, and in addition a wide range of techniques is now available for culture and microscopy to confirm these diagnoses. Such techniques include highly specific immunohistochemical markers and sensitive molecular diagnostic techniques such as the polymerase chain reaction (PCR). It is likely that with increasingly widespread availability of these investigative approaches to obstetric pathology, a greater understanding of the role of infectious agents in obstetric complications will become apparent [17].

As we have said, many of the syndromes have subtle presentations with overlapping symptomatology or essentially no symptoms at all. Clinicians therefore must maintain a high degree of suspicion when faced with such infectious complications of pregnancy [18]. Several congenital infections show the spectrum of modes of vertical transmission and severity of fetal disease encountered, in addition to the successes and limitations of the current medical interventions. Further improvements in diagnostic techniques and therapies for managing the infected fetus have occurred during the last two decades. Similarly, the widespread adaptation of new and sensitive diagnostic assays, such as the PCR, has further improved our ability to identify infectious agents as the primary cause of certain abnormal fetal conditions. Where specific diagnostic tests and therapies have proven successful in preventing or treating fetal infections, universal screening programs should be given serious consideration. Of paramount importance, however, is the active research on the development of preventive interventions for maternal infections and vertical transmission. Although specific immunotherapies, vaccines, and drug therapies hold great promise for controlling the spread of some infections, it cannot be overemphasized that some serious infectious complications of pregnancy may be avoided by simple preconception or early antenatal maternal counseling [19].

The report of transmission of blood-borne viruses, such as HIV, HBV, and HCV, from health care workers (HCW) to patients has alarmed public opinion with potential repercussions on health organization. The factors influencing the transmissibility of infection include: type of procedures performed, surgical techniques used, compliance with infection control precautions, the clinical status and viral burden of the infected HCW, and susceptibility of the patient to infection. The risk of transmission of HIV, HBV, and HCV from HCW to patients is associated primarily with certain types of surgical specialties (obstetrics and gynecology, orthopedics, cardiothoracic surgery) and surgical procedures that can expose the patient to the blood of the HCW: exposure-prone procedures.

Since the early 90's, industrialized countries have issued recommenddations for preventing transmission of blood-borne pathogens to patients during "exposure-prone" invasive procedures. With regard to HBV, there is common consent to restricting or excluding HCW tested Hepatitis B e Antigen (HBeAg) positive or HBV DNA-positive from performing exposure-prone procedures, while there are still some discrepancies in the different countries for dealing with HCV-infected personnel and in some cases also for those with HIV infection.

Efforts to prevent surgeon-to-patient transmission of blood-borne infections should focus not only on ascertaining the infection status of the HCW, but principally on eliminating the cause of blood-borne exposures, for example by the use of blunt suture needles, improved instruments, reinforced gloves, changes in surgical technique and the use of less invasive alternative procedures. These measures should be implemented in order to minimize the risk of blood exposure and consequently of virus transmission both to and from HCW to patients [20]. Thus, virus-infected medical personnel under certain circumstances might represent a risk for pregnant women. With regard to such nosocomial provider-to-patient transmissions, the pathogens Rubella Virus, HHV, and the HBV and HCV are of particular concern. In this context, one should strive to achieve optimal protection for the expectant mothers without restricting the professional activities of virus-infected members of the medical staff in an unjustified way. In this respect, it always has to be kept in mind that the risk of provider-to-patient transmissions of viruses in obstetrics and neonatology can be significantly reduced by vaccinating all personnel working in these departments against infections by the Rubella Virus, VZV, and HBV, and that additional strict adherence to so-called universal hygienic precautions will add more than an incremental benefit [21, 22]. Surgeons have the opportunity to prevent the majority of exposures by utilizing currently available technology and knowledge. Surgeons should see, use, and evaluate a variety of safety-engineered devices, because their feedback can lead to improvements in technology. Education, communication, and access to safer technology will motivate surgeons to adopt safer behavior patterns. Provided with information and tools, they can change through self-motivation [23]. Hospital-acquired infections caused by viruses are a cause of considerable morbidity and occasional mortality in critically ill neonates. The intensive care environment allows for efficient spread of viral pathogens, and secondary cases among both patients and HCW are frequently observed. The common viral causes of hospital-acquired infections in neonates include Rotavirus, Respiratory Syncytial Virus (RSV), and others [24-26].

Congenital Viral Infections

Viral infections are a major cause of fetal morbidity and mortality. Transplacental transmission of the virus, even in subclinical maternal infection, may result in a severe congenital syndrome. The past years has shed much new light on congenital infection.

A key development has been the application of PCR technology to the diagnosis of intrauterine infection. This technique appears to be the diagnostic tool of choice for CMV. Obstetric interventions may reduce vertical transmission. Education has been shown to reduce the incidence of seroconversion and HIV-positive women treated with zidovudine (ZVD) have a dramatically reduced rate of transmission to their offspring [27]. Two percent to 4% of all newborns have a major structural malformation of which only a small percentage can be explained by either aneuploidy or a single-gene disorder. No other mammal has a similar reproductive problem. This suggests that previously unrecognized viral infection accounts for a large percentage of these abnormalities by interfering with appropriate embryonic cell migration, reducing hyperplasia, or damaging the precursor structure by means of an inflammatory mechanism [28].

Infection is an important cause of stillbirth. Infection may be especially important as a cause of stillbirth occurring early in pregnancy. Identifying a specific infection as a cause of stillbirth is limited by many obstacles. Nevertheless, "good faith" efforts estimate that approximately 9% to 15% of stillbirths are caused by infections. A large variety of organisms have been associated with stillbirth, including many viruses. The two most important viral causes of stillbirth are Parvovirus and Coxsackie Virus, although a number of other viral infections appear to be causal. Other organisms that are "purported to cause" stillbirth include the HIV and others. No single strategy has been developed for effective prevention of stillbirth caused by infection. The low rate of stillbirth in most situations would require large intervention trials for hypothesis testing. Within the framework if determining epidemiological etiology, research should be initiated in the role of infectious causes [29]. Infection may cause stillbirth by a number of mechanisms, including direct infection, placental damage, chorioamnionitis, and severe maternal illness. In developed countries, between 10% and 25% of stillbirths may be caused by an infection, whereas in developing countries, which often have much higher stillbirth rates, the contribution of infection is much greater. Because infection-related stillbirth is relatively rare in developed countries, and those that do occur are caused by a wide variety of organisms, reducing this etiologic component of stillbirth much further will be difficult. However, in certain developing countries, the stillbirth rate is so high and the infection-related component so great that achieving a substantial reduction in stillbirth should be possible simply by reducing maternal infections [30].

Infection and inflammation contribute to perinatal brain damage, particularly to the white matter [31].

Cerebral palsy (CP) rates of 2 in every 1,000 births have varied little over the last 50 years, despite improvements in obstetric care. In the past, CP was thought to be due to poor obstetric care and management. However, epidemiological studies have refuted this, suggesting that there is usually an antenatal timing to the neuropathology of CP. There are many known risk factors for CP, including multiple gestation, prematurity, and low birth weight (LBW). Recently, intrauterine infection, maternal pyrexia, and the presence of thrombophilic disorders (thrombophilia) have been identified as major risk factors for subsequent CP. The interactions of viral infections during pregnancy, normal or abnormal fetal cytokine responses, and hereditary fetal thrombophilias as antenatal causes of the neuropathology of CP are now areas of research priority [32]. The etiology of CP is often unclear and because CP is a symptom complex rather than a disease, clinically defined at 4-5 years of age, it is not surprising that there are considerable problems associated with epidemiological studies of its etiology. The only reason for the CP concept is that it emanates from an insult to a growing, developing brain and a dynamic clinical picture from static pathology. Evidence suggests that 70-80% of CP cases are due to prenatal factors and that birth asphyxia plays a relatively minor role (<10%). Some antenatal risk factors are repeatedly observed to be related to CP: low gestational age, male gender, multiple gestation, intrauterine viral infections, and maternal thyroid abnormalities. Recently, intrauterine infection/inflammation with a maternal response (consisting of chorioamnionitis) and a fetal inflammatory response (consisting of funisitis or elevated interleukin-6 [IL-6] in fetal plasma) has been found to be related to white matter injury and CP. Some risk factors are associated with CP at all gestational ages, whereas others mostly affect term or preterm infants, e.g., intrauterine growth restriction (IUGR) seems to be a risk factor in term infants. There also seems to be an association between autoimmune and coagulation disorders and CP [33].

So, viral infections can cause fetal malformations and illness with serious sequelae to the infant or fetal death in utero. Determining the causative agent is important and often greatly affects the prognosis of the newborn. [34]. Rubella Virus, CMV, HSV, and HIV, for example, are capable of gaining access to the amniotic cavity and producing fetal infection, even when amniotic membranes are intact. Intrauterine invasion by viruses can be associated with maternal symptoms of infection or can be completely silent. In many instances, extensive fetal compromise with irreversible structural damage or fetal death will have occurred by the time infection is confirmed by culture or other histopathological methods.

The evidence of fetal infection may be as subtle as nascent IUGR, mildly inappropriate calcification of fetal organs, placenta, cord, and membranes, and failure to adequately develop fetal fat reserves. The evidence of infection may be as dramatic as obvious fetal malformation, severe central nervous system (CNS) structural damage, or fetal death [35].

Diagnosis of fetal infection has depended on identification of pathogens by means of microbiological cultures, immunologic techniques, and special molecular biology techniques that can identify organisms known or suspected of being associated with adverse outcomes of pregnancy. Amniotic fluid is in most cases easily and safely obtainable during the second and third trimester and can be used in several microbiological assays. These include viral cultures, quantitative assays for Ig or cytokines, and PCR for detecting microbial DNA. Unsuspected fetal viral infection is often overlooked as a possible cause of abnormalities revealed on ultrasonographic examination during pregnancy. Infectious agents can produce a wide spectrum of ultrasonographic findings. No ultrasonographic findings are pathognomonic for a particular agent.

Most affected fetuses appear sonographically normal, but serial scanning may reveal evolving findings. Common sonographic abnormalities, although nonspecific, may be indicative of fetal viral infections. These include IUGR, ascites, hydrops, ventriculomegaly, intracranial calcifications, hydrocephaly, microcephaly, cardiac anomalies, hepatosplenomegaly, echogenic bowel, placentomegaly, and abnormal amniotic fluid volume. Some of the pathognomonic sonographic findings enable diagnosis of a specific congenital syndrome (e.g., ventriculomegaly and intracranial and hepatic calcifications in CMV, eye and cardiac anomalies in congenital rubella syndrome, limb contractures and cerebral anomalies in VZV). When abnormalities are detected on ultrasound, a thorough fetal evaluation is recommended because of multiorgan involvement. Both clinical and subclinical maternal viral infections can cross the placenta, there are specific sonographic findings along with laboratory findings to detect infectious agents, and when sonographic abnormalities are detected fetal viral infections need to be considered [36]. The search for possible fetal infection consists of both direct and indirect techniques. Methods to directly demonstrate fetal infection include the cited maternal-fetal serologic studies, culture, electron microscopy, and PCR. Emerging evidence strongly suggests that prior assumptions concerning the sensitivity of both maternal and fetal-neonatal serologic studies are incorrect. Serologic studies alone are inadequate to exclude fetal infection as a cause of an ultrasonographically detected abnormality.

Indirect techniques suggestive of fetal infection include fetal hematologic and biochemical measurements. New approaches and methods for the detection of fetal infection are needed. The evaluation should be initiated antenatally. Needless delay until after delivery increases the likelihood that the diagnosis will be missed. Antenatal diagnosis provides the opportunity for therapy and often leads the practitioner to modify the obstetric and neonatal care plan [37-41].

VIRAL INFECTIONS AND ASSISTED REPRODUCTION TECHNIQUES

With the increasing demand for assisted reproduction techniques (ART), it is important to consider how to manage infection. Three main positive factors that contribute to successful in vitro fertilization (IVF) cycles are maternal age, the ovarian hyperstimulation protocol used, and the number and quality of transferred embryos. Negative factors include contamination and infection [42]. Viral infections of the genital tract may be important etiological factors for male infertility. Infectious processes may lead to deterioration of spermatogenesis, impairment of sperm function, and/or obstruction of the seminal tract. The effect of leukocytospermia on male fertility is controversial. This is probably due to different detection methods, different populations studied, and to the fact that leukocyte subtypes in semen may have different functions. In addition to potentially negative effects, leukocytes may even have protective effects on spermatozoa. Only recently have amplification methods been established to detect viruses in semen with high sensitivity and specificity. It is unclear if these infections significantly contribute to male infertility [43]. During the past 20 years, assisted reproduction has been facing a new demand from patients requiring ART: couples at risk of partner-to-partner, and MTCT of viral infections, mainly HIV-1, HCV, and HIV-HCV co-infected partners.

The general conditions and life expectancy of many patients with HIV infection are very good, and three-quarters of these individuals are in their reproductive years. For these reasons, a large number of young couples are expected to make future plans to have children. This desire is not easy to realize for serodiscordant couples, if we consider that, in order to avoid HIV virus transmission, it is necessary to encourage the condom use in vaginal and anal contacts.

On the other hand, infertile discordant HCV couples need to be included in protocols of controlled ART to avoid any risk of HCV transmission to the partner [44]. Teams practicing medically ART try to avoid viruses as much as possible. Attitudes towards chronic carriers of viruses are rapidly changing, especially for HIV patients. It is largely proven that sperm gradient preparation techniques efficiently decrease viral loads and therefore have a protective effect on contamination risk during ART. Although a few thousand ART cycles were performed in the world for this indication without contamination, it is still too early to demonstrate that this technology is fully safe. Many questions remain unresolved, such as the lack of standardized techniques for semen preparation or virus detection or the relative merits of intrauterine insemination (IUI) or intracytoplasmatic sperm injection (ICSI) to prevent HIV contamination during ART [45-47].

Notes of Antiviral Therapy and Prevention

Over the last decades, there have been major developments in basic and clinical research in the field of antiviral therapy. These have allowed the HCW to treat and prevent the morbidity and mortality of many viral infections. To this extent, he needs to know the availability of numerous antiviral compounds and begin to view them as we do antibiotics. They need to be used selectively to modify infections and prevent the morbidity and mortality associated with viral infections. Therapy of these infections is required to treat not only the patient but also to prevent infection of sexual partners and the newborn. The HCW are faced with challengers in the diagnosis, prevention, and treatment of viral STD in women. A number of antiviral compounds can be used for the treatment of acute infection. In addition, these medications have been proven to be safe and effective when administered over long periods of time to treat and suppress such viral infections. Another therapeutic way of using these antiviral medications is to reduce viral shedding in infected patients thus preventing transmission of the disease. The use of antiviral medications as postexposure prophylaxis is another area in which the clinician needs current information. The mechanism of action, the spectrum of activity, and the pharmacokinetics of these antiviral compounds are important in selecting appropriate therapy for patients. The standard of care has changed with the availability of safe and effective antiviral medications. The Food and Drug Administration (FDA), after careful and controlled clinical trials, has approved several antiviral compounds to treat viral STD [48, 49].

The history of antiviral and antiretroviral (ARV) therapy is recent compared with many other medical therapies, including traditional antibiotics in pregnancy. There are few long-term data on which to base decisions of management in pregnancy. Accessing up-to-date information is critical to optimizing the safety of care for mothers and their infants. Exposure to medications in pregnancy can be toxic to a fetus in a gestational age-dependent manner. Determination of safe medications for pregnancy must take into consideration the need for certain medications and the possibility of inadvertent exposure in early pregnancy because of unplanned pregnancies [50]. Antiviral agents are less numerous and often more toxic than antibacterial agents. Acyclovir (ACV) is commonly used for suppression and treatment of recurrent genital HSV and may be indicated for pregnant women with disseminated herpes. ZVD is indicated for pregnant women with HIV infection who have low cluster of differentiation 4 (CD4) lymphocyte counts. Ganciclovir, vidarabine, ribavirin, amantadine, didanosine (DDI), and foscarnet are rarely indicated in gynecology and are not recommended for use in pregnancy [51]. The different structure and stability of viruses requires the application of virucidal disinfection procedures in gynecology. For this purpose, disinfectants should be used which are tested according to the guidelines in a virus suspension test and in nearly all cases only a slight increase of application conditions is necessary to get equal efficacy for the disinfection or surfaces of instruments. But the application solutions of instrument disinfectants should not be used longer than one day. Experiments testing the virucidal effectivity of such solutions showed an insufficient decontamination of infectious materials already after 3 days usage [52].

Optimal protection against preventable diseases for the pregnant woman and her fetus can be provided through vaccination prior to pregnancy. When indicated, however, the benefits of immunization during pregnancy and breastfeeding may outweigh the theoretical risks of potential adverse events. Several vaccinations recommended by the Advisory Committee on Immunization Practices (ACIP) of the Centers for Disease Control and Prevention (CDC) can reduce maternal and fetal morbidity and mortality from preventable diseases. Physicians can maintain the highest standards of clinical practice by advocating for appropriate vaccinations in their female patients [53]. Vaccinations in pregnancy are an important aspect of prenatal care and of improving not only maternal health but also neonatal outcomes. Maternal immunization embraces the concepts that vaccines given to pregnant women enhance their resistance to vaccine-preventable diseases and passive antibodies that cross the placenta protect the neonate for the first 3 to 6 months of life.

It is a great public health move to get excellent protection at a small cost. Because all recommended vaccines for use in pregnancy are safe, it makes good sense to bring patients up-to-date on vaccines [54-56]. Only 2 vaccines are specifically recommended during pregnancy: influenza and tetanus, diphtheria, and acellular pertussis (Tdap). Because influenza illness disproportionately affects pregnant women compared with other populations, annual prevention of influenza illness is recommended for all women who will be pregnant during influenza season (October to May). Influenza vaccination has been recently reported to also result in decreased febrile respiratory illnesses in the newborn, likely through passive antibody transfer. Provider support for these recommendations regarding annual influenza vaccination during pregnancy is critical to ensuring vaccine delivery and improving both maternal and fetal health [57]. Vaccines have been used in pregnant women for over 200 years. Current guidelines recommend vaccination with only inactivated virus due to potential risk to mother and fetus with live vaccine. The exception is during times of pandemic or biological weapons attack, when the risk of life-threatening disease outweighs the risk of vaccination. A paucity of data is available regarding actual risk and mechanisms of live viral vaccine transfer from mother to fetus. Pregnancy-induced changes to the maternal immune system, effects of maternal infection on neonatal immunity, and the role of the placenta in transmission of infection and passive immunity to the fetus are incompletely understood [58].

Viral Sexually Transmitted Diseases

STD are among the most common infections worldwide. Spread by sexual contact, various STD directly cause much morbidity and mortality [59]. The etiology of many genital infections is still unknown or rather, an etiological relationship between a given agent and a clinical manifestation is in some infections still debated. Recent discoveries of novel etiological agents of STI may explain a lack of recovery from infections, due to the common use of antibiotic drugs to which these agents have a natural resistance [60]. Infections of the female urinary tract, cervix, vulva, and vagina produce a variety of overlapping symptoms, including vulvar pruritus, dysuria, dyspareunia, and increased or altered vaginal discharge. Recent studies have considerably improved our understanding of the etiology, pathophysiology, diagnosis, and treatment of these infections [61].

The frequency and severity of STD and their sequelae should be acknowledged by all sexually active individuals. Aspects of sexuality that place individuals at risk of STD must be reexamined. HCW must effectively inform patients and the public of these often-ill-appreciated risks in a straightforward fashion, free of judgmental and punitive attitudes. New, more-effective means of prevention, diagnosis, and treatment are being sought using research techniques in microbiology, immunology, and behavioral science. In the meantime, medical screening, treatment, and contact tracing should be carried out for patients and their sexual partners.

Sexually active individuals must be empowered with knowledge and emboldened to protect themselves and their established or potential families from these common infections. Existing means of screening and treating must be utilized fully [62].

The epidemiology of STD is a vast topic. It includes examining not only the frequency of disease but also those factors that influence the frequency. It requires taking into account not only the characteristics of the infected persons and their risk factors but also the characteristics of the causative organisms. There is a commonality between various STD that results in people frequently harboring one or more agent.

In view of this, efforts should be made to evaluate patients for inapparent disease. Another important aspect is recognizing that patients do not acquire their infection except through sexual contact, indicating that another person is involved. Therefore, for control purposes, treatment of all sexual contacts also must be addressed [63].

STD constitute a major health burden worldwide, causing pelvic inflammatory disease (PID), ectopic pregnancy, infertility, chronic pelvic pain (CPP), genital lesions, genital neoplasms, adverse pregnancy outcomes, immune system dysfunction, liver disease, and even death.

STD disproportionately affect adolescents and young adults. Of the estimated 19 million STD that occur annually each year in the United States (US), 4 million are among adolescents and 6 million among young adults. The current epidemic is complicated by the high asymptomatic carrier state associated with most STD and the often inadequate protection of condoms in preventing transmission. Sexually active individuals, particularly adolescents, must be educated on the ramifications of early onset of sexual activity and the health consequences of multiple sexual partners [64]. The economic burden imposed by STI is impressive: direct medical costs are estimated to be as high as $15.5 billion annually. Women and infants disproportionately bear the long-term consequences of STD [65].

Because pathogens spread only within the unique context of a sexual union between people when one person is infectious, the other is susceptible to new infection, and condoms are not used to prevent transmission, the epidemiological study of STI is particularly challenging. Social network analysis entails the study of ties among people and how the structure and quality of such ties affect individuals and overall group dynamics. Although ascertaining complete sexual networks is difficult, application of this approach has provided unique insights into the spread of STI that traditional individual-based epidemiological methods do not capture [66].

During the past decades, the incidence of viral STD has increased dramatically [67]. Viral STD are a major health problem for women. Over many years, the incidence of these infections has increased steadily to epidemic proportions. These infections not only cause short-term morbidity but also have been associated with significant long-term morbidity and mortality. Two of the most common viral STD are genital HSV infection and HIV infection of the female. The steady increase in the incidence of HIV infection and subsequent acquired immune deficiency syndrome (AIDS) among women requires HCW to assume an active role in detection and treatment in order to avoid transmission, to protect the health of women with HIV/AIDS, and to reduce the risk of MTCT. Because treatment with ZVD has been shown to reduce vertical transmission, routine offering of HIV testing is currently recommended for all pregnant women. The approach to testing nonpregnant patients, i.e., the choice between selective screening and routine testing, rests with the individual clinician. Testing large numbers of patients within a practice may be facilitated by the availability of an oral antibody testing system. The sensitivity and specificity of the oral test is equivalent to blood testing. Serum and oral specimens are tested by enzyme-linked immunosorbent assays (ELISA) and confirmatory Western blot assays specifically designed for use with oral samples [68]. Most of the publications reviewed focus on HPV, and a small proportion on HSV. The evidence associates cervical intraepithelial neoplasia (CIN)-1 with high oncogenic risk HPV types in less than 30% of cases, whereby CIN-2 and CIN-3 are associated with a 90% risk. However, on the basis of HPV types, four categories ["low risk" (HPV 6, 11, 42, 43, 44), "intermediate risk" (HPV 31, 33, 35, 51, 52, 58), "high risk" (HPV 16 and HPV 18)] for the associated risk for a high-grade lesion or an invasive cancer can also be defined. In practice, it appears efficient to re-evaluate patients with oncogenic types in association with low-grade cytology, as well as women with high-grade cytology or suspicious colposcopy in narrow intervals.

Several reports have suggested that HPV genital infections are multifocal. However, HPV DNA was also found in the lymph nodes and in the granulocytes of women with cervical cancer, in ovarian and endometrial tissue, in tumors of the urinary bladder, and in mammary ductal carcinoma [69].

Fertility regulation and prevention of STD are recognized pillars in fertility health work. The HIV epidemic has made it clear that there are people at risk for STD all over the world. Both STD and unwanted pregnancies are negative consequences of the same behavior, i.e., unprotected intercourse. From the perspective of the individual, the risks with unprotected intercourse vary over time and with actual life-style. To meet the needs of the individuals, the concept of contraceptive counseling needs to be expanded. Clinics where gynecologists and midwives join forces together with venerologists and social workers have been developed in Sweden. The goal for the clinics is to give an integrated message on STD and pregnancy protection [70]. Today, the notion of "safe sex" means protection from both unintended pregnancy and STD and HIV. These parallel complications of sexual activity have serious biologic and clinical sequelae that should be considered at the time of contraceptive selection. In addition, there is ongoing debate regarding potential interactions between antibiotic intervention and contraceptive steroids. Counseling and care for both family planning and infectious disease protection must be provided to all sexually active individuals. Barrier methods, especially when combines with spermicides, can reduce the risk of STD/HIV if used consistently. The combined use of oral contraceptives (OC) and condoms offers serious defense against both unintended pregnancy and STD/HIV. Intrauterine devices (IUD) also seem safe and effective in women at low risk for reproductive tract infection. Periodic screening and treatment for prevalent STD can protect the health of individuals and their sexual contacts. Finally, more research is needed on the reproductive and infectious disease repercussions of human sexuality, while counseling and care for family planning and infectious disease protection are recommended for those who are sexually active [71]. Although non-barrier contraceptive use has become a global norm, unprotected sex in relation to STI remains the norm almost everywhere. Dual protection is a form of safer sex for heterosexual couples that is more needed than practised or understood. Definitions of dual protection, found mainly in family planning literature, are very narrow. Condoms remain the mainstay of dual protection, but there is a range of options. These include non-penetrative sex and the increasing use of condoms with the back-up of emergency contraception on the part of young people.

The fact that people may fail to use dual protection consistently and correctly is not a valid reason not to promote it. It is never too late for those providing family planning and STI/HIV prevention services to start promoting condoms and dual protection. In the long-term, the development of highly efficacious and highly acceptable methods of dual protection is an urgent research priority, starting with a wider range of condoms that will appeal to more people [72]. It is important to examine the successful completed research and use it to move forward in practice to halt the almost 50% unintended pregnancy rate in the US and the continued worldwide epidemic of HIV and other STI. A significant development has been the evidence supporting the IUD as a valuable contraceptive option available to many women, including women who are HIV infected, with no increased risks of infertility or PID. Evidence exists that OC may increase cervicitis, but it is unlikely that OCP use is associated with PID. The lack of female-controlled dual method protection remains a void, but with the introduction of products such as FemCap and Reality (Wisconsin Pharmacal, Jackson, WI) condom and the continuing progress of microbicides and spermicides, the future is brighter. Clearly research into the interactions of STI and contraceptives must continue to discern how best to approach a resolution to these public health concerns that affect women and the global population [73].

Special concerns of STD for women, particularly because of its asymptomatic character, are: screening; primary prevention, e.g., abstinence, selection of sexual partners, restriction of sexual activities, use of barriers (condoms, vaginal spermicides, diaphragm in conjunction with spermicides), vaccines, and the role of the gynecologist in STD prevention. There is an increased risk of cervical cancer. Infection is lifelong for HSV and HIV and malingering for chronic hepatitis B. Genital HPV and HSV infections cannot be identified serologically. The fetus can be fatally or severely affected by STD. As the spectrum of STD has broadened to include many infections that are not readily cured, prevention of STD has become more important than ever.

Primary prevention methods include abstinence, careful selection of sexual partners, condoms, vaginal spermicides, and a vaccine for HBV and HPV. Condoms will protect against STD only if they are used consistently and correctly, while vaginal spermicides may also reduce risk of certain STD. HCW should routinely counsel women on methods to reduce risk of STD. Abstinence is the only effective prevention for STD. Likelihood of infection may be reduced by limiting partners, but how partners are chosen and knowledge of infection is a more important determinant.

Partners need to be asked about current symptoms, history of STD, multiple partners, and history of known STD partners, as well as past history of homosexual activity, intravenous drug use, hemophilia, and previous exposure to high-risk persons for STD. Visible genital warts or lesions, wartlike growths, ulcers, or rash need explanations. Avoidance of oral anal and digital anal activity reduces transmission of Hepatitis A Virus (HAV). Any mechanical barrier that remains intact should reduce the risk of STD: barriers specifically covering the cervix are excellent. Condom use is effective when used as follows:

1) at the onset of sexual activity;
2) without petroleum jelly or baby oil on latex;
3) with care of fingernails which may tear holes;
4) with complete withdrawal of the penis before complete detumescence; and
5) with a withdrawal hold at the base of the penis.

Spermicides, such as nonoxynol-9 (nonylpenoxypolyethoxyethanol, N-9), are effective against STD. Diaphragm use with spermicide may be effective because of the spermicide. There is a reduced risk of transmission of HSV or HPV to a partner. Vaccines are only available for HBV and HPV. Obstetrics and gynecology residency training in STD is unavailable in 4 out of 5 medical schools, and gynecologists are ethically obligated to accurately inform about STD diagnosis and treatment [74]. Vaginal sponges offer women control over protection against both pregnancy and STD, including HIV. Spermicide-impregnated sponges combine the actions of a physical barrier that blocks the cervix with a material that absorbs the ejaculate and a spermicide. Commercially available spermicides contain 1-5% of N-9, shown to inhibit organisms responsible for genital herpes and HIV. On the other hand, N-9 is associated with a significantly higher risk of ulcerative genital diseases and vulvitis. A lower dose of N-9 appears to avert vaginal irritation without compromising contraceptive efficacy. Use of chlorhexidine (CH), a spermicide less irritating to mucosal cells than N-9 but active against HIV in vivo and in vitro, has been investigated. Also promising are initial findings regarding the Protectaid contraceptive sponge with F-5 gel. Epidemiologic studies and clinical trials should provide quantitative estimates of the level of protection offered by barrier methods and identify the method that combines the highest protection, ease of use, and user acceptability [75]. The inconvenience of current methods limits their acceptability and leads to higher user failure rates.

New methods, such as female condoms, nonlatex male condoms, and new cervical caps have been developed: the Reality polyurethane vaginal pouch has already received conditional FDA approval for use in the US. The material used in a FDA-approved nonallergenic glove has been tested for its effectiveness as a condom. In addition, the FemCap, a cervical cap that had a life table probability of failure within 1 year of 4.8%, is available. It is important for clinicians to be informed of new options becoming available for those patients who may be good candidates for these barrier methods. Reproductive health providers have long overlooked barrier and spermicide contraceptives, but they are rather effective when used consistently and correctly, have relatively few side effects, and protect against STD and HIV. The mean percentage of women who have an unplanned pregnancy during the first year, if they have correctly and consistently used condoms is 2%, 3% for spermicides, 6% for cervical cap and diaphragm, 6% for nulliparous users of the sponge, and 9% for parous users of the sponge. If they do not use these methods and/or spermicides properly, however, failure rates increase 3-7 times. New barrier methods and spermicides should help people overcome obstacles, e.g., sensitivity or allergy to latex. One condom manufacturer has developed nonlatex male condoms for those who are sensitive or allergic to latex or the chemicals added to latex during the manufacturing process. Another manufacturer has altered the male condom by adding a silicone-lubricated pouch of latex to fit loosely around the glans penis, thereby reducing sensation loss. A new barrier method is the cervical cap which fits and covers the cervix snugly. Female condoms empower women to protect themselves against pregnancy, STD, and HIV. They should be available to the US market soon.

Some research indicates that spermicide use with barrier methods poses a risk of UTI, but the benefits exceed the risk. Barrier and spermicide methods appear to protect against cervical cancer and pregnancy complications [76]. It is conceivable that women using OC do not develop as much tubal damage as women not using OC because of a modified immunological reaction. A study carried out in Europe showed a statistically significant protective effect against PID of the levonorgestrel (LNG)-containing IUD as compared with the copper-containing Nova-T. A case/control study of 1028 women in Chicago in 1970 noted admission for PID during the following 7 years of only 1 woman who had been sterilized compared to 9 controls. A case/control study examining risk factors for CIN in 103 women with biopsy-confirmed CIN-2 or CIN-3 did not find an increased risk with either OC or IUD use after adjusting for other known risk factors.

After adjustment for age and education, the odds ratio (OR) for diaphragm use was 0.3 and the OR for condom use was 0.5.

Thus, hormonal contraception and tubal ligation give protection to the upper genital tract but not to the cervix [77]. Although OC are the most reliable contraceptive method, they have limited anti-STD properties and their relationship with STD remain unclear. Various mechanisms explain a protective role of OC against STD.

However, in no way can OC be considered a safe anti-STD contraceptive method, when compared to specific barrier methods, which provide both contraception and anti-STD protection. It is concluded that although OC possess some anti-STD properties, mainly in the prevention of PID, they should be used in combination with a barrier method [78]. The needs for contraception are increasing world-wide as more women desire protection from unwanted pregnancies. Since the incidence of STD has increased in many countries, consultation for contraception should be provided together with that on STD. Each woman may choose the contraceptive method according to her needs but she should also be informed about the beneficial and negative effects of the method in preventing STD [79, 80].

The worldwide epidemic of STD presents a major public health challenge to medical practitioners and educators as they seek to implement preventive educational strategies in the adolescent population. The serious consequences of many STD and the insufficient impact of condom promotion in this high-risk group have led to increasing recognition that sexual intercourse is medically unwise for young adolescents. As a result of this recognition, some educators have proposed that adolescent sexuality education focus on the explicit teaching of noncoital sexual activities, sometimes called outercourse. Noncoital sexual activities will positively impact the rising incidence of STD and unplanned pregnancy in teenagers [81]. Intercourse during menses is an acceptable sexual behavior that is practiced by 3-30% of sexually active women. This pattern of sexual behavior may contribute to transmission of some STD. Yet, intercourse during menses is probably not associated with increased risk for PID. The above-mentioned susceptibility for increased risk for STD in women engaged in sexual intercourse during menses could be explained by the sexual behavior itself and/or by hampered response of innate immune system during menses. Still, while counseling couples about intercourse during menses, its potential advantages should be weighed against possible disadvantages [82]. Premature sexual intercourse results in high figures of adolescent pregnancy and abortion, as well as in increased risk of STD.

Lack of information on the prevention of STD and poor hygiene in both boys and girls are also main reasons for increased morbidity because of STD during adolescence. Contraceptive behavior during adolescence varies between countries and communities. It seems, however, that the condom and OC are popular contraceptive methods. Ineffective methods such as periodic abstinence, coitus interruptus, and withdrawal before ejaculation are in use. On the other hand, compliance of adolescents on contraception is poor. The above are additional causes for increasing rates of adolescent pregnancies. Countries providing sexual education programs in schools present lower rates of pregnancy and abortion. Adolescent pregnancy is safe if a careful follow-up is accepted by the teenager. A significant number of homeless youth are homosexuals or lesbian adolescents. Most of them are at high risk for HIV infection, AIDS, and STD. It is concluded that sexual education programs are absolutely necessary to offer adolescents the knowledge on the complications of premature sexual activity, as well as prevention of the undesired pregnancy and STD [83]. Clinicians treating adolescent girls should address the general lack of knowledge about the risks and consequences of STD. They should be prepared to offer confidential and comprehensive counseling, screening, and treatment according to established guidelines. Office policies that protect adolescent confidentiality are an important component in providing effective care. Adolescence is a period during which lifelong health behaviors are established. It provides a critical opportunity for promoting responsible behaviors and reducing risks through health promotion and prevention strategies [84].

Of the many perspectives from which one can view teenage sexual activity, the most evident are as a normal developmental milestone in the life of the adolescent, or as risk-taking and possibly health-compromising behavior. Since unfortunately, knowledge about sexuality, reproduction, and contraception is often acquired after sexual activity has begun, the prevention of pregnancy and STD should be given high priority in health care and in education. The role of sex education has been a controversial issue for years and communication within the family the teenager's decision to use contraception is often difficult both for the parents and for the adolescent. In the areas of adolescent sexual behavior, sex education, contraception, and counseling, it is imperative and of paramount importance that the health-care system focus on this target group [85].

Women with disabilities can and do contract STD. However, because of access barriers, attitudinal misconceptions, and lack of awareness of their risk status, these infections may go under or undiagnosed.

The treatment of STD in women with disabling conditions presents diagnostic and therapeutic challenges to clinicians, because symptoms may be confusing and may mimic manifestations of underlying disorders. Women with spinal cord injury may be at risk for the development of autonomic activation as a sign of STD.

To enhance compliance with medication regiments, the limitations of the patient should be considered. Furthermore, women with disabilities are at high risk for sexual abuse. Therefore, the presence of an STD may be of special concern. Developing good communication with the patient will enable the clinician to work with her to sort out symptoms, design therapeutic regiments, and to help protect her from abuse [86]. Sexual assault is a common occurrence that carries significant physical and mental health morbidity. Some of the most common concerns expressed by sexual assault victims can be allayed by addressing the risks of rape-related STI. Although exact risks cannot be accurately quantified, it is important that health-care professionals provide counseling as well as prophylaxis and/or treatment as indicated. Screening and treatments should follow established guidelines, and follow-up care is indicated to confirm successful prevention or treatment. Continued support, surveillance, and medical attention should be offered as needed [87]. Domestic violence and HIV infection are problems of great public health worldwide, especially sub-Saharan Africa and much of the developing countries. This is due to their far reaching social, economic, and public health consequences. The two problems have gender inequality and gender power imbalances as the driving force behind the "epidemics". HIV infection is mainly acquired through heterosexual relations, which themselves are greatly influenced by socio-cultural factors, underlying which are gender power imbalances. Unfortunately, gender relations, and gender issues in general, have not been given much emphasis in the medical perspective, especially in efforts for prevention and control of HIV infection. There is thus a need to mainstream gender relations in reproductive health [88].

In both men and women, STD-associated genital infections may cause permanent damage to the reproductive tract resulting in sub- or infertility. In men, the wide zone between sterility and normal fertility makes it difficult to demarcate the precise role of infection on post-infection fecundity, but it seems less important than in women. Of independent importance for infertility, ectopic pregnancy, and time between PID and first intrauterine pregnancy are number of infections, severity of the infections, contraception at the index laparoscopy, age, and delayed treatment. STD-associated in-subfertility is acquired and, hence, preventable [89].

STD may have a significant impact on the pregnant woman and her fetus and neonate. Infection at various stages of pregnancy may result in severe maternal disease, congenital defects, premature delivery, or neonatal infection. The clinician caring for pregnant women must be aware of the multitude of STD and their potential risks during pregnancy [90].

Knowledge of the symptoms and physical examination features, methods of diagnosis, indications for screening, and appropriate treatment options are essential for obstetric/gynecologic HCW [91]. STD grouped together are one of the most common medical complications of pregnancy. They can have serious adverse effects on the health of both the pregnant mother and her baby. The increasing prevalence of many STD and the advent of HIV-related problems emphasize the need for STD awareness in the care of pregnant women [92]. Screening for HPV, HBV/HCV, and HIV should be considered in all pregnant women. Recognition of viral STD, followed by appropriate counseling and management, will avoid most neonatal viral infection [93].

The STD threaten the reproductive health of women in many ways, ranging from premature births through congenital infections and death.

An understanding of the natural history of these diseases permits timely interventions which can mitigate the perinatal damage caused by these infections substantially.

Ideally, primary prevention or safer sex will be adopted by sexually active women, thereby reducing the morbidity not only for their offspring but for themselves as well. Antiviral therapy is not yet available for minimizing any hazard of fetal exposure to HPV, HSV, HIV, and HBV/HCV infections [94]. The prevalence of maternal infections may vary in different populations, and others might arrive at different estimates about the percentage of infants colonized and, concerning those infants colonized, about the percentage with adverse outcomes.

Additionally, many women are colonized or infected simultaneously with several organisms, and this may result in different projections of morbidity and mortality rates. New information is generated continually describing the relationship between various maternal colonizations and preterm birth, and screening and treatment protocols for several diseases may reduce the prevalence of adverse outcomes.

Therefore, the prevalences of various adverse pregnancy outcomes are only approximations and may change as new information becomes available. Nevertheless, it is reasonable to estimate the relative effect of various maternal STD on adverse pregnancy outcome.

By comparing the effect of direct transmission of sexually transmitted organisms on adverse outcomes with the effect on overall outcome through an increase in the rate of preterm births, we should be able to use this type of analysis to establish some basis for allocation of resources to future research as well as intervention programs aimed at reducing STD-related adverse outcomes of pregnancy [95].

Treatment of STD begins with prompt and accurate diagnosis. Several new diagnostic techniques allow more rapid or easier testing, however sometimes at a cost [96]. Home-based screening for STI has been shown to be a feasible approach for men and women from a variety of settings, including high-risk, low-income, and resource-poor communities. In recent studies, the testing rate with home-based screening was up to 11 times greater than the testing rate with clinic-based screening. For most individuals, self-collection and testing of urine or vaginal specimens at home was considered to be easy, acceptable, and often preferred over testing at a clinic. There is limited evidence with regard to the cost-effectiveness of home-based versus clinic-based screening for STI. However, a study from the US concluded that home-based screening is cost-saving. Improvements in screening rates for STI can be achieved with home-based screening methods. Making low-cost home test kits available may encourage at-risk young individuals with less access to clinic care, who may not otherwise be screened, to self-test for STI [97].

Guidelines for the treatment of patients with STI are developed by the CDC after consultation with a group of professionals knowledgeable in the field. All recommended and alternative regimens are drawn from the most recent treatment guidelines. Clinicians have the opportunity and obligation to provide education and counseling to patients. Prevention messages should be tailored to the individual patient with consideration given to her specific risk behaviors [98]. Barriers to STD control include cultural aspects, difficulties in changing sexual behavior, asymptomatic disease in women, and expensive and inaccessible tests for diagnosis. The classical clinical approach based on etiologic treatment has never been achieved by developing countries. The international community has been searching for new approaches. Syndromic management and mass treatment are strategies recently found as useful. Then, the current approach to STD management must include: prompt attention to every patient seeking care for STD, early diagnosis and treatment, delivery of short term treatment at the clinic, education on STD/HIV, screening for other STD with pre- and post-test counselling, counseling on risk reduction, provision of condoms, and integration of STD services with family planning, prenatal, and gynecological services [99].

Considerable efforts have been made to improve the syndromic approach to STD management in developing countries, especially amongst women but the poor performance of the algorithm for managing vaginal discharge limits the effectiveness of this strategy. The facilitating role of the HIV has been the main impetus to STD control rather than reduction of morbidity in women, especially pregnant women and their children. There are no easy solutions but action on several fronts, with more attention to core groups, men, and adolescents is indicated [100].

STI are relatively common during pregnancy, especially in indigent, urban populations. Education, screening, treatment, and prevention are important components of prenatal care for women at increased risk for these infections. Treatment of these STI is clearly associated with improved pregnancy outcome and reductions in perinatal mortality [101].

The serious implications of the STD pandemic that currently challenges educators, medical practitioners, and governments suggest that prevention strategies, which primarily focus on barrier protection and the management of infection, must be reevaluated and that initiatives focusing on primary prevention of behaviors predisposing individuals to STD risk must be adopted. HIV/AIDS, HPV, and genital herpes illustrate the pervasive presence of STD and their serious consequences for individuals and national infrastructures.

Although risk reduction and treatment of existing infection is critical, the promotion of optimal life-long health can be achieved most effectively through delayed sexual debut, partner reduction, and the avoidance of risky sexual behaviors [102].

Escalating rates of STD in many areas of the world necessitate a re-evaluation of current public health STD preventive programmes. Pervasive long term sequelae for many STD afflicted people and the emerging threat, caused by the HIV/AIDS pandemic, to some national infrastructures, suggests that ongoing initiatives focusing primarily on risk reduction through barrier protection have not met their desired objective.

Recent strategies to promote non-coital sexual involvement as a means of achieving STD reduction fail to address the transmission of infection that may occur through alternative non-intercourse sexual activities. The demonstrated success of the innovative, comprehensive ABC strategy shows that while risk reduction and treatment of existing infection remain important, the promotion of optimal health may be achieved more effectively through broad based comprehensive and adaptable programmes [103, 104].

HUMAN IMMUNODEFICIENCY VIRUS

AIDS cripples the immune system, making the patient susceptible to a variety of infections and disorders. AIDS is caused by direct blood contact with a transmissible agent, now known as the HIV (Figure 1) [105]. Women account for half of the global HIV/AIDS infections. Heterosexual contact is the leading risk factor in women. Over 50% of patients are significantly immunosuppressed at the time of diagnosis [106]. Infection with HIV results in a chronic, persistent infection that usually progresses slowly from an asymptomatic state to full-blown AIDS. A great deal of information has been learned in the past decades, yet many questions remain unresolved. Much more research is needed into the conditions surrounding the perinatal transmission of HIV. Many women who give birth to a child with AIDS are themselves asymptomatic for HIV infection during pregnancy and at delivery. Thus, routine prenatal HIV screening programs must be ensured. Such screening programs must provide pretest and post-test counseling with consent and confidentiality.

Seroprevalence studies conducted during the perinatal period or at birth using newborn blood samples will provide important epidemiologic data for further research investigations as well as continued estimates of the prevalence of HIV infection. As the epidemic continues and the true prevalence rates are determined, additional resources for public health care, housing, insurance, and foster care for children will be needed. The number of women who are infected is increasing at an alarming rate. Every opportunity to increase public awareness about the AIDS epidemic and modes of transmission must be exploited if we are to impact on the spread of HIV infection. Prospective studies of pregnant HIV-positive women and pediatric follow-up can provide a wealth of data about AIDS and disease progression in both the mother and the infant. Even if some children do not develop AIDS, the possibility of permanent effects of in utero exposure to the virus still exists. Even if a vaccine is developed in the near future, the impact of this deadly virus will have repercussions for many years to come [107]. The increasing number of women with AIDS or with serologic evidence of exposure should alert practicing obstetricians and gynecologists to expect to encounter symptomatic or asymptomatic patients who have been exposed to the HIV [108]. Like the Influenza Virus, HIV can change its protein coat rapidly. The victim can appear perfectly healthy and still spread the disease. In countries with low maternal mortality, it could become the most common cause of maternal death. If people are to adopt safe sex practices, they must be convinced that they are at risk, that a lethal disease can be asymptomatic but ineffective for many years. They must know that safety practices, including the use of condoms, and perhaps especially spermicidally lubricated condoms, offer worthwhile protection. If any link in this chain is broken, individuals will not adopt such voluntary practices. There are no known political or geographical barriers to human copulation: now is the time to act, particularly in countries with a low or no prevalence of AIDS. Obstetricians must fight AIDS with the same commitment to preventative medicine that they bring to good obstetrics and good family planning [109].

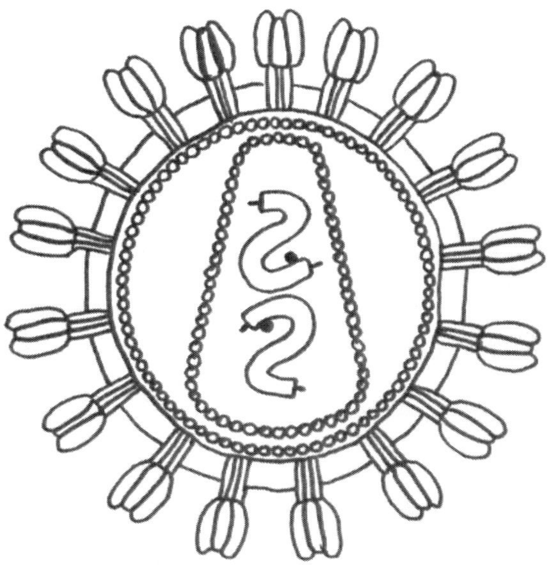

Modified from en.wikipedia.org.

Figure 1. Human Immunodeficiency Virus (HIV).

There is hardly any other disease where differences of opinion are as dramatic as they are in AIDS. Safely established epidemiologic data are interpreted most controversially and heatedly discussed.

Gynecology and obstetrics are no exception: here, too, scientific discussion is marred by emotional overtones. Special attention is focused on the problems of the incubation time (3 months to more than 19 years), where in contrast to other diseases it is not the time of manifestation but the final stage of the disease that counts.

That an infection may even be transmitted via intact mucosa is a newly established fact. Routes of infection can also be, besides those already known, saliva, gynecological (vaginal and rectal) specula and possibly a direct iatrogenic infection. The problem of the incidence of MTCT during pregnancy has not yet been clarified.

According to latest results, the probable quota of infected children (without treatment) is about 40%. Pregnancy care must include the offer of HIV testing. This is in fact mandatory, especially in women with enhanced risk of infection. If the doctor omits this information, he is liable to be sued for damages. Even in late pregnancy stages, testing is still meaningful (vaccination recommendations, newborn and infant care).

Special precautionary measures are recommended for parturition [110]. The CDC and the American College of Obstetricians and Gynecologists (ACOG) have recommended that pregnant women who are at increased risk for AIDS be tested for antibodies to HIV. When this recommendation is implemented, some clinicians who undoubtedly have had limited experience with patients infected with HIV will be responsible for the care of pregnant women found to be asymptomatically infected with HIV. There is, therefore, a need for information that will ensure that adequate counseling is provided and that appropriate medical and infection control measures are instituted. As a result of increased screening of at-risk populations, obstetricians with limited experience with AIDS will find themselves caring for pregnant women infected with the HIV [111].

HIV-1, the causative virus in AIDS, is epidemic in a Central Africa belt from Gabon to the East coast, and from Uganda to Zimbabwe, with the highest prevalence in the lakes and highlands of Central Africa. HIV-2 causes a milder disease in Western Africa centered in Senegal. HIV infections occur primarily in young adult men aged 30-34, women aged 20-24, infants and children under 4, and a few girls. Transmission patterns vary widely depending on sexual customs in the ethnically diverse continent. Prevalence tends to be high in cities and among subgroups such as prostitutes, where promiscuity is restricted. Where female sexual permissiveness exists, seropositivity is high in women generally. Besides sexual behavior, risk factors for HIV in Africa also include uncircumcised man, OC, STD causing genital ulceration, and Chlamydia infection.

Transmission to neonates occurs, especially if the mother has advanced AIDS, but transmission by breast milk is uncertain. Transmission by blood transfusion is common because transfusion are up to 10 times as common in Africa as in the West, especially in obstetrics and pediatrics.

Clinically, HIV infections present as Herpes Zoster in 95% of Africans, and commonly as slim disease: weakness, fever, chronic watery diarrhea, and weight loss of unknown cause. Associated infection are vulvovaginal candidiasis (VVC), cryptosporidiosis, isosporiasis, tuberculosis, and salmonellosis. Other presenting symptoms are unusual sites of lymphadenopathy, cough, and sepsis. Diagnosis can be made by the World Health Organization (WHO) clinical case definition, or be screening tests, which are now more reliable for African patients than formerly. In Africa, AIDS can cause destitution and disgrace for families, and will probable severely affect progress made national economies because of deaths of young productive adults [112]. Apart from number of exposures, if any, several factors influence the efficiency of HIV transmission during sex. Acute HIV infection, with extraordinarily high semen viral load, in conjunction with concurrent partnerships maximizes this efficiency.

Delaying sexual debut and avoiding HIV exposure among biologically and socially vulnerable youth is critical. Reducing unintended pregnancies keeps girls in school and prevents vertical (also possibly horizontal) transmission. Female condoms, especially newer versions, are an under-exploited prevention technology. Control of STI, which facilitate HIV acquisition and transmission, remains important, especially among the most at-risk populations.

Pathogens, such as HSV type 2, which contribute most to HIV transmission in Southern Africa must be targeted, although the importance of bacterial vaginosis and Trichomonas vaginalis is under-recognized. Also, heavy episodic alcohol use affects sexual decision-making and condom skills.

Moreover, prevailing social contexts, partly a consequence of poor leadership, constrain the behavioral “choices” available for girls and women. Priority health sector interventions for preventing HIV are: male and female condom programming, prevention and control of STI, outreach to most vulnerable populations, HIV testing in all patient-provider encounters, male circumcision, and the integration of HIV prevention within sexual and reproductive health services. Future interventions during acute HIV infection and microbicides will reduce women’s biological vulnerability. Far-reaching measures, such as sexual equity and alcohol control, create conditions necessary for achieving sustained prevention results. These are, however, contingent on stronger, more informed cultural and political leadership [113]. HIV/AIDS impacts on every aspect of reproductive health and presents considerable challenges to healthcare systems. Fertility is particularly valued in Africa and voluntary childlessness is unusual.

AIDS results in a reduction in both fecundity and fertility, as well as compromising the outcome of pregnancy. The stigma of childlessness is quite profound and impacts both social life and social standing within the community, particularly of the women who are affected. Unfortunately, treatment for infertility is often inadequate and, because of limited resources, is frequently denied to HIV-positive couples. Undoubtedly, the challenges in dealing with the HIV/AIDS pandemic in Africa are enormous. However, appropriate solutions are available and these need to be put in place. It is essential that the management of the HIV patient is holistic and takes all needs, including that of fertility, into account [114]. Sex work remains an important contributor to HIV transmission within early, advanced and regressing epidemics in sub-Saharan Africa, but its social and behavioral underpinnings remain poorly understood, limiting the impact of HIV prevention initiatives. Female sex workers (FSW) commonly have limited economic options, many dependents, marital disruption, and low education. Their vulnerability to HIV, heightened among young women, is inextricably linked to the occupational contexts of their work, characterized most commonly by poverty, endemic violence, criminalization, high mobility, and hazardous alcohol use.

These, in turn, predict behaviors such as low condom use, anal sex, and co-infection with other STI. Sex work in Africa cannot be viewed in isolation from other HIV-risk behaviors such as multiple concurrent partnerships, there is often much overlap between sexual networks. High turn-over of FSW, with sex work duration typically around 3 years, further heightens risk of HIV acquisition and transmission. Targeted services at sufficiently high coverage, taking into account the behavioral and social vulnerabilities, are urgently required to address the disproportionate burden of HIV carried by FSW on the continent [115].

Gynecologic care should be directed toward early identification and aggressive treatment of infectious and neoplastic processes that may take a more fulminant course in immunosuppressed women. Dealing with women's contraceptive needs highlights the problem of preventing STD through contraceptive technology. Public health policies and recommendations will be of no avail without an educated and supportive medical community. Both AIDS surveillance data and surveys on the seroprevalence of HIV indicate that HIV infection through heterosexual transmission is showing a trend of dramatic increase among US women. In women, especially pregnant women, AIDS has a more fulminant course than in men and there is a shorter survival time from diagnosis to death.

Gynecologists may be the first source of medical contact among asymptomatic HIV-positive women, and primary care providers should aware of unusual gynecologic manifestations of HIV infection. Protracted herpes infection, refractory VVC, and widespread condylomata often represent early warning signs of an underlying immunocompromised state. Women with impaired cellular immunity are at greater risk of genital HPV and neoplasia. Deficient cellular immunity also facilitates activation of latent infections such as CMV, HSV, and HPV. PID is found in a disproportionately high number of HIV-infected women, although it is unknown whether the inflammation is secondary to the AIDS virus or a co-factor. Genital ulcers both increase the risk of HIV seroconversion and enhance the infectiousness of women already HIV-positive. HSV and other gynecologic conditions are likely to be more fulminant in presentation, more protracted in course, and resistant to conventional therapy in HIV-infected patients.

To facilitate the early identification and treatment of these conditions, Papanicolaou (Pap) smears should be taken every 4-6 months in infected women and there should be liberal use of colposcopy. OC users should be advised to switch to condom/N-9 use to reduce the potential for disease transmission and accelerated progression [116].

Gender-specific manifestations, such as cervical neoplasia and vaginal moniliasis, appear to pursue a more aggressive course in HIV-infected women. Little is known about the pharmacokinetics of drugs for HIV and related infections. OC may alter the metabolism of some drugs used in HIV-infected women. Little is currently known regarding the natural course of HIV infection in women. Women infected with HIV should be followed-up frequently with specific attention paid to the reproductive system. Additional studies should be conducted to determine the impact of HIV on gender-specific diseases [117]. Genital infections by other pathogens may be the first clue to the diagnosis. With progressive immunodeficiency, such infections may follow a protracted course or become recurrent, often requiring maintenance therapy [118].

Gynecologists have an obligation to become informed about the transmission, clinical manifestations, and management of HIV. Women with HIV infection are at increased risk of lower genital tract neoplasia with extensive cervical, vaginal, and vulvar lesions. There is also a strong association between HIV infection and STD involving genital ulcerations. In fact, herpes, warts, and VVC may be the initial clinical presentation of HIV infection.

Estradiol levels may fall in seropositive women, but, in general, menstruation and ovulation are maintained. Latex condoms remain the only contraceptive choice for HIV-infected women. Sufficient data have not been accumulated on the effectiveness of the female condom, but it has the potential of giving women in developing countries in particular greater control over HIV prevention. Condom use is essential even if both partners are HIV-positive since the acquisition of different HIV strains can accelerate disease progression [119]. After the advent of highly active ARV therapy (HAART), a decrease occurred in the mortality rate, which now seems to have stabilized. One of the consequences of this current situation is that more and more HIV-infected women are now reaching menopause. Therefore, factors often investigated in seronegative women need to be evaluated in middle-aged, HIV-positive women. In midlife, HIV-positive women will experience the onset of menopause, while concomitantly they may also be affected by metabolic complications related to the HIV infection and to HAART. Conditions related to middle-aged women with HIV such as menstrual disorders, gynecologic surgery, age at menopause, menopausal symptoms, reproductive hormones, cognitive function, bone mineral density (BMD), cardiovascular disease (CVD), and lipid and glucose metabolism in middle-aged women with HIV may be aggravated by the HIV infection and by HAART [120, 121]. HAART has improved the life span of people living with HIV and AIDS. Advances in scientific knowledge and management of the HIV-positive pregnant woman have also led to reduction in the risk of MTCT of HIV. The gynecological and reproductive health needs and care of the HIV-positive woman are poorly appreciated, suboptimal, and largely neglected, with potential to negatively affect their quality of life (QOL) and efforts at control of the HIV epidemic. The HIV-positive woman suffers increased frequency and severity of pelvic infections and cervical premalignant and malignant lesions. Relapses and treatment failures of these conditions are common among these patients. Infertility and contraception are also challenges to the HIV-positive woman. Gynecological and reproductive health care is an integral part of the comprehensive health care needs of the HIV-positive woman. In addition to ARV treatment, HIV positive women should be provided regular screening for STI, cervical cytology, counseling and services for infertility and contraception. Appropriate attention to the gynecological and reproductive health needs of the HIV-positive woman will improve her general health status and quality of life and contribute to reduction in the incidence of HIV infection [122]. The increased use of screening tests has led to the identification of large numbers of women with HIV.

Consequently, there is an increased role for obstetrician-gynecologists in caring for infected women. Women infected with HIV are living longer, healthier lives and, therefore, the need for routine gynecologic care has increased [123].

Gynecologic disease is commonly encountered in women infected with the HIV. The clinical course of CIN, invasive cervical cancer, PID, syphilis, and VVC may be altered by HIV infection and may be refractory to standard treatment, especially with increasing degrees of immune suppression. Careful screening for gynecologic disease and vigilant surveillance for treatment failure are important in the care of women infected with HIV [124]. A panel of leading Italian specialists in infectious diseases, obstetrics, and gynecology met in a national consensus workshop on women facing HIV to review critical aspects and discuss recommendations for selected key questions on four issues:

1) women and HAART: access to care and adherence to therapy, side effects and drug-drug interaction;
2) HIV-infected pregnant women: prevention of MTCT;
3) desire for children among women living with HIV: ART; and
4) STD and genital disturbances.

The method of a nominal group meeting was used, and recommendations were graded for their strength and quality of evidence using a system based on the one adopted by the Infectious Diseases Society of America (IDSA) [125].

Women with advanced HIV infection are at a risk for opportunistic infections (OI). OI lead to significant morbidity and cost. Some of OI may impact women more significantly than men, that is, HPV infection and cervical cancer. OI during pregnancy can increase the risk of MTCT of HIV and some OI, such as HCV [106]. The issue of TORCH testing in pregnant women infected with the HIV virus remains confusing, even more so than it is in the non-HIV-infected gravida. Unfortunately, the data presented make the recommendations of how to test for these various infections in pregnancy that much more difficult. Patients who are newly diagnosed as being HIV-infected and referred for prenatal care or who have not had TORCH testing probably should be tested.

Thus, the prenatal patient with newly diagnosed HIV infection should be tested for Toxoplasma gondii IgG antibodies. If positive for IgG antibodies, IgM antibodies should be obtained in an attempt to rule out acute T. gondii infection.

Patients who test negative do not require any further testing until after the pregnancy unless they are severely immunocompromised and show signs and symptoms of toxoplasmosis. Antibodies (IgG) to CMV should be obtained in the HIV-infected gravida who is at high risk for CMV disease, i.e., patients with CD4+ T cell counts less than 100/mm^3. Unfortunately, the previously described problems with antibody detection make this testing less than ideal. Thus, it is not routinely recommended in the HIV-infected pregnant patient who presents for prenatal care except for those at risk of disease reactivation. As for HSV testing, there is no value in routinely testing patients prenatally for evidence of the disease. Finally, syphilis testing in the HIV-infected gravida is of major importance. Once tested, the patient who tests negative and who remains at risk for infection should probably be retested in the third trimester. Patients who are found to have the disease and who are treated need to be tested serially to rule out re-infection or treatment failure [126].

Sexual transmission of HIV-1, in the absence of co-factors, is poorly efficient. Data support that HSV type-2 (HSV-2) may increase a woman's susceptibility to HIV-1. Potential mechanisms by which HSV-2 serves as an HIV-1 enhancing co-factor include:

1) initiation of a clinical or subclinical mucosal inflammatory response;
2) alteration of innate mucosal immunity; and
3) weakening or breaching the protective genital epithelia.

No clinical trial has examined prevention of primary HSV-2 infection to eliminate the major morbidities of this recurrent disease and as a strategy to reduce HIV-1 transmission. Topical administration of potent antivirals can achieve local concentrations that are orders of magnitude higher than those obtained with oral administration.

Simultaneous prevention of sexual acquisition of HSV-2 and HIV-1 via topical ARV agents will have a synergistic impact on both epidemics [127]. HCV) infection is common in HIV infected individuals in the US and in Western Europe. The improved prognosis for HIV-infected people has increased the desire of parenthood. There is no evidence to support advising against pregnancy in HIV-HCV co-infected women [128].

HIV infection primarily affects women during their reproductive years, and the co-existence of gynecological infections is not surprising, given the fact that HIV is mainly acquired via heterosexual contact. Most gynecological infections are themselves sexually acquired, and have the potential to increase the risk both of acquiring and transmitting the HIV.

As most STI are asymptomatic, there is a need to improve methods of diagnosis and algorithms for early detection of STI. HIV infection, however, particularly advanced disease, may alter the clinical presentation, course, and response to conservative treatment for some of the STI [129]. VVC is one of the most common fungal infections that recur frequently in HIV infected women. Symptoms of VVC are pruritis, discomfort, dyspareunia, and dysuria. Vulval infection presents as a morbiliform rash that may extend to the thighs. Vaginal infection is associated with white discharge, and plaques are seen on erythematous vaginal walls. Even though rarely or never resulting in systemic fungal infection or mortality, left untreated these lesions contribute considerably to the morbidity associated with HIV infection. Prevention and treatment of this condition is an essential part of maintaining the QOL for these individuals. No randomized controlled trials (RCT) were found addressing treatment of VVC in HIV positive women. In comparison to placebo, fluconazole was found to be an effective preventative intervention. However, the potential for resistant Candida organisms to develop might impact the feasibility of implementation. Direction of findings suggests that clotrimazole and Lactobacillus improved the prophylactic outcomes when compared to placebo. There is a need to evaluate drugs and drug regimens for VVC treatment and prophylaxis in HIV positive women through RCT. Development of resistance to azoles remains under-studied and more work must be done in this area, so as to determine whether routine prophylaxis for VVC is at all needed or whether adequate HAART would be sufficient to prevent recurrent VVC. The viral load in vaginal secretions with or without treatment or prophylaxis has not been studied, this is very relevant to the spread of HIV [130]. Among the now pandemic STI, Chlamydia trachomatis is the predominant bacterial pathogen. The female genital tract is the primary site for heterosexual transmission of both C. trachomatis and HIV-1. Infection with C. trachomatis, and with a variety of other STI, increases the risk for transmission of HIV-1, although the mechanisms for this finding remain unclear. In vitro modeling has been used to assess the mechanisms by which infection with genital C. trachomatis serovars might increase the transmission of HIV-1 across the female genital tract. C. trachomatis infection of an immortalized endocervical epithelial cell line (A2EN) increases the cell surface expression of the HIV-1 alternative primary receptor, galactosyl ceramide (GalCer), and of the HIV-1 co-receptors, chemokine receptor type 4 (CXCR4) and type 5 (CCR5). C. trachomatis infection also increases the binding of HIV-1 to A2EN cells, and, subsequently, increases levels of virus in co-cultures of HIV-exposed A2EN and susceptible MT4-R5 T cells.

Finally, in vivo endocervical cell sampling reveals a dramatic increase in the number of CD4+, CXCR4, and/or CCR5 positive T cell targets in the endocervix of C. trachomatis positive women when compared to those who are C. trachomatis negative. This combination of in vitro and in vivo results suggests several mechanisms for increased transmission of HIV-1 across the endocervices of C. trachomatis-infected women [131]. PID and HIV infection are frequently coincident. The diagnosis of PID can be more difficult to make in HIV-infected than in uninfected women.

In general, HIV-infected women with PID have a good response to standard intravenous antibiotic therapy. However, surgical therapy is more frequently required for HIV-infected women with PID, especially those with more severe degrees of immunosuppression, than for uninfected women [132].

HIV infection has been associated with progressive deterioration of the immune system and the development of OI and various malignancies. As more experience has been accumulated on the nature and complications of AIDS, the gynecological implications of neoplasia developing in the HIV-positive patient became apparent. A type of cervical malignancy that takes a very aggressive course is being increasingly reported. Other lower genital tract tumors such as vaginal and vulvar neoplasia are also more prevalent in HIV-positive women and a closer follow-up is probably indicated in these patient population. Gestational trophoblastic disease (GTD) in AIDS patients has also been reported to be more resistant to chemotherapy and may have a grave prognosis. Finally, nongynecological malignancies such as non-Hodgkin's lymphoma (NHL) and Kaposi's sarcoma may have their first site of appearance in the genital organs, thus simulating gynecological tumors [133]. Among HIV-positive women, those who are more severely immunosuppressed appear to be at higher risk for CIN, also known as squamous intraepithelial lesions (SIL). Women who are HIV-positive also are more likely than HIV-negative women to have multifocal lower genital tract neoplasia. Cervical cancer is one of the most important AIDS-related malignancies in women. Cancer and intraepithelial neoplasia of the lower genital tract can be persistent, progressive, recurrent, and difficult to treat in HIV-positive women. The most effective method for treating SIL has not been determined. Regular performance of Pap smears in HIV-positive women is of critical importance, as is careful examination of the entire lower genital tract. Also, women with high-grade intraepithelial or cervical cancer should be tested for HIV [134]. HIV and HPV are both sexually transmitted viruses with many risk factors in common. Studies have found that HIV-seropositive women are at least five times as likely to be infected with HPV as seronegative controls.

In immunocompromised HIV-seropositive women, the risk of CIN is almost as high as in women with SIL on their Pap smear. Some studies have shown the false-negative rate of cervical cytology in HIV-seropositive women to be very high, although others have shown it to be comparable with the rate in seronegative controls. However, given the prevalence of CIN in this population, even a "normal" false-negative rate may result in many missed CIN lesions. Among HIV-seropositive women and especially among those who are immunocompromised, CIN is more likely to progress and recur after treatment. Recurrence rates may reach 87% 36 months after treatment in markedly immunosuppressed women. Cryotherapy is especially ineffective in these patients. Vulvar condyloma and vulvar intraepithelial neoplasia (VIN) are much more prevalent in HIV-seropositive women and especially in those who are markedly immunosuppressed or who have been immunosuppressed for a prolonged period of time. Immunocompromised women should be followed with cytology and colposcopy of the cervix and vulva, although those with normal immune systems may be followed with cytology alone. Because the rates of recurrence and progression are so high after treatment of these women, they should be followed with colposcopy and cytology every 6 months [135]. All HIV-infected women should be screened at least annually for cervical cancer with cervical cytology. All patients with any abnormality in the Pap smear should be referred for colposcopic evaluation. Patients with documented high-grade dysplasia should be treated. All patients must be observed closely after treatment for recurrence. Treatment with agents such as imiquimod or 5-fluorouracil (FU) may help to decrease recurrence rates. Patients who are diagnosed with cervical cancer should be treated with surgery or concurrent chemotherapy and radiation as determined by extent of disease and health status. It appears that HAART may have a positive impact on cervical dysplasia and cancer. Thus, all HIV-infected patients should be managed optimally on HAART. Hopefully, as patients live longer and healthier on HAART, they will be more compliant with cervical cancer screening, and cervical cancer will become an increasingly rare disease [136].

Cancer of the cervix is the second most common cause of cancer-related death in women worldwide, and in some low resource countries accounts for the highest cancer mortality in women. The highest burden of the HIV/AIDS epidemic is currently in sub-Saharan Africa, where more than half of the people infected are women who have no access to cervical cancer screening. The association between HIV and invasive cervical cancer is complex, with several studies now clearly demonstrating an increased risk of pre-invasive cervical lesions among HIV-infected women.

However, there have not been significantly higher incidence rates of invasive cervical cancer associated with the HIV epidemic. The highest numbers of HIV-infected women are in poorly-resourced countries, where the natural progression of HIV disease in the absence of HAART sometimes results in deaths from OI before the onset of invasive cervical cancer [137]. The recurrence rate of CIN after conization in HIV-infected women ranges from 20% to 75%. No conclusions can be drawn about the impact of CD4 cell counts on the recurrence rate. Available evidence suggests that standard excisional treatments for CIN are associated with high rates of recurrence in HIV-positive women. Despite the fact that the evidence is limited because of the few number of eligible studies, this issue should be considered in the management of HIV-positive patient with CIN [138]. HAART seems to have little, if any, beneficial effect on the natural history of intraepithelial lesions in HIV-positive women. Despite this fact, HAART does increase the life expectancy of HIV-positive women. Therefore, it remains important to closely monitor HPV-related disease in women with HIV who are receiving HAART, particularly in regions of the world where cervical screening is not available routinely [139]. HIV-infected women in different geographic regions (such as Zambia, Brazil, Rochester NY) appear to be infected with less prevalent types of high-risk HPV as compared to the general population who, across all continents, are more commonly infected with types 16 and 18. Secondly, integration of HPV DNA into the host genome is no longer thought to be a necessary cause of malignant transformation of cervical cells. However, rate of integration appears to differ by the type of HPV. In fact, the types of HPV which appear to be more common in cervical dysplasia of HIV-infected women are the same types which are more likely to require integration for malignant transformation. Finally, HPV types found in HIV-infected women are relatively common and likely to persist. The most common among these types belong to the alpha-7 and -9 species which are the most carcinogenic species. Given that current vaccines target high-risk HPV-16/18, the findings from the above mentioned studies may have important implications for the design of HPV vaccines that target the types of HPV associated with disease risk in HIV-infected women. HPV typing and assessment of the physical state (whether it is integrated or episomal) appear to be two valuable parameters for the prognostic evaluation of dysplastic lesions of the uterine cervix. This, however, has not yet been assessed in HIV-infected women. Recent data about the immune response in HPV/HIV co-infection may lead to understanding potential mechanisms for less virulent HPV causing malignant transformation in HIV-infected women [140].

There is a paucity of recent data on the effect of HAART on HPV infection and its related anogenital abnormalities/cancer. Review articles on the molecular biology of HPV in HIV infection outline why, despite HAART, anogenital tumors may continue to increase in this population. Studies continue to confirm the high prevalence of HPV infection and to define the different HPV types correlated with anogenital cytologic abnormalities, an important area in light of the development of an effective type-specific HPV vaccine. Anogenital HPV infection remains highly prevalent and persistent in HIV-infected individuals. HIV is associated with a wide diversity of HPV types and a high prevalence of anogenital cytologic abnormalities. The incidence of anogenital HPV-related cancers remains high in the HAART era, raising concerns of HPV infections as a rising health burden among HIV-infected individuals. Interventions aimed at preventing HPV infections with vaccinations need to be evaluated in HIV-infected individuals [141].

HIV infection appears to alter the natural history of HPV-associated oncogenesis, but its impact on gynecology has only recently been defined: the CDC designated moderate and severe cervical dysplasia, as well as cervical carcinoma in situ (CIS), as a category B defining condition, and invasive cervical cancer as a category C defining condition of AIDS in 1993 (Table 1). Anal HPV infection and anal SIL have been found to be highly prevalent among HIV-positive homosexual men, and recent preliminary data suggest a relatively high prevalence among HIV-positive women as well. Moreover, HPV infection and associated lesions are also observed in body sites other than the anogenital area, particularly the skin and the oral cavity [142]. Studies assessing geographic variations in HPV types and prevalence in cervical dysplasia and cancer in HIV-infected women suggest that although HPV types 16 and 18 dominate, multiple other HPV types may play a role in carcinogenesis. Anal dysplasia and cancer incidence continues to rise in the HAART era.

However, data on outcomes following therapy for anal dysplasia (infrared coagulator, high-resolution anoscopy-guided ablation) and anal cancer (chemoradiation and possibly intensity-modulated radiation therapy) have been encouraging. Oral HPV may be associated with lower genital tract HPV infection and may have implications in the development of oropharyngeal cancer. As HIV-infected patients in the HAART era continue to have high rates of cervical and anal cancer, it is important to continue screening efforts and treatment of preinvasive disease. Treatment options for anal dysplasia and anal cancer in HIV-infected individuals are expanding and may lead to decreased morbidity and mortality.

Table 1. Centers for Disease Control and Prevention (CDC) classification system for Human Immunodeficiency Virus (HIV) infection

1993 Revised Classification System for HIV Infection and Expanded Surveillance Case Definition for Acquired Immune Deficiency Syndrome (AIDS) Among Adolescents and Adults
Criteria for HIV infection for persons ages >13 years: a) repeatedly reactive screening tests for HIV antibody (e.g., enzyme immunoassay [EIA]) with specific antibody identified by the use of supplemental tests (e.g., Western blot, immunofluorescence assay [IFA]); b) direct identification of virus in host tissues by virus isolation; c) HIV antigen detection; or d) a positive result on any other highly specific licensed test for HIV. Cluster of differentiation (CD)4+ T-Lymphocyte categories: Category 1: ≥500 cells/ml Category 2: 200-499 cells/ml Category 3: <200 cells/ml Clinical categories: Category A: consists of one or more of the conditions listed below in an adolescent or adult (≥13 years) with documented HIV infection. Conditions listed in Categories B and C must not have occurred. • Asymptomatic HIV infection • Persistent generalized lymphadenopathy • Acute (primary) HIV infection with accompanying illness or history of acute HIV infection Category B: consists of symptomatic conditions in an HIV-infected adolescent or adult that are not included among conditions listed in clinical Category C and that meet at least one of the following criteria: a) the conditions are attributed to HIV infection or are indicative of a defect in cell-mediated immunity; or b) the conditions are considered by physicians to have a clinical course or to require management that is complicated by HIV infection. Examples of conditions in clinical Category B include, but are not limited to:

Table 1. (Continued)

1993 Revised Classification System for HIV Infection and Expanded Surveillance Case Definition for Acquired Immune Deficiency Syndrome (AIDS) Among Adolescents and Adults
• Bacillary angiomatosis • Oropharyngeal candidiasis (OPC, "thrush") • Vulvovaginal candidiasis (VVC): persistent, frequent, or poorly responsive to therapy • Cervical dysplasia (moderate or severe)/cervical carcinoma in situ (CIS) • Constitutional symptoms, such as fever (38.5°C) or diarrhea lasting >1 month • Oral hairy leukoplaki (OHL) • Herpes zoster ("shingles"), involving at least two distinct episodes or more than one dermatome • Idiopathic thrombocytopenic purpura (ITP) • Listeriosis • Pelvic inflammatory disease (PID), particularly if complicated by tubo-ovarian abscess (TOA) • Peripheral neuropathy (PN) For classification purposes, Category B conditions take precedence over those in Category A. For example, someone previously treated for OPC or persistent VVC (and who has not developed a Category C disease) but who is now asymptomatic should be classified in clinical Category B. Category C: includes the clinical conditions listed in the AIDS surveillance case definition. For classification purposes, once a Category C condition has occurred, the person will remain in Category C. Conditions included in the 1993 AIDS surveillance case definition: • Candidiasis of bronchi, trachea, or lungs • Esophageal candidiasis (EC) • Invasive cervical cancer* • Disseminated or extrapulmonary coccidioidomycosis • Extrapulmonary cryptococcosis • Chronic intestinal cryptosporidiosis (>1 month's duration) • Cytomegalovirus (CMV) disease (other than liver, spleen, or nodes) • CMV retinitis (with loss of vision) • HIV-related encephalopathy • Herpes Simplex Virus (HSV) infection: chronic ulcer(s) (>1 month's duration) or bronchitis, pneumonitis, or esophagitis • Disseminated or extrapulmonary histoplasmosis

1993 Revised Classification System for HIV Infection and Expanded Surveillance Case Definition for Acquired Immune Deficiency Syndrome (AIDS) Among Adolescents and Adults
• Chronic intestinal isosporiasis (>1 month's duration) • Kaposi's sarcoma • Burkitt's lymphoma (or equivalent term) • Immunoblastic lymphoma (or equivalent term) • Primary lymphoma in brain • Disseminated or extrapulmonary Mycobacterium avium complex (MAC) or M. kansasii • Mycobacterium tuberculosis, any site (pulmonary* or extrapulmonary) • Disseminated or extrapulmonary Mycobacterium, other species or unidentified species • Pneumocystis carinii pneumonia (PCP) • Recurrent pneumonia* • Progressive multifocal leukoencephalopathy (PML) • Recurrent Salmonella septicemia • Toxoplasmosis of brain • Wasting syndrome due to HIV Definitive diagnostic methods for diseases indicative of AIDS: • Cryptosporidiosis, isosporiasis, Kaposi's sarcoma, lymphoma, PCP, PML, Toxoplasmosis, cervical cancer: microscopy (histology or cytology) • Candidiasis: gross inspection by endoscopy or autopsy or by microscopy (histology or cytology) on a specimen obtained directly from the tissues affected (including scrapings from the mucosal surface), not from a culture • Coccidioidomycosis, cryptococcosis, CMV, HSV, histoplasmosis: microscopy (histology or cytology), culture, or detection of antigen in a specimen obtained directly from the tissues affected or a fluid from those tissues • Tuberculosis, other mycobacteriosis, salmonellosis: culture • HIV encephalopathy (dementia): clinical findings of disabling cognitive or motor dysfunction interfering with occupation or activities of daily living, progressing over weeks to months, in the absence of a concurrent illness or condition other than HIV infection that could explain the findings. Methods to rule out such concurrent illness and conditions must include cerebrospinal fluid (CSF) examination and either brain imaging (computed tomography [CT] or magnetic resonance [MR]) or autopsy • HIV wasting syndrome: findings of profound involuntary weight loss of greater than 10% of baseline body weight plus either chronic diarrhea (at least two loose stools per day for ≥30 days), or chronic weakness and documented fever (for ≥30 days, intermittent or constant) in the absence of a concurrent

Table 1. (Continued)

1993 Revised Classification System for HIV Infection and Expanded Surveillance Case Definition for Acquired Immune Deficiency Syndrome (AIDS) Among Adolescents and Adults
illness or condition other than HIV infection that could explain the findings (e.g., cancer, tuberculosis, cryptosporidiosis, or other specific enteritis) • Recurrent pneumonia: recurrent (more than one episode in a 1-year period), acute (new X-ray evidence not present earlier) pneumonia diagnosed by both: a) culture (or other organism-specific diagnostic method) obtained from a clinically reliable specimen of a pathogen that typically causes pneumonia (other than P. carinii or M. tuberculosis), and b) radiologic evidence of pneumonia. Cases that do not have laboratory confirmation of a causative organism for one of the episodes of pneumonia will be considered to be presumptively diagnosed. Suggested guidelines for presumptive diagnosis of diseases indicative of AIDS: • EC: recent onset of retrosternal pain on swallowing and OPC diagnosed by the gross appearance of white patches or plaques on an erythematous base or by the microscopic appearance of fungal mycelial filaments from a noncultured specimen scraped from the oral mucosa • CMV retinitis: a characteristic appearance on serial ophthalmoscopic examinations (e.g., discrete patches of retinal whitening with distinct borders, spreading in a centrifugal manner along the paths of blood vessels, progressing over several months, and frequently associated with retinal vasculitis, hemorrhage, and necrosis). Resolution of active disease leaves retinal scarring and atrophy with retinal pigment epithelial mottling • Mycobacteriosis: microscopy of a specimen from stool or normally sterile body fluids or tissue from a site other than lungs, skin, or cervical or hilar lymph nodes that shows acid-fast bacilli of a species not identified by culture • Kaposi's sarcoma: a characteristic gross appearance of an erythematous or violaceous plaque-like lesion on skin or mucous membrane (Note: presumptive diagnosis of Kaposi's sarcoma should not be made by clinicians who have seen few cases of it) • PCP: a history of dyspnea on exertion or nonproductive cough of recent onset (within the past 3 months), chest X-ray evidence of diffuse bilateral interstitial infiltrates or evidence by gallium scan of diffuse bilateral pulmonary disease, arterial blood gas (ABG) analysis showing an arterial oxygen partial pressure (pO_2) <70 mmHg or a low respiratory diffusing

1993 Revised Classification System for HIV Infection and Expanded Surveillance Case Definition for Acquired Immune Deficiency Syndrome (AIDS) Among Adolescents and Adults
capacity (<80% of predicted values) or an increase in the alveolar-arterial (A-a) oxygen tension gradient, and no evidence of a bacterial pneumonia • Recurrent pneumonia: recurrent (more than one episode in a 1-year period), acute (new symptoms, signs, or X-ray evidence not present earlier) pneumonia diagnosed on clinical or radiologic grounds by the patient's physician • Toxoplasmosis of brain: recent onset of a focal neurologic abnormality consistent with intracranial disease or a reduced level of consciousness, evidence by brain imaging (CT or MR) of a lesion having a mass effect or the radiographic appearance of which is enhanced by injection of contrast medium, and serum antibody to toxoplasmosis or successful response to therapy for toxoplasmosis • Pulmonary tuberculosis: when bacteriologic confirmation is not available, other reports may be considered to be verified cases of pulmonary tuberculosis if the criteria of the Division of Tuberculosis Elimination (DTBE), National Center for Prevention Services (NCPS), CDC, are used.

[*] Added in the 1993 expansion of the AIDS surveillance case definition.

1994 Revised Classification System for HIV Infection in Children <13 Years of Age
Diagnosis of HIV infection in children[*]: a) A child <18 months of age who is known to be HIV seropositive or born to an HIV-infected mother and: • has positive results on two separate determinations (excluding cord blood) from one or more of the following HIV detection tests: - HIV culture - HIV polymerase chain reaction (PCR) - HIV antigen (p24) or • meets criteria for AIDS diagnosis based on the 1987 AIDS surveillance case definition. b) A child ≥18 months of age born to an HIV-infected mother or any child infected by blood, blood products, or other known modes of transmission (e.g., sexual contact) who: • is HIV-antibody positive by repeatedly reactive EIA and confirmatory test (e.g., Western blot or IFA) or • meets any of the criteria in a) above.

Table 1. (Continued)

1994 Revised Classification System for HIV Infection in Children <13 Years of Age
Diagnosis of HIV infection in perinatally exposed children (PREFIX E): a) A child who does not meet the criteria above who: • is HIV seropositive by EIA and confirmatory test (e.g., Western blot or IFA) and is <18 months of age at the time of test; or • has unknown antibody status, but was born to a mother known to be infected with HIV. Diagnosis of HIV infection in seroreverter children (SR): a) A child who is born to an HIV-infected mother and who: • has been documented as HIV-antibody negative (i.e., two or more negative EIA tests performed at 6-18 months of age or one negative EIA test after 18 months of age); • has had no other laboratory evidence of infection (has not had two positive viral detection tests, if performed); • has not had an AIDS-defining condition. *This definition of HIV infection replaces the definition published in the 1987 AIDS surveillance case definition. Clinical categories for children with HIV infection: Category N (not symptomatic): children who have no signs or symptoms considered to be the result of HIV infection or who have only one of the conditions listed in Category A. Category A (mildly symptomatic): children with two or more of the conditions listed below but none of the conditions listed in Categories B and C. • Lymphadenopathy (≥0.5 cm at more than two sites; bilateral = one site) • Hepatomegaly • Splenomegaly • Dermatitis • Parotitis • Recurrent or persistent upper respiratory infection (URI), sinusitis, or otitis media Category B (moderately symptomatic): children who have symptomatic conditions other than those listed for Category A or C that are attributed to HIV infection.

1994 Revised Classification System for HIV Infection in Children <13 Years of Age
Examples of conditions in clinical Category B include but are not limited to: • Anemia (<8 g/dl), neutropenia (<1,000/mm³), or thrombocytopenia (<100,000/mm³) persisting ≥30 days • Bacterial meningitis, pneumonia, or sepsis (single episode) • Persisting (>2 months) OPC ("thrush") in children >6 months of age • Cardiomyopathy • CMV infection, with onset before 1 month of age • Recurrent or chronic diarrhea • Hepatitis • Recurrent HSV stomatitis (more than two episodes within 1 year) • HSV bronchitis, pneumonitis, or esophagitis with onset before 1 month of age • Herpes zoster ("shingles") involving at least two distinct episodes or more than one dermatome • Leiomyosarcoma • Lymphoid interstitial pneumonia (LIP) or pulmonary nodular lymphoid hyperplasia (PNLH) complex • Nephropathy • Nocardiosis • Persistent fever (lasting >1 month) • Toxoplasmosis, onset before 1 month of age • Disseminated varicella (complicated chickenpox) Category C (severely symptomatic): children who have any condition listed in the 1987 surveillance case definition for AIDS, with the exception of LIP. Conditions included in clinical Category C for children infected with HIV*: • Multiple or recurrent serious bacterial infections (i.e., any combination of at least two culture-confirmed infections within a 2-year period), of the following types: septicemia, pneumonia, meningitis, bone or joint infection, or abscess of an internal organ or body cavity (excluding otitis media, superficial skin or mucosal abscesses, and indwelling catheter-related infections) • Esophageal or pulmonary (bronchi, trachea, lungs) candidiasis • Disseminated coccidioidomycosis (at site other than or in addition to lungs or cervical or hilar lymph nodes) • Extrapulmonary cryptococcosis • Cryptosporidiosis or isosporiasis with diarrhea persisting >1 month • CMV disease with onset of symptoms at age >1 month (at a site other than liver, spleen, or lymph nodes)

Table 1. (Continued)

1994 Revised Classification System for HIV Infection in Children <13 Years of Age
• Encephalopathy (at least one of the following progressive findings present for at least 2 months in the absence of a concurrent illness other than HIV infection that could explain the findings): a. failure to attain or loss of developmental milestones or loss of intellectual ability, verified by standard developmental scale or neuropsychological tests; b. impaired brain growth or acquired microcephaly demonstrated by head circumference measurements or brain atrophy demonstrated by CT or MR imaging (serial imaging is required for children <2 years of age); c. acquired symmetric motor deficit manifested by two or more of the following: paresis, pathologic reflexes, ataxia, or gait disturbance • HSV infection causing a mucocutaneous ulcer that persists for >1 month or bronchitis, pneumonitis, or esophagitis for any duration affecting a child >1 month of age • Disseminated histoplasmosis (at a site other than or in addition to lungs or cervical or hilar lymph nodes) • Kaposi's sarcoma • Primary lymphoma in brain • Small, noncleaved cell (Burkitt's) lymphoma or immunoblastic or large cell lymphoma of B-cell or unknown immunologic phenotype • Disseminated or extrapulmonary M. tuberculosis • Disseminated Mycobacterium, other species or unidentified species (at a site other than or in addition to lungs, skin, or cervical or hilar lymph nodes) • Disseminated MAC or M. kansasii (at site other than or in addition to lungs, skin, or cervical or hilar lymph nodes) • PCP • PML • Recurrent Salmonella (nontyphoid) septicemia • Toxoplasmosis of the brain with onset at >1 month of age • Wasting syndrome in the absence of a concurrent illness other than HIV infection that could explain the following findings: a) persistent weight loss >10% of baseline or c) downward crossing of at least two of the following percentile lines on the weight-for-age chart (e.g., 95th, 75th, 50th, 25th, 5th) in a child ≥1 year of age

1994 Revised Classification System for HIV Infection in Children <13 Years of Age
or
d) $<5^{th}$ percentile on weight-for-height chart on two consecutive measurements, ≥30 days apart
plus
a) chronic diarrhea (i.e., at least two loose stools per day for >30 days)
or
b) documented fever (for ≥30 days, intermittent or constant)
*Diagnosis criteria according to the 1987 AIDS surveillance case definition.

Adapted from CDC, 2001.

Trials assessing safety and immunogenicity of the HPV quadrivalent vaccine in people with HIV have started enrollment, and if successful, may prevent many HPV-associated cancers [143].

The incidence of VIN nearly doubled between 1973 and 1987. In one study, VIN has been reported to occur 29 times more frequently in HIV-infected women than in a control group of self-identified non-HIV-infected women. Because women with HIV are now living longer, they face an increased possibility of the development of these infections along with the long-term sequelae and the risk of transformation to cancer. Treatment of VIN is guided by the size and location of the lesion, the grade of the dysplasia, and identification of coexisting disease in other sites. One of the most difficult management and education issues encountered following women with HIV disease and lower genital tract neoplasia is that the best mode of treatment for VIN has yet to be determined. Screening of the entire lower genital tract, including the vulva for dysplasia, is recommended for early detection and timely initiation of management [144]. Vulvar cancer in young HIV-seropositive women may be associated with other HPV-related diseases and immunosuppression, as evidenced by low CD4 counts and the presence of antecedent AIDS-defining illnesses [145]. The optimal treatment of advanced vulvar cancer in HIV positive patients remains unclear given the small number of cases reported in the literature. Lessons from the anal cancer literature may help inform the care of vulvar cancer patients given the comparable high prevalence of this disease in the patients infected with HIV [146].

Kaposi's sarcoma has become a common manifestation in people with AIDS, especially men. A few reports of Kaposi's sarcoma in women with AIDS have involved nongenital areas. However, of the few patients with genital Kaposi's sarcoma reported in the US, none was believed to be HIV-positive.

Genital Kaposi's sarcoma associated with HIV has been reported in other parts of the world. This report should alert HCW to include Kaposi's sarcoma in the differential diagnosis of vulvar lesions [147]. Since it was first claimed in 1995 that hCG inhibits HIV-associated Kaposi's sarcoma, focus has been lost on establishing a credible hypothesis to explain a novel action ascribed to hCG, which is, after all, a pregnancy hormone. After 7 years, no real progress has been made, and there remains no consensus as to which component of hCG preparations is responsible for inducing apoptosis of HIV-associated Kaposi's sarcoma. It would certainly seem apparent that many basic experiments on hCG species have been overlooked in the studies that have been published. Furthermore, the much wider literature concerning the association of hCG with promoting oncogenesis has been ignored [148]. HIV infection may predispose patients to extensive metastatic choriocarcinoma and influence the course of treatment. It has been proposed that HIV infection be considered a poor prognostic risk for gestational trophoblastic neoplasias [149].

Science has made great strides in understanding the management of the many gynecologic conditions that affect HIV-positive women with an increased frequency. As HIV-infected women's life expectancy continues to lengthen, new treatments are necessary for recurring conditions, such as lower genital tract neoplasias. The medical field has much to learn about the interaction between sex steroids, HIV-infection, and the immune system. As knowledge grows, clinicians will be better equipped to counsel women about contraceptive issues, pregnancy, and menopause [150]. The advent of HAART has promoted a reduction in mortality due to HIV. Thus, more women are living longer after receiving a diagnosis of HIV infection. With an increase in survival, topics related to the menopausal transition in HIV-infected women have emerged, such as age at menopause, BMD, and menopause-related symptoms. To this end, several studies have investigated age at menopause in HIV-infected women [151]. In the foreseeable future, HIV-infected women who acquired disease during the peak years of the epidemic are expected to survive to experience menopause and even years beyond. The HIV epidemic may be viewed as "mature", as its earlier victims become part of the geriatric population. Research about the process of menopause in HIV-infected women and, conversely, about HIV infection in women undergoing menopause is currently limited. Existing research suggests that the process of menopause is affected by HIV infection, inasmuch as infected women appear to experience menopause at an earlier age, with greater symptomatology, and with different reproductive hormone profiles compared with HIV-uninfected women.

HIV infection also appears to affect BMD, CVD, and cognition, with some age-related interactions. Lifestyle and demographic factors have pervasive importance for both HIV infection and the menopause in women. Clinicians should appreciate the potential role of HIV infection in caring for menopause-aged women [152]. This increased survival has led to concerns about the long-term implications of HIV disease and its treatment. Women with HIV infection appear to lose ovarian function earlier in life than women without HIV infection. They also have evidence of reduced BMD and increased cardiovascular risk. Moreover, many of these increases in risk factors are present even prior to the menopausal transition. All of these risks, present at midlife, augur poorly for future health and describe a substantially increased burden of disease likely to accrue to HIV-infected women as they enter older age groups. Further compounding the adversity faced by the HIV infected, the demographics of women most vulnerable to this disease include adverse social and economic influences, both of which worsen their long-term prognosis. For example, drug use and poverty are related to more severe menopausal symptoms and chronic stress is related to worse psychological and cardiovascular risk. An understanding of how menopause interacts with HIV infection is therefore most important to alert the clinician to perform surveillance for common health problems in postmenopausal women, and to address directly and appropriately symptomatology during the menopausal transition [153].

Because of the long incubation period from initial infection to AIDS diagnosis, the majority of young adults with AIDS were probably initially infected as adolescents. HIV seroprevalence studies of adolescents show a male-to-female ratio approaching 1:1, with many HIV-infected adolescent women identifying none of the standard risk. Factors such as sexual and drug experimentation, risk taking, and sense of invulnerability so characteristic of adolescence put adolescents at special risk for HIV. There is no published information on if or how clinical manifestations of HIV disease in adolescents might differ from those seen in adults. Medical care should be broad-based and should include access to clinical trials for new drug treatments. General knowledge levels about AIDS are high among US adolescents, but behavioral changes have lagged behind. All adolescents should be targeted for intensive education about HIV along with interventions designed to enhance their general coping, communication, and decision-making skills [154]. The obstetrician/gynecologists may be responsible for the primary reproductive healthcare, prenatal care, and pregnancy options counseling of the adolescent with HIV.

Important knowledge includes the stages of HIV infection, biologic and behavioral risk factors for HIV acquisition in youth, HIV counseling and testing procedures, and the reproductive healthcare issues in HIV-positive adolescents [155].

The percentage of AIDS cases among women, particularly women of color, in the US is increasing yearly. Despite this increase, there has been a relatively steady decline in the number of AIDS cases occurring perinatally. Regardless of the reasons HIV-infected couples choose to become pregnant, studies indicate that providing support, such as contraceptive counseling and ART, can improve the health outcome in the face of HIV-related challenges. Issues specific to ARV therapy, including viral resistance, pregnancy outcomes, and adverse fetal effects, complicate the treatment of perinatal HIV. Postpartum case is yet another area that requires special consideration when supporting HIV-infected parents and children. The growing body of data on pregnancy and HIV may indicate a rising commitment to research of and support for the unique challenges HIV-infected families face [156]. Risk testing for HIV serostatus is unlikely to detect more than 20% of HIV-positive pregnant women because risk factors target intravenous drug users and the sexual behavior of men. Pregnancy does not seem to have a major impact on the progress of HIV disease, but could be detrimental particularly in the later stages of the disease. Especially in developing countries, where HIV-positive patients are more likely to be of poor nutritional status and burdened with a number of other infections such as malaria and tuberculosis, there is a higher risk of preterm labor, small-for-dates babies, and chorioamnionitis in pregnancy. The risk of vertical transmission is increased when viral loads are high, the general maternal condition is poor, and delivery is preterm. Rates in Papua New Guinea appear to be following the higher rates which have been reported from Africa. Gynecological conditions found in association with HIV infection, including PID, VVC, and cervical neoplasia, may be resistant to treatment and tend to recur. Contraception for HIV-positive women may be more important to them than prevention of viral transmission: Depo-Provera and tubal ligation have special benefits in this regard, especially when both partners are seropositive. HIV infection in association with psychiatric disturbance might be an indication for termination of pregnancy [157].

The continued high rates of unintended pregnancies and the unrelentless expansion of the AIDS epidemic, especially in less developed countries, warrant the development of novel strategies to help individuals avoid these risks. Dually active compounds displaying contraceptive and microbicidal anti-HIV properties constitute one such strategy.

Sharing the same anatomical and functional context, sperm fertilization and genital infection by HIV offer an opportunity for simultaneous intervention. Some of the molecules and mechanisms used by sperm to fertilize the oocyte are similar, if not identical, to those used by HIV while infecting host cells. An example of common structures is the lipid membrane surrounding the spermatozoon and the HIV core. Disruption of its architecture by surface-active compounds exerts both spermicidal and virucidal activity. A more specific alteration of lipid rafts (membrane microdomains enriched in cholesterol and glycosylphosphatidylinositol [GPI]-anchored proteins) by beta-cyclodextrins also results in similar effects. During fertilization and infection, both sperm and HIV interact with their target cell receptors through chemical charges, hydrophobic forces, and carbohydrate recognition. Anionic polymers such as cellulose sulphate and polystyrene sulphonate (PSS) inhibit sperm and HIV cell binding. Because some of the molecules involved in this interaction, e.g., heparin sulphate proteoglycan, are also used by other pathogens to infect their target tissues, polyanions exert broad antimicrobial activity as well. During fertilization and infection, sperm and HIV, as well as other microbes, use signal transduction molecules and mechanisms such as adenyl cyclase/cyclic adenosine monophosphate (cAMP)-dependent kinase, calcium, and tyrosine phosphorylation, whose inhibition has been shown to impair sperm function and HIV replication. These commonalities at the level of sperm and HIV structure, cell binding, and fusion processes, and signaling pathways therefore provide the biological framework to develop bifunctional inhibitors with both antimicrobial and contraceptive properties [158]. Important considerations in choosing a family planning method for women infected with HIV-infected women will respond to standard therapy, but require multiple courses of treatment or use of innovative treatment methods. All HIV-infected women deserve careful evaluation for and treatment of gynecologic diseases. The US Centers for Disease Control's revised (1993) case definition for HIV infection now includes several gynecologic diseases. Clinical category B illnesses (attributable to or complicated by HIV) include persistent, frequent, or poorly responsive VVC, moderate or severe CIN, and PID. Clinical category C illnesses (AIDS-defining) include chronic HSV ulcers and invasive cervical cancer. Until data on the impact of contraceptives on the clinical course of HIV are available, a combination of barrier and hormonal methods or tubal ligation is recommended. All HIV-infected women deserve careful, nonjudgmental evaluation for gynecologic disease and contraception [159]. Over 50% of the 33.3 million HIV-positive persons are women within the reproductive age group.

With increasing availability and use of HAART, the prognosis, life expectancy, and QOL of infected persons has improved. HIV-positive women, like their uninfected counterparts, may desire to plan pregnancies, limit their families, or avoid pregnancy. The effective use of contraception by HIV-positive clients can contribute significantly to reduction in both sexual and vertical transmission of the virus. HIV-positive clients can use most of the available contraception methods including barrier, hormonal, IUD, and sterilization.

However, some ARV drugs interact with hormonal contraceptives with potentials for reduction in efficacy. Dual protection with concomitant use of a more effective contraceptive method and male or female condom to prevent HIV and STI is the standard.

It is necessary to make provision for contraceptive service as part of comprehensive care for the HIV-positive client [160].

As the HIV epidemic evolves, heterosexual intercourse is increasingly risky: the risk of infection in exposed young women is 4- to 7-fold higher than in young men and nearly half a million newborns annually have HIV. Risk of transmission of HIV varies from 1 in 200 to 1 in 10 000 coital incidents, depending in part on the integrity of the vaginal epithelium. Consistent use of male condoms has been proven to reduce horizontal transmission of HIV by 80% among HIV-serodiscordant couples. Hormonal contraception may increase the risk of HIV acquisition in high-risk women such as commercial sex workers, but not in women at low risk of HIV. While hormonal contraception did not affect progression of disease in two cohort studies involving 370 women, in a RCT among women not receiving ARV medication, clinical disease accelerated in the OC group (13.2/100 woman-years) compared with the copper IUD group (8.6/100 woman-years, hazard ratio [HR] 1.5, 95% confidence interval [CI] 1.04-2.1).

Hormonal contraception does not interfere with antiviral drug effectiveness. All the available reversible contraceptive methods can generally be used by women at risk of HIV infection and by HIV-infected women [161]. In the Women's Interagency HIV Study, there did not appear to be an association between hormonal contraception use and HIV-1-RNA levels. There was a small increase in CD4 cell counts among hormonal users of doubtful clinical significance [162]. Hormonal methods of contraception are safe, acceptable, and effective in preventing unwanted pregnancies. Many published studies have examined the impact of hormonal contraception on

HIV disease acquisition and transmissibility. Far fewer have investigated the relationship between hormonal contraception and HIV disease progression.

Several clinical studies suggest an overall effect but are not definitive, and the mechanisms behind HIV disease progression are unclear. Animal and immunological data suggest that immunomodulation by hormonal contraceptive methods may affect the immune response to HIV infection [163]. Moreover, there is concern that coadministration of ARV drugs may alter contraceptive efficacy. Several studies of combined OC pills (COC) identified decreased serum estrogen and progestin levels when coadministered with certain ARV drugs. The contraceptive efficacy of injectable depot medroxyprogesterone acetate (DMPA) and the LNG intrauterine system (IUS) were largely unaffected by ARV, while data on the contraceptive patch, ring, and implant were lacking. HIV-positive women should be offered a full range of hormonal contraceptive options, with conscientious counseling about possible reduced efficacy of COC and the contraceptive implant when taken with ARV. DMPA and the LNG-IUS maintain their contraceptive efficacy when taken with ARV [164]. There are safety concerns regarding the use of IUD and IUS in HIV-infected women. Although studies are limited, IUD appear to be safe for use by most HIV-infected women [165].

Growing numbers of women and men who are HIV infected and aware of their serostatus, want to have children. Gynecologists are involved in the dilemmas of counseling those couples about reproductive decisions. No rational argument can abolish the desire of many young women to have children in the face of the life-threatening infection. The clinical and immune status of the would-be mothers and her partner's serostatus must be considered. For seronegative women with HIV-infected partners, after confirming that seroconversion is not occurring, the partner's clinical and immune status must be evaluated.

The risk of transmission through unprotected intercourse increases with the degree of immune suppression in the partner. The couple's stability and the woman's motivations for becoming pregnant must also be carefully evaluated. About one third of such discordant couples separate after the birth of their child. For selected couples who have clearly decided to attempt pregnancy, the objective of reproductive counseling is to reduce their risk of heterosexual transmission. An alternative is the "natural" method, consisting in having unprotected intercourse only during ovulation [166]. In a study, HIV type 1 seropositive men that were not on ZDV therapy and were in early disease stage (>200 CD4+ cells/mm^3) had normal semen parameters as defined by WHO criteria. In contrast, untreated men in advanced disease stage ($\leq$200

CD4+ cells/mm^3) had significant reductions in sperm concentration and total sperm count and an increased percentage of abnormal sperm forms.

Men receiving ZDV ARV therapy, regardless of disease stage, had normal semen parameters similar to those of untreated early disease stage patients. Seminal white blood cell (WBC) concentrations were not affected significantly by disease progression but were reduced in patients receiving ZDV. Most HIV-1-infected men had semen parameters consistent with fertility. Disease progression was associated with reduced semen quality, but this effect appeared to be abrogated by ZDV therapy. ZDV was also associated with a significant reduction of WBC numbers in semen. As seminal WBC are principal HIV-1 host cells in ejaculates of HIV-1-infected men, this effect could explain recent laboratory and epidemiological evidence that ZDV therapy is associated with a reduced prevalence of HIV-1 in semen and a lower rate of sexual transmission [167].

For a number of years the localization of HIV-1 in male genital tract tissues and secretions has been intensively investigated using a variety of microscopy techniques including immunocytochemistry, in situ hybridization (ISH), in situ PCR, and electron microscopy. These studies have failed to demonstrate an association between HIV-1 and either testicular germ cells or spermatozoa [168, 169]. The likelihood of HIV infection/association with viable mature sperm is low [170]. Anyway, the use of IVF-ICSI to avoid disease transmission in HIV-1 serodiscordant couples desiring children appears to be safe and yields high rates of pregnancy. However, success is influenced by the woman's age [171]. Various ART have been used to reduce or eliminate infectious elements known to be present in semen so that isolated spermatozoa can be safely inseminated or used for ICSI into oocytes. Presently, several European centres and a few US groups offer assistance to HIV seropositive men and their seronegative partners by performing either IUI or IVF. Although the data remain observational, sperm washing techniques appear to be relatively safe and effective, offering HIV-serodiscordant couples an opportunity to have children [172]. The need for fertility services in the HIV-positive population has thus increased and may be employed for management of infertility and protection from transmission or acquisition of HIV infection. As such, preconception counseling, sexual health, and fertility screening have become routine in the management of HIV-positive couples. The option of care include adoption, self insemination with husband sperm, embryo donation from couples who have been verified to be HIV negative, insemination with donor sperm, timed unprotected intercourse (TUI), and sperm washing combined with IUI and ART including IVF or ICSI. Access to these fertility services by HIV-positive clients should be facilitated as part of efforts to promote their reproductive health and rights [173].

Yet, few programs in the US permit unrestricted access to ART for HIV-seropositive patients. Some of these individuals have conventional problems causing infertility. Many others are attempting to minimize viral transmission to their spouse or offspring. European centers remain far ahead of those in the US in advancing techniques and offering services to safeguard the uninfected while providing effective, affordable care to the HIV-seropositive patient [174, 175].

HIV is becoming increasingly common among childbearing women. Through federally recommended testing programs, obstetricians can identify pregnant women in their practices who are HIV infected. Hence, obstetricians must be prepared to face the social, ethical, and medical dilemmas brought on by HIV infection in pregnancy [176]. Although coexistent HIV infection and pregnancy are still rare in most communities, as the prevalence of HIV and AIDS continues to rise, the practicing physician can expect to see this more frequently. The internist plays a crucial role in educating these patients as to the importance of "safe sex" practices and pregnancy prevention. As with any complex medical problem, once pregnant, these patients are best managed with a team approach, involving the obstetrician, internist, neonatologist, and social worker. Perinatal transmission of HIV has become an important mode of acquisition, which results in the birth of severely ill infants who succumb early to their disease and who often are abandoned in the hospital nursery for the duration of their short lifetime. Consequently, prevention of perinatal transmission is a primary goal. Several recent studies of the seroprevalence of HIV in pregnant women have shown high rates of infection. Landesman et al. report a seroprevalence of 2% when cord blood samples were tested in a blinded fashion in an inner city municipal hospital in Brooklyn, New York. At this time, there is no evidence that HIV infection or AIDS adversely affects fertility. Perinatal transmission of HIV infection occurs in 33-50% of affected pregnancies. Circumstantial evidence suggests that pregnancy adversely affects the course of disease [177]. HIV infection may impair a large portion of the human immune response. Infection of CD4+ T cells results in depletion of this population, leading to dysfunction of T-cell-dependent activities. Numerous other immune functions are directly or indirectly impaired, including the function of CD8+ T cells and decreases in total lymphocytes, IL-2 secretion, IL-2R expression, proliferative response to mitogens, natural killer (NK) activity, antibody-dependent cell-mediated cytotoxicity (ADCC), and several other measures. Immune alterations seen in normal pregnancy include decreases in CD4 and T cells, the proliferative response to mitogen, IL-2 secretion, and NK activity.

These changes are largely cellular and usually are not apparent clinically. Normal pregnant women are immunocompetent. When pregnancy is complicated by asymptomatic HIV infection, the obstetric outcome does not seem to be adversely affected. Preliminary studies show that the course of HIV disease may not be adversely affected in these women, but this matter is the subject of intense investigation [178]. The role of the placental tissue in the perinatal transmission of HIV is still far from being understood. Significant data regarding transplacental infection have been collected, but differences in technique have led to controversy. It appears clear that many Hofbauer cells are CD4+ and can become infected with HIV. Less certain but probable is infection of trophoblasts themselves. Whether infection is CD4-mediated or via cell-cell fusion is not established. Transplacental traffic of virus and cells remains a little-studied possibility. Further data are needed regarding the fascinating concept of the placenta as a modulator of infection [179].

Many aspects of HIV infection in pregnancy remain unclear. Subsets at increased risk for perinatal transmission, adverse pregnancy outcome, and development of symptomatic HIV infection need to be identified. For instance, relative risks (RR) may be quite different in asymptomatic HIV infected patients with T4 lymphocyte counts >200 cells/mm^3 compared to those with either symptoms of HIV infection or T4 cell counts <200 cells/mm^3. Antiviral therapy with agents, such as azidothymidine (AZT), reduces the risk of transplacental and intrapartum HIV transmission. Obstetricians will be involved increasingly in providing care to HIV-infected patients and educating patients in order to prevent HIV infection [180]. Human immunodeficiency virus infections complicating pregnancy have become a major public health problem worldwide. Infected women may transmit the virus to offspring and longitudinal studies have reported this risk to be from 13% to 40%. Differences in reported transmission risks are likely to be related to maternal plasma viremia, maternal immunologic responses, or both. Studies of ARV therapy and immune-based therapy to reduce the risk of perinatal transmission are needed.

In addition to these fetal concerns, management in pregnancy needs to address maternal health-care needs and HCW's concerns regarding the risk of occupational exposure. Appropriate maternal management includes serial assessments of maternal T-lymphocyte function and consideration of prophylactic and therapeutic treatment options proven effective in nonpregnant adults [181]. The incentive to undergo prenatal HIV counseling and testing is related not only to fetal concerns, but also to the potential benefit of early and comprehensive therapy for women.

Treatments that should be considered for use during pregnancy include the ARV agent ZDV and prophylactic agents to prevent Pneumocystis carinii pneumonia, the most common OI seen in patients progressing to AIDS. Assessment of the risks and benefits of these treatments during pregnancy is complex and requires discussions between physician and patient [182]. Management involves supportive multiagency care, easy and effective communication, an awareness and understanding of other issues (which may be more important to the mother than her HIV infection), and specialists with both experience and an up-do-date knowledge base [183].

Although lymphocyte counts may drop during pregnancy, HIV infection does not appear to increase the risk of obstetric complications and poor pregnancy outcome.

Although most pregnant women with HIV are asymptomatic, progression of disease, including the development of OI, may occur during gestation. Serious bacterial infections are not common unless the CD4 count is <300 cells/mm^3. Transmission of HIV to the neonate complicates approximately 30% of affected pregnancies [184]. MTCT has been reported to occur during pregnancy (in utero), at delivery, or postpartum (breastfeeding). There are a multiplicity of variables or cofactors that may influence such transmission. Among the obstetric factors reported to be more strikingly associated with MTCT are preterm delivery, LBW, and birth order in twin pregnancies. Perhaps the most controversial issue in obstetric management is the association of mode of delivery and transmission. Some large studies and meta-analyses have found a protective effect of cesarean section (CS) varying from OR of 0.8 to 0.56.

Unfortunately, those large studies have not included the duration of rupture membranes in their analyses. When such a variable (duration of ruptured membranes) is taken into account, the protective effect of the CS may disappear. The impact of such obstetric variables on transmission can be explained by the hypothesis that a significant proportion of the perinatal transmission occurs intrapartum and is related to the dose exposure (time and concentration) of the presenting part to the genital tract virus load and to the maternal blood virus load. Although prospective studies are underway to elucidate the effect of CS on transmission, the results are academic if recent potent antiviral agents are demonstrated to reduce or minimize the viral load in blood and in cervicovaginal secretions. Meanwhile, the current management of the delivery process should have as a goal the reduction of the presenting part to the cervicovaginal secretions by preserving the intactness of the membranes and by the proper use of invasive procedures when clinically indicated [185].

Along with increasing knowledge of factors that put infants at risk for MTCT (e.g., maternal-viral load, HIV-disease state, prematurity, and prelabor rupture of membranes [PROM]), there are new approaches to reducing the likelihood of such transmission (e.g., ZDV treatment). Additional means of reducing transmission may become available in years to come. In this context, prenatal identification of HIV-infected women is vital. Finally, appropriate use of early diagnostic tests in HIV-exposed infants will allow effective use of prophylactic and therapeutic means [186].

The pace at which our knowledge and treatment of the HIV has advanced has been staggering. A disease that was unknown three decades ago, that was untreatable only two decades ago, and whose rate of MTCT was immutable just 20 years ago, is now readily diagnosed, treated with increasing effectiveness, and blocked from transmission in the large majority of cases.

None of these advances can be provided to patients unless their physicians actively screen patients and, for those identified as HIV infected, assure them of access to the latest therapies [187].

High levels of maternal viral load and more advanced maternal disease are associated with a greater risk of vertical transmission of HIV. Antepartum and intrapartum maternal treatment with ZDV and postpartum neonatal ZDV treatment decreases the risk of transmission by two-thirds, at least in patients with earlier stages of the disease. Breastfeeding is a source of postpartum HIV transmission and may double the total transmission rate. ZDV should be used in pregnancy to decrease the viral load and reduce transmission of HIV to the fetus.

Other antiviral agents should be used during pregnancy if indicated, although current information is lacking about their effects on the fetus and any potential benefits in decreasing vertical transmission of HIV. Breastfeeding should be avoided. It is believed that 50% of vertical transmission occurs during labor and delivery through exposure to secretions and blood. HIV is also transmitted through breast milk.

A literature review revealed several postulated determinants of vertical transmission, such as maternal, obstetric, infant, and viral factors. In addition, it is recommended that HIV-positive pregnant women undergo assessment of viral load and degree of immunosuppression, that infected women be treated with oral ZDV during pregnancy and intravenous ZDV during labor, that combination therapy be considered when appropriate, and that patients be counseled about the risk of transmission during invasive prenatal testing [188].

There is sufficient evidence indicating a higher vertical HIV-1 transmission rate in the last trimester and during labor compared with the first trimester.

ARV therapy either single or in combination given to the mother during the last trimester and delivery can reduce the viral load in the maternal circulation. Vertical HIV-1 transmission during delivery can be minimized by appropriate timing and route of delivery. Elective CS before the onset of labor with an intact bag of forewaters provides the least mother-to-fetus microtransfusion compared to other modes of delivery. Since an effective combination of HIV-1 Ig and HIV-1 vaccine given to the HIV-1 exposed newborns to prevent HIV-1 transmission similar to the viral hepatitis B model is not firmly established at present, postexposure ARV prophylaxis and nonbreastfeeding are advocated for infants born from the HIV-1 infected mothers. In cases of advanced stage of maternal HIV-1 infection, and in developing areas where malnutrition prevails, an adequate supply of essential micronutrients is proposed as an adjunctive measure to reduce HIV-1 perinatal transmission [189].

Because of the constant evolution of the interventions, the public policies also need constant revisions. The effectiveness of elective CS has both positive and negative aspects which merit consideration. Newer approaches, such as HAART, which have shown to decrease the AIDS mortality, have also shown zero transmission in small cohorts. Shorter and cheaper interventions are also somewhat effective and are good alternatives to resource poor countries [190]. Evidence suggests that more aggressive ARV therapy for the mother, which allows suppression of viral loads to undetectable levels, may be safe and may provide significant additional benefits. However, treatment needs to be individualized, weighing the possible teratogenic risks against the benefits of decreased transmission. Multiple prospective cohort studies support elective CS as an additional means to decrease vertical transmission, but its role in relation to other therapies has not been determined. As in nonpregnant patients infected with HIV, prevention of OI and adequate psychosocial support are essential [191]. The number of perinatal AIDS cases in the US decreased dramatically from 1985 to 1997. This public health success can be attributed to collaboration among researchers, clinicians, HIV-positive pregnant women, and advocacy groups, and to much greater knowledge about how HIV is transmitted from mothers to their infants. ARV regimens used to prevent transmission include the AIDS Clinical Trial Group (ACTG) Study 076 AZT regimen, abbreviated regimens, and combination therapy. The safety of anti-HIV drugs during pregnancy has not been well documented. Modified obstetrical practices, such as avoiding fetal scalp electrodes as well as artificial rupture of membranes, play a role in preventing HIV transmission during birth [192].

In many developing countries, because the prevalence of maternal HIV infection is high (more than 30% in some sub-Saharan African countries) and the resources commonly used to prevent transmission in developed countries are generally not available, MTCT is a devastating problem. Countries already experiencing infant mortality rates 10- to 20-fold greater than those in developed countries can expect a doubling of infant and childhood mortality due to HIV.

Those infants who escape infection themselves can expect to be orphaned in early childhood. Low-cost antiviral therapy can reduce transmission substantially, but many countries do not have the infrastructure to screen pregnant women for HIV and appropriately treat the mothers and infants. In developing countries, reduction in MTCT is feasible, but will require substantial additional resources and a well-functioning obstetric care system [193]. The transformation of the HIV epidemic over the last 30 years has been remarkable. With access to appropriate therapies, clinicians can now offer infected women a much improved prognosis as well as a very high likelihood of birthing children who will be HIV uninfected. However, these advances are purchased through the use of complicated, expensive medical regimens (HAART) that are associated with a litany of toxicities and risks. In caring for HIV-infected pregnant women and prescribing these medications, obstetricians must always bear in mind their dual responsibilities, providing optimal care to the mother and reducing the likelihood of MTCT of HIV. To accomplish those goals, the physician must first monitor the patient's immunological and virological status including resistance testing. The results of those tests will guide the clinician in choosing when to initiate therapy and in deciding whether to use regimens directed solely at transmission interruption or those that will simultaneously treat the mother's infection. When using HAART, physicians must be cognizant of the pregnancy-specific risks associated with some of the component agents.

The core goal of all medical therapy is to bring the patient's viral load to an undetectable level. When that goal is reached, the chance of transmission to the child is minimized, the need for a CS is reduced, and the patient's prognosis is optimized.

However, if a woman is not pregnant, then the initiation of therapy can be delayed because long-term adherence with medications can be difficult, side effects are not uncommon, and prognosis is not adversely affected so long as the CD4 count and the viral load remain in a reasonable range. None of the advantages cited above can be achieved unless all women have their HIV status determined as early in pregnancy as possible [194].

The HIV global epidemic is having a devastating effect on women of reproductive age: women aged 15-24 years are 2.5 times more likely to be infected than young men in the same age group. Further, MTCT accounts for almost two-thirds of the new infections that occur in children world-wide, annually. MTCT of HIV-1 varies widely and is dependent on obstetric practices, mode of delivery, breastfeeding, and the level of the viral load in the mother. ARV in pregnancy is prescribed for two main reasons:

1 women who need ARV medication for their own health; and
2 women who do not need treatment, or do not have access to treatment are offered prophylaxis to prevent MTCT, using one of a number of ARV regimens known to be effective.

HIV infection is also associated with significant maternal morbidity and mortality. Clinicians caring for HIV-infected women need to update their knowledge continuously to provide optimal care [195]. HIV infection during pregnancy is a condition that requires multidisciplinary care. Care must be rendered that is appropriate for both the mother and the fetus. Prevention of MTCT of HIV is of paramount concern. To prevent transmission, universal testing for HIV infection in pregnant women is ideal. In the US and other developed countries, great strides have been made toward decreasing the risk of HIV transmission to infants to <2% with use of a combination of HAART during the antepartum period and during labor and delivery, scheduled CS when appropriate, avoidance of breastfeeding, and 6 weeks of ZDV prophylaxis for infants. The continuation of ARV therapy after delivery depends on the needs of the mother with regard to treatment of her own health. In resource-limited countries, where simplified and shortened courses of ARV regimens have been used, reduction in MTCT has also been shown, although not as effectively as that with HAART. In these settings, exclusive breastfeeding for 6 months is recommended to reduce the risk of postnatal transmission [196-198].

Several potential means of preventing vertical transmission of HIVare under study. Although the perinatal use of ARV agents can prevent some of these infections, those agents are neither uniformly effective nor universally available. A significant portion of vertical transmission may be an intrapartum phenomenon, potentially amenable to obstetric interventions, such as CS or vaginal virucides. The utility of these obstetric interventions will be determined in large part by the timing of vertical transmission.

HIV can be transmitted during the intrapartum period [199]. Cumulative data on serological testing of newborns and infants have shown that:

1) maternal and newborn anti-HIV-1 IgG titers are high at delivery, which may explain the persistence of antibody in the infants of seropositive mothers;
2) in some situations, serial HIV-1 antibody testing may identify infected infants; and
3) detection of anti-HIV-1 IgA or IgM is specific for infection but the sensitivity of this assay may be compromised in certain situations, such as when infected infants are hypogammaglobulinemic or when the rise and fall of HIV-1-specific IgM synthesis following acute infection has been completed before delivery of the infant.

Cumulative data on PCR, viral culture, and tests for antigen in newborns and infants have shown that:

1) among all age groups, viral culture is probably the most specific test available for detection of HIV-1, as PCR and the p24 antigen test may (though rarely) give false-positive results;
2) the sensitivity of these tests increases in the order of antigen, culture, and PCR, with relatively insensitive results in the first 3 months of life for all of these tests;
3) the sensitivity of all of these tests improves and approximates 90% to 100% when infants over 6 months of age are tested; and
4) data regarding the sensitivity, specificity, and usefulness of these virological assays in infants under 3 months of age are very scant and inconclusive [200].

In 2008, between 129,000 and 194,000 of the 430,000 pediatric HIV infections worldwide were attributable to breastfeeding. Yet in many settings, the health, economic, and social consequences of not breastfeeding would have dire consequences for many more children.

Two shifts have been suggested in perspective. The first is to evaluate prevention of MTCT of HIV interventions more holistically, to include the psychosocial and economic consequences as well as the biomedical ones. The second shift in perspective should be one that contextualizes postnatal prevention of MTCT efforts in the cascade of maternal health services.

Prevention of MTCT efforts include extended postnatal ARV prophylaxis, exclusive breastfeeding promotion, counseling, breast milk pasteurization, breast milk banking, novel techniques for making breast milk safer, and optimal breastfeeding practices. The research efforts will maximize the number of healthy, thriving, HIV-free children around the world [201].

Obstetrician-gynecologists provide comprehensive primary and preventive care for women and are ideally suited to provide HIV screening for their patients [202]. Women now comprise approximately half of all HIV-infected individuals and the epidemic of pediatric HIV disease continues unabated in the developing world. The issue of MTCT has been a major concern for public health officials since the early years of this epidemic. Not uncommonly, the first opportunity to ascertain the HIV status is when a woman presents to a hospital in labor. Rapid HIV tests can provide fast results, allowing time for the provider to offer ARV therapy.

Several effective ARV regimens are now available for the intrapartum patient whose rapid HIV test comes back as positive. ARV therapy should be initiated as soon as possible after a positive rapid HIV test result and prior to standard confirmatory testing. Rapid screening for HIV infection and antiretroviral regimens can reduce the risk of perinatal transmission from the intrapartum patient whose rapid HIV test comes back positive [203]. Rapid HIV testing of women in labor whose status is not known allows the prompt treatment of mother and baby to reduce transmission risk. The feared clinical resistance in the mother after treatment with a single dose of nevirapine (NVP) has been confirmed. Strategies are required to minimize this resistance and allow the use of NVP for treatment of the mother.

There are new findings of mitochondrial toxicity in babies who have been exposed to ARV medicines during pregnancy or delivery, but the clinical implications are not clear. Long-term follow-up of exposed children is required. Resource-poor countries are starting to use multiple drugs to further reduce transmission to the infant. These efforts are reducing the rates of transmission to the level found in affluent countries. Improvements in treatment continue to reduce the risk of HIV MTCT in resource-poor countries, but subsequent maternal resistance continues to be a problem since treatment for the mother's health is now possible. The long-term effects on the infant are still not understood [204]. There has recently been a renewed interest in mandatory antenatal HIV testing in pregnancy. There is emerging data that the risk of HIV MTCT is associated with late initiation of therapy during pregnancy and a diminishing importance of intrapartum ZDV in women with an undetectable viral load at delivery.

Publications, predominantly from cohort studies, continue to demonstrate no difference in HIV transmission rates in women with undetectable viral loads according to the mode of delivery but do confirm an increase in morbidity associated with CS.

New studies of continuation of ARV prophylaxis to infants with ongoing exposure to HIV-infected breast milk are encouraging although may be associated with increased toxicity and resistance. There is an urgent need to continue research to better understand optimal antenatal screening policy, optimal ARV therapy within available resources, preferred mode of delivery considering morbidity and HIV transmission, and finally, new methods to protect breastfed children from infection [205].

Public health efforts need to continue addressing testing at the earliest opportunity, the psychosocial issues which impact negatively on the care of HIV-positive individuals, and ways to reduce stigmatization associated with this viral illness [206]. In fact, besides a specialized medical treatment, women with a drug addiction and HIV-positive pregnant women require intensive psychosocial care. HIV-infected people are still isolated and suffer from the social stigmata. Their essential needs for sexuality and children of their own are often ignored or even condemned because of irrational fears about HIV, which continue despite rapid medical improvements. The life-expectancy for example has increased since the inauguration of protease inhibitors. Vertical transmission of HIV is below 2% through medical treatment in pregnancy, elective CS and renunciation of breastfeeding. Drug-addicted pregnant women are given the opportunity to change their life in order to care for their children appropriately. The basis for this is a substitution with levomethadone and elimination of the use of other drugs. The addicted women often can reduce the dosage of levomethadone during the course of their pregnancy and sometimes can cease totally.

Normally they are highly motivated and thus can ease the withdrawal symptoms of their newborns following delivery. By establishing a reliable social net during pregnancy mothers learn to recognize the demands of their children after birth and thus emotional and cognitive deficits can be prevented [207]. As more experience has accrued regarding HIV infection in women and HIV infection in pregnancy, there has remained a gap in our understanding of the psychosocial effects of HIV infection upon the pregnant women. There is limited information regarding psychologic and sociologic effects of HIV infection upon pregnancy and vice versa, there is sufficient indication of a relationship between stressors related to each of these and the potential for a deleterious affect upon the pregnancy.

These stresses often include the determination whether to disclose or not disclose their serostatus [208]. These women must navigate the complexities of two health concerns (HIV infection and pregnancy) and the complexities of two health care provision systems (obstetrics and infectious disease). Depression is not uncommon in pregnant women and has been identified as a robust predictor of non-adherence to ART and implicated in difficulty utilizing prenatal care [209].

Management of women with HIV infection or AIDS should follow the established guidelines for ARV therapy and prevention and treatment of opportunistic complications of HIV infection. Women with child-bearing potential should be treated as medically indicated for other HIV-infected patients, including during pregnancy. In fact, preliminary results of ACTG 076 indicated that ZDV therapy during pregnancy reduces vertical transmission of HIV about threefold [210]. However, the full impact of HIV infection and AIDS on women's health and the optimal management of symptomatic and asymptomatic cases have yet to be delineated. The urgency to establish effective management protocols is underscored by the fact that AIDS has recently become the leading cause of death for minority women in many urban areas. The administration of antepartum and intrapartum ZDV (AZT) has advanced efforts to minimize perinatal transmission and produced promising results. However, important issues pertaining to prevention of HIV infection in women, mandatory testing of women of reproductive age, and the management of HIV-positive women during the interconceptional period remain controversial.

Addressing HIV throughout the continuum of reproductive health is a major priority and a concern of all HCW. Women's health care must assume the lead in counseling all women about their risk of HIV, ensuring that HIV-positive women make informed decisions about their reproductive health and that HIV-negative women modify high-risk behavior to avoid becoming infected. Since obstetricians and gynecologists, nurse practitioners, and midwives are often the first care providers whom at-risk and HIV-infected women contact, they must be able to identify, assess, and optimally manage these patients [211]. ZDV therapy seems to be effective for reducing vertical transmission of HIV infection and preventing paediatric AIDS. Besides those cases in which it is indicated, ZDV plays an important role in safeguarding maternal well-being. Even though no data indicating teratogenic effect of this drug exist, its use during the first trimester should be limited to those cases where it is absolutely indicated.

All undergoing this therapy should be informed that no information regarding the long term effects of this drug are available yet.

Further controlled studies are necessary if this drug is to be used in those cases where it could actually be of benefit [212]. In a series of scenarios to quantify the benefits of maternal-neonatal ZDV administration for the prevention of vertical HIV transmission against the potential risks of drug-induced complications in uninfected children, the impact of different estimates for the QOL decrement from any adverse ZDV effect in HIV-uninfected children was assessed, and threshold values for this estimate were established, i.e., critical values below which withholding ZDV would be the preferred choice. A decision analysis model was created with use of a Markov cohort simulation, for evaluating both survival and quality of life for two hypothetical cohorts of HIV-exposed neonates: one with in utero and neonatal exposure to preventive ZDV therapy and the other not exposed. The model included the probability of congenital HIV infection with and without ZDV treatment (estimates derived from ACTG 076), the yearly probability of death with and without congenital HIV infection, a range of probabilities of adverse effects from ZDV use, and a range of ages in life when any adverse effect would manifest. Across a wide range of estimates for multiple contingencies, ZDV use was associated with a greater number of quality-adjusted life years than was non-use. Only in implausible, pessimistic scenarios (i.e., a high incidence of profound adverse effects beginning early in life) would withholding ZDV be the rational choice for an asymptomatic HIV-infected pregnant woman [213].

With the approval of new ARV agents, monotherapy with ZDV, although still standard for prevention of MTCT of HIV, has become inadequate therapy for treatment of the mother. Clinicians must now consider alternative therapeutic strategies in spite of a dearth of experience in the setting of pregnancy [214]. The safety and efficacy of the newer therapeutic agents have yet to be established during pregnancy. However, the need to maintain maternal health mandates that clinicians understand the benefits and limitations of ARV therapy beyond ZDV [215]. ZDV was the first agent approved for treatment of HIV disease, and since its widespread availability in 1987, the pharmacokinetic disposition and clinical effects of ZDV have been extensively evaluated. In addition to its utility as a component of a multidrug combination regimen for the treatment of adult and pediatric HIV-1 infection, it is the only agent approved by the FDA for the prevention of HIV-1 MTCT.

The effectiveness of ZDV for the prevention of HIV-1 MTCT has been demonstrated in several studies.

The optimal time during gestation to initiate ZDV therapy and the relative importance of the intrapartum and newborn components is the focus of both current interventional and observational studies. Until more information is available from these trials, the combined maternal/newborn ZDV regimen studied in ACTG 076 remains the recommended treatment regimen of choice in the US [216]. Recent advances in HAART have reduced AIDS mortality remarkably. But as longer use of these combination regimens makes evident, unexpected side effects are now reported that might reflect gender-based differences in occurrence. Controversy still exists in relation to the level of HIV-1 quantification in men and women and its association with disease progression. Women have been reported to have lower viral loads with equal progression or higher progression with equal viral loads. This finding has not been consistent in all studies. Psychosocial variables, such as poverty, lack of care, and young age, adversely affect more women than men. If the viral dynamics are thought to be different, then the response to treatment might be as well. So far, the effectiveness of HAART has been seen equally among men and women. Barriers to adherence, such as caregiving burdens, multiplicity of roles and fear of disclosure, might disproportionately affect women. By far, the best news is that the survival of both men and women has improved with the newer therapeutic advances [217]. The use of combination ARV therapy during pregnancy has enabled us to decrease perinatal HIV transmission to less than 1%, in areas with adequate resources. Questions remain regarding the safety of these medications for the mother, fetus, and child. Recent publications present conflicting data about associations between ARV and prematurity and other adverse pregnancy outcomes, and if HAART is necessary for all pregnant women. The pharmacokinetics of some ARV medications are altered significantly during pregnancy: placental transfer to the fetus is variable. The well-documented benefit of HAART for preventing MTCT generally outweighs the potential risks to the fetus, infant, and mother. However, potential adverse effects are of concern, and questions remain as to the optimal treatment strategy [218]. It is essential that women admitted for preterm labor have a confidential review of maternal history and prenatal record for HIV serostatus. Combination ARV therapy should be continued during tocolysis of preterm labor and, if tocolysis fails, through delivery. Counseling and rapid HIV testing should be performed in the intrapartum or postnatal periods if the woman's serostatus has not been determined. Women identified as being HIV infected who are in labor should be treated with:

1) ZDV in labor and for 6 weeks to the neonate;
2) NVP single dose to the mother in labor and single dose to the neonate;
3) ZDV-lamivudine (3TC) in labor and to the neonate for 1 week; or
4) NVP (as above) and the ZDV regimen (as above).

CS should be recommended to all women when the most recent viral load is ≥1000 copies/ml or is unknown [219]. The package insert for NVP cautions use in HIV-infected women (including pregnant women) with CD4 counts ≥ 250 cells/μl. However, recent studies showed that the CD4 count of pregnant women receiving ARV therapy was not predictive of NVP toxicity. Initiating NVP-based ARV therapy during pregnancy at CD4 ≥ 250 cells/μl increases toxicity risk and should be avoided, necessitating urgent revision of current guidelines supporting this practice.

Those charged with the care of HIV-infected pregnant women should make frequent use of the Public Health Service (PHS) Website (http://www.aidsinfo.nih.gov), which provides a regularly updated, practical, and thorough guide to management of patients who have HIV [220].

Almost three decades have elapsed since researchers identified HIV as the cause of AIDS, with current estimates from the Joint United Nations (UN) Programme on HIV and AIDS (UNAIDS) that 33.4 million adults were living with HIV/AIDS in 2008. Two-thirds of this burden of disease is in Sub-Saharan Africa, and 60% of those infected are women. The disease still remains incurable and current prevention strategies including abstinence, male/female condom use, and male circumcision are only partially effective. New strategies to curb the epidemic are urgently needed. Scientists are diligently exploring HIV prevention methods that are safe, effective, and affordable.

These new biological interventions include oral pre-exposure prophylaxis using oral ARV drugs, ARV treatment in HIV-infected persons to reduce transmission, and topical ARV-based microbicide formulations [221]. Oral ARV pre-exposure prophylaxis in high-risk individuals may be a reliable tool in preventing the transmission of HIV. Presently, there is no reliable evidence to support the use of any ARV agent for HIV chemoprophylaxis. The use of ARV agents for HIV chemoprophylaxis cannot be recommended at present. To assess the value of ARV agents for HIV chemoprophylaxis, well-conducted trials with the statistical power to answer questions about pre-exposure prophylaxis efficacy and safety in various populations and risk groups are advocated. These trials also should evaluate other important issues of concern, such as drug safety, adherence, drug resistance, and the effect of pre-exposure prophylaxis on risk behavior [222].

New preventative methods are:

1) a natural microbicide: intravaginal lime or lemon juice has been used for centuries as a traditional contraceptive. The juice can also kill HIV in the laboratory, but clinical trials are needed to see if vaginal application is acceptable, safe, and effective;
2 intravaginal estrogen: monkeys can be protected from Simian Immunodeficiency Virus (SIV) infection by keratinizing the vagina with topical estrogen. If women take the OC pill vaginally it retains its contraceptive efficacy, and the estrogen it contains should thicken the vagina and protect against HIV infection. Clinical trials are needed;
3 male circumcision: removal of the inner foreskin removes the main site of HIV entry into the penis, resulting in a sevenfold reduction in susceptibility to infection. The practice needs to be promoted;
4 post-coital penile hygiene: wiping the penis immediately after intercourse with lime or lemon juice or vinegar should kill the virus before it has had a chance to infect. A clinical trial of efficacy is needed; and
5 photoVoice: asking schoolchildren in developing countries to photograph their impressions of HIV/AIDS is a powerful way of getting them to discuss the subject openly, and develop their own preventative strategies [223].

There is an urgent need to expand the range of interventions to prevent HIV transmission and acquisition, especially those that can be controlled by women. Microbicides, defined as antimicrobial products that can be applied topically for the prevention of HIV and other STI, may offer one of the most promising preventive interventions, because they could be inexpensive, readily available, and widely acceptable. The first microbial product to be clinically evaluated contained N-9, a nonionic surfactant, as the active agent [224, 225].

The use of human mucosal tissue models is an important tool advancing our understanding of the specific mechanisms of sexual HIV transmission. Despite 30 years of study, major gaps remain, including how HIV-1 transverses the epithelium and the identity of the early immune targets (gate keepers). Because defining HIV-1 transmission in vivo is difficult, mucosal tissue is being used ex vivo to identify key steps in HIV-1 entry and early dissemination. Elucidating early events of HIV-1 infection will help us develop more potent and specific HIV-1 preventatives such as microbicides and vaccines.

Mucosal tissue has been incorporated into testing regimens for ARV drugs and monoclonal antibodies. The use of mucosal tissue recapitulates the epithelium and immune cells that would be exposed in vivo to virus and drug [226]. Cytokine patterns are potential biomarkers of vaginal inflammation, which are needed for the safety evaluation of topical microbicide products for the prevention of sexually transmitted HIV-1 infection.

In order to be effective, the vaginal anti-HIV-1 microbicides should avoid proinflammatory responses that facilitate transepithelial viral penetration and replication. Pro-inflammatory and anti-inflammatory cytokines play bi-directional roles in HIV-1 pathogenesis, transmission, susceptibility and resistance. Previous research has shown that many of these key mediators of mucosal barrier function (e.g., IL-1, IL-1 receptor antagonist, IL-6, tumor necrosis factor [TNF]-alpha, TNF-receptor II, transforming growth factor [TGF] beta, IL-8, IL-10, IL-12, macrophage inhibitory protein [MIP] 1, etc.) can be detected in the vaginal secretions of healthy or infected individuals using non-invasive sampling techniques.

It has been showed that vaginal formulations, temperature, and matrix-specific factors in the vaginal fluids may interfere with cytokine detection, and therefore specific protocols must be validated for various collection procedures and cytokine assays.

These results suggest that combined patterns of cytokine dynamics rather than individual measurements might distinguish proinflammatory product-related effects in microbicide safety trials. More research is needed to establish cytokine mucosal baselines and modulation by genetic factors, sexual intercourse, menstrual cycle, exercise, hormones, stress, and infections before guidelines can be established for clinical trial enrolment criteria, the prediction of side/adverse events and ultimately microbicide benefit prognostication [227]. Primary prevention of HIV continues to pose an important challenge in the US. Recent clinical trials conducted in Kenya, South Africa, and Uganda have demonstrated considerable benefit of male circumcision in reducing HIV seroincidence in males.

These results have ignited debate over the appropriateness of implementing routine provision of neonatal circumcision in the US for HIV prevention. The applicability of the scientific data from Africa to this country must be carefully considered before rational policy recommendations regarding routine neonatal circumcision can be made as a strategy to prevent the spread of HIV in the US [228]. The development of multiple indication (multipurpose) prevention technologies (MIPT) is driven by overlapping relationships in the area of female reproductive health.

Of particular interest is the application of intravaginal rings (IVR) for the delivery of two drugs simultaneously, to prevent one STI and pregnancy, or two STI. IVR are currently available commercially for contraception and have been developed for release of microbicides to prevent sexual transmission of HIV-1. Novel IVR are capable of releasing relatively large amounts of drugs such as tenofovir, along with those that contain independent delivery elements, such as pods, that can be used to release drugs at independent rates. The field of MIPT remains one of potential. There is yet to be a proven microbicide effective at preventing sexual transmission of HIV-1. Development of MIPT in the near term will proceed under the assumption that one or more ARV drugs will eventually be proven successful. IVR have already demonstrated success in the area of contraception. Prevention of sexual transmission of HIV-1 and HSV-2 (or suppression of recurrence) remains an attractive MIPT target. In the long term, development of MIPT will require validation of surrogate end points, particularly for prevention of HIV-1 transmission [229].

Occupationally acquired HIV infection appears to be an uncommon event, with prospective studies thus far reporting an incidence of 0.6% or less. Strategies for preventing transmission of HIV infection in an obstetric/ gynecologic setting are a matter of appropriate barrier protection, good infection control technique, and a large measure of common sense [230]. In professionally conditioned HIV infections of medical personnel, blood has so far been the only source of infection that is of any importance. Hence, measures to prevent such infections must primarily aim at avoiding any contact with blood from HIV-infected patients. Since the HIV status of the patients and possibly also other infections transmitted by blood (hepatitis) are often unknown, the following protective measures must be applied in all patients as a matter of routine. Fundamentally, gloves must always be worn when coming into contact with blood, body fluids, mucosa, and non-intact skin. In operative procedures and deliveries, barrier methods must be employed to protect the eyes, nose, mouth, and skin, as well as technical procedures during surgery and organizational measures to prevent any possible injuries or lesions caused by operative interventions and to reduce the number of persons exposed to risk. So far, needle pricks have been the most frequent mode of infection. Hence, used cannules should be treated with utmost care: do not return them into their protective cover but throw them directly into solid waste containers. After contamination, blood and other body fluids should be eliminated immediately. In case of massive contamination with material containing HIV, chemoprophylaxis should be given careful consideration [229].

The CDC have made recommendations designed to decrease the transmission of blood-borne pathogens and have been given the force of law by the Occupational Safety and Health Administration (OSHA). Despite prospective data documenting contamination rates and effect preventive measures, for unknown reasons many physicians and other HCW continue to ignore preventive practices [231]. Two trials of safer needles show that their new design reduces the number of needlesticks. However, hospitals are moving slowly toward adopting the new products. The new needles are designed with features to reduce the incidence of HCW being infected via accidental sticks, which account for 39% of all cases of occupational infection [232]. Physician denial of exposure is common. Prompt identification of exposure, including rapid testing of index patients of unknown HIV status, combined with prompt initiation of prophylactic medication, may reduce transmission by 81% [233].

The risk of HIV-infected or otherwise impaired practitioners infecting or injuring their patients is very low, but is of proper concern to patients, practitioners, and healthcare facilities. Practitioners' general legal and ethical duties to protect patients includes protection against their own liability to present risk of harm. Healthcare facilities have similar duties of care to protect patients, for instance by proper selection and management of personnel, but may also bear indirect or vicarious ("no fault") legal liability for injuries due to the negligence of the personnel they engage. Impaired practitioners should disclose their status to licensing and health facility authorities. They are entitled to non-discriminatory employment opportunities, but may be licensed and approved to practice under conditions that appropriately protect patients. When impaired practitioners practice within such approved conditions, modern courts hold that they have no legal duty to volunteer disclosure of their status to their patients [234].

Resolutions of ethical controversies related to HIV screening, counseling, and research may come from achieving greater clarity about the ultimate goals of obstetric and gynecologic care [235]. Identifying pregnant women's HIV infection status provides them with the opportunity to seek appropriate treatment and to take measures to prevent vertical and horizontal transmission. Prenatal screening program options include targeting at-risk women, testing on a voluntary basis, or mandating prenatal HIV screening. When examining these options, the number of cases identified, programmatic costs, long-term health care costs, and legal implications must all be considered. Research indicates that targeting at-risk women misses a significant percentage of seropositive women, although programmatic costs may be lower.

It is difficult to ascertain the difference between voluntary and mandatory programs with respect to the number of cases identified and treated. As a result, long-term savings are difficult to calculate. Mandatory programs would have the greatest direct costs and place the greatest burden on the woman's constitutional rights. By making HIV counseling and testing a routine component of prenatal care, voluntary programs could achieve the benefits of prenatal HIV screening without violating the woman's civil liberties [236]. Universal testing with patient notification and right of refusal ("opt-out" testing) is recommended by most national organizations and federal agencies. Although opt-out and opt-in testing (but not mandatory testing) are both ethically acceptable, the former approach may identify more women who are eligible for therapy and may have public health advantages. It is unethical for an obstetrician-gynecologist to refuse to continue providing health care for a patient solely because she is, or is thought to be, seropositive for HIV. HCW who are infected with HIV should adhere to the fundamental professional obligation to avoid harm to patients. Physicians who believe that they have been at significant risk of being infected should be tested voluntarily for HIV [237-253].

HUMAN PAPILLOMAVIRUS

HPV are simple, nonenveloped, double-stranded DNA viruses, which are responsible for an enormous global burden of genital disease (Figure 2). The majority of HPV belong to the genus alpha-papillomavirus, which can be further subdivided into species and then strains. Approximately 200 strains of HPV have been identified, and the whole genomes of approximately 100 strains have been discovered and completely sequenced. Between 13 and 18 HPV strains have been characterized as conferring a high oncogenic risk, with 12 of these strains belonging to the HPV species 7 (HPV-18, -39, -45, -59, -68) and species 9 (HPV-16, -31, -33, -35, -52, -58, -67). While strains belonging to the same species are phylogenetically related, they may differ biologically. HPV has been strongly associated with malignancy in the female lower genital tract. Oncogenic HPV types 16 and 18 are responsible for a majority of cervical cancers and can also cause low- and high-grade cervical lesions (CIN 1, 2, 3) as well as high-grade vulvar or vaginal intraepithelial neoplasia (VIN or VaIN 2/3). Nononcogenic types HPV 6 and 11 also contribute to the overall burden of HPV disease, giving rise to CIN 1, anogenital warts, cutaneous lesions, and respiratory papillomatosis.

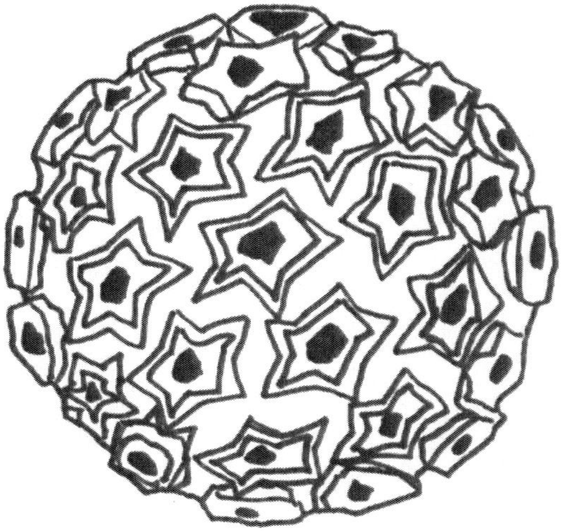

Modified from it123rf.com.

Figure 2. Human Papillomavirus (HPV).

Because squamous-cell carcinoma (SCC) of the cervix is preceded by a spectrum of easily detectable and treatable premalignant changes, it is very preventable [254-256]. Studies have shown a strong association between certain HPV and the development of cervical carcinoma and its precursor lesions. The oncogenic potential of Papillomaviruses has been clearly demonstrated in both laboratory animals and cultured cells. Furthermore, susceptibility to certain HPV has been associated with a recessive genetic defect that results in SCC of the skin. HPV are difficult to study, however, because of the lack of an animal model, difficulty in developing a tissue culture system permissive for their replication, and a lack of understanding of their biology. Current understanding of the natural history of anogenital neoplasia may provide insights into the mechanisms the host uses to cope with potentially oncogenic HPV. Recent advances in our understanding of viral pathogenesis have provided insights into the natural history of HPV infection and subsequent development of neoplasia. A more thorough understanding of the molecular mechanisms responsible for viral oncogenesis will facilitate the development of novel preventive and therapeutic strategies to prevent and treat HPV-associated cervical neoplasias.

Strategies under current investigation are focusing on the induction of effective humoral and cell-mediated immunity, the expression of HPV gene products, and cofactors that interact with HPV gene products to affect cell transformation. As a result of these investigative efforts, prophylactic HPV capsid vaccines and other gene therapies have become clinically available [257, 258]. Important strides in understanding the virus have been made, particularly in the following areas: modes of transmission and risk factors associated with transmission, the oncogenic potential of specific viral types and the mechanism by which they cause cancer, and the spectrum of infection, ranging from asymptomatic carrier states to overt warts, preneoplastic lesions, and invasive cancer. Sophisticated new tests for the detection of HPV that hold great promise for improved screening for cervical cancer precursors and invasive cancer and for the triage of abnormal cervical cytology also have been developed. Understanding the immunology of HPV has allowed the development of new and more effective treatment modalities for HPV infection and the development of primary prevention modalities, including HPV vaccines [259].

The incidence of cervical cancer in the US has decreased more than 50% in the past 30 years because of widespread screening with cervical cytology. In 1975, the rate was 14.8 per 100,000 women. By 2008, it had been reduced to 6.6 per 100,000 women. Mortality from the disease has undergone a similar decrease from 5.55 per 100,000 women in 1975 to 2.38 per 100,000 women in 2008. The American Cancer Society (ACS) estimates that there have been 12,170 new cases of cervical cancer in the US in 2012, with 4,220 deaths from the disease. Cervical cancer is much more common worldwide, particularly in countries without screening programs, with an estimated 530,000 new cases of the disease and 275,000 resultant deaths each year. When cervical cancer screening programs have been introduced into communities, marked reductions in cervical cancer incidence have followed. New technologies for cervical cancer screening continue to evolve as do recommendations for managing the results.

In addition, there are different risk-benefit considerations for women at different ages, as reflected in age-specific screening recommendations. The ACS, the American Society for Colposcopy and Cervical Pathology (ASCCP), and the American Society for Clinical Pathology (ASCP) have recently updated their joint guidelines for cervical cancer screening, and an update to the US Preventive Services Task Force (USPSTF) recommendations also has been issued [260]. HPV is a highly prevalent, STI responsible for significant morbidity and mortality.

High-risk HPV types are now known to be necessary in the etiology of cervical cancer and to lead to both high-grade and low-grade cervical lesions. They are also implicated in a substantial portion of anal, penile, and head and neck precancers and cancers. HPV 16 and 18 are the most common HPV types found in cervical cancer and are responsible for approximately 70% of these cancers. In contrast, low-risk HPV types, the most common of which are HPV 6 and 11, cause genital warts, low-grade cervical lesions, and recurrent respiratory papillomatosis (RRP), but they do not cause cervical or other HPV-related cancers. Infection is most common in young, sexually active populations, and an estimated three fourths of adults will be infected with HPV during their lifetime. Cervical screening programs exist in the US and other developed countries to identify and treat precancerous cervical lesions, but they do not reach all women and are costly. Until recently, no highly effective primary prevention strategy to reduce the risk of HPV acquisition existed. However, a quadrivalent HPV vaccine, which protects against the most common high-risk and low-risk HPV infections (HPV 16, 18, 6, and 11), and a bivalent HPV vaccine that protects against high-risk HPV types 16 and 18 are now available. If implemented widely, vaccination against HPV promises to dramatically reduce HPV-associated morbidity and mortality [261]. A Markov model constructed as part of a systematic review of cervical cytology conducted at the Duke University Evidence-based Practice Center (Durham, North Carolina) incorporated states for HPV, low- and high-grade SIL, and cervical cancer stages I-IV to simulate the natural history of HPV infection in a cohort of women from ages 15 to 85 years. The base-case model resulted in a lifetime cervical cancer risk of 3.67% and a lifetime cervical cancer mortality risk of 1.26%, with a peak incidence of 81/100,000 at age 50 years. Age-specific distributions of precursors were similar to reported data. Lifetime risk of cancer was most sensitive to the incidence of HPV and the probability of rapid HPV progression to high-grade lesions (two- to threefold variations in risk). The model approximates the age-specific incidence of cervical cancer and provides a tool for evaluating the natural history of HPV infection and cervical cancer carcinogenesis as well as the effectiveness and cost-effectiveness of primary and secondary prevention strategies [262].

Cervical cancer is the second most common cancer in women worldwide and the leading cause of cancer deaths in developing countries. While incidence and mortality rates of cervical cancer have fallen significantly in developed countries, 83% of all new cases that occur annually and 85% of all deaths from the disease occur in developing countries. Cervical cancer is the most common cancer among women in sub-Saharan Africa.

The incidence is on the increase in some countries. Knowledge and awareness of this disease on the continent are very poor and mortality still very high. Facilities for the prevention and treatment of cervical cancer are still very inadequate in many countries in the region. Governments in sub-Saharan Africa must recognize cervical cancer as a major public health concern and allocate appropriate resources for its prevention and treatment, and for research. Indeed, cervical cancer in this region must be accorded the same priority as HIV, malaria, tuberculosis, and childhood immunizations [263]. Analysis of the burden of HPV in the Extended Middle East and North Africa (EMENA) region highlights an unexpectedly high prevalence of HPV, with rates of HPV ranging from 0% to 25% in low-risk women with normal cytology and up to 98% in those with genital warts and preinvasive and invasive lesions. In addition, cervical cancer screening practices are, at best, opportunistic in most countries of the region. Therefore, the observed change in social and sexual behavior in the EMENA population, particularly in youths, could lead to an increase in HPV and its related diseases, especially cervical cancer. There is the need for the introduction and standardization of screening practices in the region. Moreover, surveillance studies are needed to enable the identification of HPV type distribution and to determine the potential impact of the introduction of HPV vaccines. These socio-epidemiological data are of marked value to health care decision and policymakers in prioritizing available public health interventions [264].

HPV itself is both ubiquitous and markedly heterogeneous but can nevertheless be classified as either a high-risk type or a low-risk type based upon its frequency of detection in cervical cancer. Given that the association between HPV and cervical cancer is causal, the classification of this virus has been strengthened by large-scale epidemiologic studies and is widely accepted across many disciplines. It is evident, however, that cervical cancer is frequently associated with multiple HPV types. Therefore, it is crucial to distinguish causal types of HPV (drivers) from noncausal types (passengers) in cervical lesions [265]. HPV infection of the cervix affects the developing immature metaplastic cells of the transformation zone. Cervical neoplasia can be viewed as the interaction of high-risk HPV and immature metaplastic epithelium. Once maturity is reached, there is minimal risk of subsequent development of cervical squamous neoplasia. Exposure to HPV is an extremely common event, especially in young sexually active women. Yet, despite frequent HPV exposure at that phase of life in which the cervical transformation zone is at its most vulnerable, established expressed disease is relatively uncommon.

Most studies in which the natural history of CIN is not altered by cervical biopsy reveal a progression rate from low to high grade CIN of less than one third. Where viral type is taken into account, however, the progression rate from normal but high risk HPV-infected cervical epithelium to CIN 2 or 3 is higher. Despite this, most cervical abnormalities will not transform into invasive cancer, even if left untreated. The variance between the high rate of HPV infection, the intermediate rate of CIN, and the relatively low rate of cervical cancer establishes a stepwise gradient of disease of increasing severity with decreasing prevalence. In an immunocompetent host, HPV infection alone does not appear to be sufficient to induce the step from high grade CIN to invasion. Epidemiological studies indicating that HPV infection with oncogenic viral types is far more common than cervical neoplasia suggest the necessity of cofactors in cervical carcinogenesis. The long time-lag between initial infection and eventual malignant conversion suggests that random events may be necessary for such conversion, and the spontaneous regression of many primary lesions suggests that most patients are not exposed to these random events. Potential cofactors include cigarette smoking, hormonal effects of OC and pregnancy, dietary deficiencies, immunosuppression, and chronic inflammation. In those women who develop cervical cancer, malignant progression is rarely rapid, more commonly taking many years or decades. Malignant progression has been documented in patients who presented initially with only low-grade HPV-induced atypia.

On the other hand, progression may be a misnomer, as "apparent" progression may really represent adjacent "de novo" development of higher grade CIN. Although most cervical cancers contain high-risk HPV types, up to 15% of such cancers test negative for HPV, raising the possibility that a few, usually more aggressive, cervical cancers may arise from from a non-viral source [266]. Although the majority of sexually active adults will be infected with HPV at least once in their lives, it is sexually active women less than 25 years of age who consistently have the highest rates of infection. Besides youth and gender, common risk factors for HPV infection and clinical sequelae of infection include high number of sexual partners and coinfection with C. trachomatis or HSV. Most HPV infections are cleared by the immune system and do not result in clinical complications. Clinical sequelae in cases of low-risk HPV infection consist of genital warts, and clinical manifestations of high-risk HPV infection include abnormal Pap test results, low-grade SIL (L-SIL), high-grade SIL (H-SIL), and cervical cancer. L-SIL, H-SIL, and cervical cancer carry significant morbidity and/or mortality, while genital warts and abnormal Pap test results are often significant sources of psychosocial distress.

Currently, there are neither effective means of preventing HPV transmission nor cures for clinical manifestations: infection can only be prevented via complete sexual abstinence, while treatment for clinical sequelae such as genital warts and cytologic abnormalities consists of removing the problematic cells and watching for recurrence. This method consumes significant health care resources and is costly.

New prophylactic HPV vaccines promise to dramatically reduce the incidence of HPV infection, genital warts, and cytologic abnormalities [267]. After taking HPV into account, smoking habit appears to be the most significant environmental risk factor, and the risk of this malignancy increases significantly with intensity and duration of smoking. Women with HIV infection experience a higher incidence of CIN and invasive cervical cancer. Among HIV+ women, the HAART increases the regression rate of CIN, but the majority of these lesions do not regress to normal.

As far as OC, a systematic review of 28 studies found that, compared with never pill users, the RR of cervical cancer increased with increasing duration of OC use. The results were similar for SCC and adenocarcinoma, and the RR decreased after pill discontinuation. However, by weighing risks and benefits, the WHO does not recommend any change in OC practice. There is no correlation between hormone replacement therapy (HRT) and cervical cancer. Experimental data have shown that estradiol and progesterone can modulate the host immune response to HPV 16. Prophylactic vaccination in conjunction with cervical screening is the best prevention strategy for cervical cancer [268].

The most common manifestation of sexually transmitted HPV infection is a nonpapilliferous hyperplasia in the transformation zone. Such subclinical HPV infections closely resemble CIN and were previously misdiagnosed as such. In essence, the triage of the abnormal Pap smear amounts to the differentiation between benign warty proliferation, minor-grade dysplasia, and full-thickness intraepithelial neoplasia. Hence, a clear understanding of the morphologic expression and natural history of different types of HPV infection is now essential to the rational management of patients with lower genital tract neoplasia [269]. Pathologic and epidemiologic studies performed over the past five decades have provided evidence that the development of SCC of the cervix is a multistep process involving a precursor preinvasive stage. Infection by a variety of HPV types may result in active viral intranuclear replication without integration into the cellular genome. This episomal form of infection is manifested morphologically by the development of mild dysplasia, CIN 1 with koilocytosis, and acanthosis.

Approximately 20 different HPV types have been associated with CIN 1 lesions, whereas high-grade dysplasia and CIS (CIN 2 and 3) are associated with only a few viral types (mainly HPV 16, 31, 33, and 35). Low-grade lesions are differentiated and have a low risk of progression to cancer, whereas high-grade lesions are characterized by nearly complete or complete loss of squamous maturation and a higher risk of progression to invasive cancer. Based on the biologic dichotomy of an infectious and a neoplastic process and the segregation of HPV types into two groups, a modification of the CIN classification into low-grade and high-grade SIL in accordance with the Bethesda System has been proposed. The value of identifying HPV DNA by such molecular techniques as Southern blot analysis, ISH, and the PCR in the early detection of preinvasive lesions has been determined and their routine use is at present recommended [270]. The spectrum of genital HPV infections comprises clinical, subclinical, and latent disease in addition to HPV-associated neoplasia. The definition of subclinical and latent HPV infection is still incomplete and awaits clarification by highly sensitive HPV detection systems that preserve the morphology of the tissue. Genital HPV infect the human body mainly by sexual transmission, but other pathways of HPV transmission may be possible as suggested by:

1) high prevalences of antibody reactivity in children;
2) lack of association of HPV seropositivity with sexual activity;
3) presence of HPV DNA in oral cavity scrapings of children and adults; and
4) development of RRP among children exposed to HPV 6 or 11 during birth.

Successful infection depends on the infection site and the immunological state of the host: susceptibility to genital HPV seems highest for the squamous epithelium of the lower genital tract. HPV DNA is also present in extragenital sites but this is rarely accompanied by clinical or subclinical lesions. The molecular basis for this specific tropism is unknown. The immune response in HPV-infected tissues is characterized by depletion of T helper/inducer cells or Langerhans cells and an impaired immunological function of NK cells or the infected keratinocyte. Epidemiological studies indicate that individuals with cell-mediated immunodeficiencies are at increased risk for genital HPV infections. Regression or persistence of subclinical and latent genital HPV infections as analyzed in longitudinal investigations show a constant come-and-go of HPV presence.

In an infected individual, complete clearing of the virus seems rather exceptional. With respect to progression, the biological potential of cervical HPV infections is characterized by an increased risk for development of HPV-associated neoplasia, especially in lesions infected with high-risk HPV types (e.g., HPV 16 and 18).

Demographic data of genital HPV infections are very variable due to differences in the HPV detection assays used and in the populations examined. The prevalence of subclinical and latent genital HPV infections appears to be at least three times higher compared with clinical HPV infections. This rate increases by a further 3-5-fold when patients are examined several times. Seroreactivity against genital HPV types may be due to an active infection or the result of contact with HPV earlier in life [271].

The natural history of infection is one that enables the virus to remain immunoevasive within the cervical epithelium and persist for decades. Many studies have provided important information on why some women clear infection and why others do not. The infectious process of HPV may be affected by many cofactors, adding to the complexity of disease development. Vaccination against oncogenic HPV along with cervical screening are two methods that have been developed to provide protection and eliminate the overall burden of disease in women [272]. The natural history of HPV-related disease still is poorly understood. Screening of apparently healthy populations suggests that most HPV exposure results only in latent infection, that is, there is no active HPV DNA replication, but the HPV copy number is held at a steady state because viral replication parallels cell division. Unfortunately, knowledge of the cell-virus interaction and the host-immune response has not yet provided an effective medical therapy.

Rather, the management of HPV-induced disease remains rooted to the strategy of repeated local destruction. The physician should work methodically through a series of strategic decisions before committing to a management plan [273].

The data on the etiological factors may enable us to suggest a synergism between the various factors associated with the pathogenesis of cervical cancer. Infection of the cervix by HPV 16/18 may result in persistence of viral DNA. The persistent HPV-DNA undergoes disruption at the E2 region, when integrated into the host genome. The transcriptional products E6 and E7 oncoproteins bind to and cause the degradation of tumor protein 53 (p53) and retinoblastoma (Rb) tumor-suppressor gene (TSG) products. It is possible that, at that point, other cofactors may be involved in the progression toward a precancerous or cancerous condition.

Those cofactors may include cigarette smoking, by introducing co-carcinogens to the tissue or by suppressing the local or systemic immune resistance similar to the effect of depressed immune resistance seen in AIDS or immunosuppression of transplant patients, hormones, by enhancing growth of HPV and transformation of HPV infected cells, low serum vitamin levels, leading to decreased tissue resistance, or other infections causing local inflammation and the production of free radicals. CIN develops, leading eventually to cervical cancer [274].

However, it is known that the carcinogenesis is a multistep process. Changes in the cytogenetic equilibrium, such as chromosomal imbalances, allelic loss, and structural aberrations, happen during the transformation from normal epithelium to cervical cancer. Numerous studies support the hypothesis that HPV infection is associated with development of malignant or pre-malignant changes of the lower genital tract. However, there is little clinical evidence that HPV detection would allow prediction of development of cervical cancer. Regarding the "human aspect" of carcinogenesis, there are efforts to detect markers that predict the risk of progression [275]. Recent studies have indicated that the E6 and E7 gene products play a critical role in cervical carcinogenesis. The E6 and E7 products interfere with the p53 and Rb protein (pRb) functions, respectively, and deregulate the cell cycle. The HPV DNA is integrated into the host's chromosomes with disruption of the E2 gene. This disruption promotes the expression of E6 and E7, leading to the accumulation of DNA damage and the development of cervical cancer. The study of the immune response against HPV has been hampered by the lack of a cell culture system for the virus. A breakthrough was made by the discovery that a major capsid protein late (L) 1 self-assembles into virus-like particles (VLP) when expressed in eukaryotic systems. VLP-based vaccines are in commerce, and DNA vaccines for the HPV surface protein genes are under development. The E7 and E6 oncoproteins are attractive targets for cancer immunotherapy because their expression is required to maintain the oncogenicity of cervical cancer cells. Cancer immunotherapy for cervical cancer with vaccinations of E7 peptides or dendritic cell-based immunotherapy is moving toward clinical trials [276].

Research exploring the E6-p53 and E7-pRb model has resulted in the identity of the viral gene's actions on numerous cellular proteins and processes normally involved in cell growth and proliferation. Specially, several findings have established the various ways by which the HPV-infected cell may escape controls governing cell growth and proliferation, including the fidelity of the host cell's genome and apoptosis.

A large body of knowledge already generated in this area supports the view that high-risk HPV types have the ability to transform cells into a malignant phenotype. Such ability, however, is not sufficient to actually and inevitably produce cervical carcinoma, as indicated by the frequent spontaneous clearance of HPV infection and the long delay between the onset of persistent infection and emergence of the malignancy. Delay in the participation of cofactors has been suggested as explanation in this regard. However, it remains unclear how and when cofactors or factors that are innate in the HPV-infected cells launch the host cells into an irreversible progression to carcinoma [277]. The expression of human papillomavirus 16 E6-E7 oncogenes results in chromosomal aneuploidy, favoring the integration of high-risk HPV genomes into cellular chromosomes. The integration of HPV 16 may not always be required for the progression to the invasive phenotype unlike HPV 18 DNA. Such integration sites are randomly distributed over the whole genome. The genetic susceptibility of codon 98 of the fragile histadine triad has been elucidated. The interaction between HIV and HPV are complex and favor the persistence and progression of cervical disease. Future research should pave the way for therapeutic vaccine development [278]. The identification and functional verification of host proteins associated with HPV E6 and E7 oncoproteins may provide useful information for understanding cervical carcinogenesis and the development of cervical cancer-specific markers. In addition, proteomic profiling of altered proteins by anticancer drugs on cervical cancer cells may contribute to providing the fundamental resources for investigation of disease-specific target proteins, elucidation of the novel mechanisms of action, and development of new drugs. The advent of proteomics has provided the hope of discovering novel biological markers for use in the screening, early diagnosis, and prediction of response to therapy [279].

Cervical cancer is a multistep process with accumulation of genetic and epigenetic alterations in regulatory genes, leading to activation of oncogenes and inactivation or loss of TSG. In the last decade, in addition to genetic alterations, epigenetic inactivation of TSG by promoter hypermethylation has been recognized as an important and alternative mechanism in tumorigenesis. In cervical cancer, epigenetic alterations can affect the expression of HPV as well as host genes in relation to stages representing the multistep process of carcinogenesis [280]. HPV-associated apoptosis can be primarily attributed to some early proteins, such as E2, E5, E6, E7, and so on. Though these proteins have a low molecular size, they are capable to interact with a series of host cellular regulation proteins to induce or inhibit apoptosis.

The oncoproteins E6 can inhibit the apoptosis mainly through p53 pathway. The E5 protein can protect cells from TNF-related apoptosis. The E2 protein have regulatory functions in viral transcription and induction of apoptosis. The oncoprotein E7 plays the role in both apoptosis activation and inhibition. In addition, the HPV full-length E2 proteins involve in activating or repressing the transcription of E6/E7, so as to regulating the apoptosis caused by E6 and E7. HPV early proteins can interfere with apoptosis and trigger gynecopathias for women [281].

The immune mechanisms following HPV infections are barely characterized. However, the association of serum antibodies to HPV proteins with HPV-related diseases is now well-established. Antibodies to some early viral proteins but also to virus capsids (as measured by using VLP) are found in a significant proportion of patients with benign and malignant HPV-related diseases. A small number of patients, however, are devoid of detectable antibodies. It is not clear whether the missing immune response is of any biologic significance for the patient or merely reflects differences in antigen presentation during the course of infection. Clearly, the relatively low sensitivity of serologic assays renders them unsuitable for diagnostic purposes. However, certain combinations of assays may reach a higher predictive value, and hence a particular disease may be diagnosed by a pattern of positive (and negative?) reactions. The humoral immune response in patients with subclinical infections is less well characterized, but such studies are currently being performed in different laboratories [282]. Both cellular and humoral immune responses are essential for the clearance of HPV-associated cervical lesions.

There is increasing evidence that the immune system plays a pivotal role in determining the outcome of HPV infection. Viruses and associated neoplastic cells are proposed to have evolved mechanisms to avoid immune attack. T-cell-mediated immune responses against oncogenic HPV are believed to play a central role in cervical carcinogenesis. The presence of HPV-specific cytotoxic T lymphocytes (CTL) in a majority of human cervical cancer patients provides an approach for further study of their functional role in modulating this malignancy. Tumor-infiltrating lymphocytes (TIL) develop as manifestations of the recognition and defense against malignant cells by the host immune system. Cancer cells may overcome immune surveillance, either by downregulating the proliferation of HPV-specific CTL, or altering the effector compositions of immune cells against HPV infections. TIL in the tumor microenvironment can be functionally inhibited and lose the ability of clonal proliferation as a result of depressed expression of IL-2Ralpha.

The upregulation of inhibitory signaling relates to the modulation of the virus- and/or tumor-specific immune responses. Alteration of host genetic susceptibility may also lead to abnormal immune response as a general genomic instability resulting from virus persistence. Induction of HPV-specific immune responses is anticipated as an intimate point for the treatment of cervical neoplasia [283]. The innate immune responses involving macrophages, NK cells, and NK T cells may play a role in the first line of defense against HPV infection. In the second line of defense, adaptive immunity via CTL targeting HPV 16 E2 and E6 proteins appears to eliminate cells infected with HPV 16. However, HPV can evade host immune responses. First, HPV does not kill host cells during viral replication and therefore neither presents viral antigen nor induces inflammation. HPV 16 E6 and E7 proteins downregulate the expression of type-1 IFN in host cells. The lack of co-stimulatory signals by inflammatory cytokines including IFN during antigen recognition may induce immune tolerance rather than the appropriate responses. Moreover, HPV 16 E5 protein downregulates the expression of human leukocyte antigen (HLA)-class 1, and it facilitates evasion of CTL attack. These mechanisms of immune evasion may eventually support the establishment of persistent HPV infection, leading to the induction of cervical cancer. Considering such immunological events, prophylactic HPV 16 and 18 vaccine appears to be the best way to prevent cervical cancer in women who are immunized in adolescence [284].

People with deficient cell-mediated immunity have an increased susceptibility to viral infections and certain cancers, particularly large cell lymphomas and cancers of the skin and anogenital region. All are linked to viral origins. Neoplasms in the immunodeficient patient often occur at a relatively young age, involve multifocal locations, and tend to persist, recur, and progress rapidly. Anogenital neoplasms show a strong association with HPV infection and also persist, extend, and progress, in spite of standard therapy. Since standard therapy of anogenital HPV infection and neoplasia is often not effective in immunodeficient patients (and others with an anogenital neoplastic syndrome), special treatment is required. 5-FU chemosurgery, followed by maintenance 5-FU therapy, is effective and provides field suppression against recurrent HPV infection and neoplasia, with minimal damage to affected organs. After removal of all detectable HPV infection or neoplastic lesions, immunodeficient patients require close surveillance of the entire anogenital tract. Immunodeficient patients are an in-vivo human laboratory in which to study the natural history of HPV and its oncogenic effects on the anogenital tract.

The theory of HPV oncogenesis is supported by the evidence gathered from these patients [285]. Ano-genital neoplasia is about 20 x more common in renal transplant patients than the general population. Neoplasms in the immunosuppressed are more morbid and mortal because: patients are younger, tumors are more undifferentiated, they have more and larger foci, more sites are involved, neoplasms tend to persist, recur, and progress, and there are more complications from treatments. Intraepithelial neoplasia engenders some morbidity. Invasion is rarer, but when it occurs, it is always morbid, and all too often mortal. Invasive ano-genital cancer is primarily preventable because the lower genital and anal tracts are accessible to inspection, cytologic screening, endoscopy, and biopsy. Prime prevention is avoiding infection with HPV. Next best is detecting HPV/intraepithelial neoplasia early with frequent inspection, cytology, and liberal biopsies, and then removing any condylomas or intraepithelial neoplasia that develop [286].

Although HPV appears to be essential to the transformation of these epithelial cells, it is not sufficient, and a variety of cofactors and molecular events must take place between when an HPV infection occurs and a cervical cancer or its precursor develops. Steroid contraception has been postulated to be one mechanism whereby HPV exerts its tumorigenic effect on cervical tissue. Steroids are thought to bind to specific DNA sequences within transcriptional regulatory regions on the HPV DNA to either increase or suppress transcription of various genes. Although some earlier studies were reassuring as no increased incidence of cervical cancer was observed, subsequent research has shown a causative association, especially among long-term users. The role of steroids was further enhanced by the discovery of hormone receptors in cervical tissue. Some earlier studies of OC steroids found no increased risk, even after controlling for other risk factors, including smoking and number of partners. However, prospective studies have shown a greater progression of dysplasia to CIS with more than 6 years of oral steroid contraceptive use. Similar findings were also evident from other work, including the Royal College of General Practitioners (RCGP) OC Study. The WHO Collaborative Study of Neoplasia and Steroid Contraceptives showed a RR of 1.2 for invasive cancer in users of the long-acting progestational contraceptive, DMPA. However, in users of more than 5 years duration, an estimate of 2.4 was reported. The upstream regulatory region (URR) of the HPV type 16 viral genome mediates transcriptional control of the HPV genome and is thought to contain enhancer elements that are activated by steroid hormones. It has been shown that steroid hormones bind to specific glucorticoid-response elements within HPV-DNA.

Experimental evidence has revealed that high-risk type HPV 16 are able to stimulate the development of vaginal and cervical SCC in transgenic mice exposed to slow-release pellets of 17 beta-estradiol in the presence of human keratin-14 promoter. SCC developed in a multi-stage pathway only in transgenic mice and not in nontransgenic mice. The early (E) 6 oncoprotein of HPV 16 has been shown to bind to the p53 tumor suppressor gene and stimulate its degradation by a ubiquitin-dependent protease system. Steroid hormones are thought to increase the expression of the E6 and E7 HPV 16 oncogenes, which in turn bind to and degrade the p53 gene product, leading to apoptotic failure and carcinogenesis. However, the molecular basis of this remains to be proven [287]. A new analysis from eight studies conducted by the International Agency for Research on Cancer (IARC) and a systematic review of cervical cancer and the use of hormonal contraceptives are two recent major epidemiological links strongly suggesting the increased risk of cervical cancer (up to twofold), but only for women who were both long-term users (5 years or more) and who had persistent HPV infections of the cervix. These findings seem biologically plausible, but weighing the various risks and benefits, the WHO does not recommend any change in OC use or practice [288].

Based on the available molecular, clinical and epidemiologic data, a subset of HPV are unequivocally the etiologic agents for cervical cancers and their precursors. Different mucosotropic HPV have varying neoplastic potential. However, the great majority of cervical HPV have oncogenic potential. Since oncogenic HPV-induced epithelial transformation to a high-grade lesion or cancer is rare relative to the rate of infection, the term high risk is discouraged. HPV's interaction with host cells has two principal biologic consequences:

1) all anogenital HPV induce low-grade squamous lesions, which are the morphologic correlate of a productive infection; and
2) rarely, HPV induce a proliferative epithelial phenotype that pathologists recognize as a high-grade lesion and that is the proximate cytohistologic precursor of invasive cervical carcinoma.

HPV biology and issues of practical clinical management should be reflected in the classification systems used for cytologic and histologic diagnosis. The molecular identification of HPV (HPV testing) potentially may be very useful for primary screening or secondary triage of patients with certain lesions.

However, the technology available to the practicing clinician is still evolving. Optimization of type spectrum, sensitivity, specificity and ease of use is under development. Data regarding these factors as well as a clear cost-benefit analysis are sparse or pending in several large trials. Until such data are available, caution in clinical implementation of HPV testing is warranted [289].

Vulvar pathology is located at the border between dermatology and gynecology. The gynecologist is concerned by VIN lesions as patients meet them for that problem. He makes distinction with dermatologic lesions so as to refer proper patients to dermatologists. A recent classification of VIN has a major interest. One individualizes two kinds of precancerous lesions. The first one is lichen sclerosis with dermatologic treatment by dermocorticoids and the other etiology is HPV infection with frequent association with cervical localization. Gynecologists are more familiar with this second etiology. Thus, they have to:

1) check for VIN;
2) know their appearance and how the diagnosis can be made by biopsy;
3) precise the etiology;
4) appreciate the severity of the disease; and
5) discuss which treatment is indicated: destruction or surgery [290].

The incidence of HPV-related VIN is increasing worldwide. This is associated with an increasing incidence of invasive vulvar cancer in young women. Undifferentiated VIN has an invasive potential. A subset of very young patients with pigmented lesions and spontaneous regression has been described. Differentiated VIN is HPV-negative and affects older women, who are at risk of invasive cancer. Chromosomal changes and angiogenesis may play a role in carcinogenesis. Immunocompromised women bear a substantial risk of VIN. These facts demand the awareness of both women and physicians, because there is evidence of diagnostic delays in patients with vulvar cancer. The standard treatment is surgical excision, which may be combined with laser treatment in extensive disease. The standard modalities of treatment for VIN, surgical excision and laser ablation, are both sub-optimal, associated with high rates of disease recurrence. There is a need for non-surgical treatment options for VIN: topical antiviral agents and photodynamic therapy (PDT), by altering the local immunological parameters, have the potential to clear both VIN and HPV [291, 292].

The pathogenesis of vulvar and cervical cancer are thought to be similar and to be related to a sexually transmitted agent, which, in recent years, has been demonstrated to be HPV. These two neoplasms differ dramatically in age distribution and relationship to precursor lesions, making a common etiology unlikely. The apparent discrepancies can be explained by a hypothesis that implicates HPV as an etiologic factor for the majority of cervical carcinomas but for only a small proportion of vulvar carcinomas.

Most vulvar carcinomas occur in older women and are not related to HPV, whereas a subset of vulvar carcinomas occur in young women and are related to this virus. Characterization of two distinct types of vulvar carcinoma may clarify associated risk factors and may have important implications in the clinical management of this disease [293]. SCC of the vulva is a rare disease: the incidence is 1-2 per 100,000 women per year. Among women more than 75 years of age, the incidence is at least ten times higher. The cause of vulvar carcinoma is not known. In contrast to what has been stated for many years, in recent case-control studies no evidence was found that diabetes mellitus, obesity, vascular diseases, nulliparity, an early menopause, and syphilis are risk factors for developing a vulvar carcinoma. The factors that play a role in the etiology of vulvar carcinoma are: vulvar dystrophy, a history of genital HPV-infection, a history of cervical neoplasia, advanced age, smoking, and a compromised immunity. Usually, for the development of a vulvar carcinoma, more than one of the above mentioned factors have to be present [294]. HPV DNA is more common in vulvar cancers of young women who smoke than in older nonsmokers. Patients with HPV-negative tumors are at an increased risk of recurrence and death from vulvar cancer [295]. HPV is thought to cause some vulval SCC by degrading p53 product. Evidence on whether HPV-negative vulval SCC results from p53 mutation is conflicting. Data suggest that HPV-independent vulval carcinogenesis does not exclusively require disruption of p53, p53 disruption may work synergistically with loss of heterozygosity (LOH) at specific loci and p53-positive VIN should be checked carefully for the presence of occult invasion [296]. Vulvar cancer continues to rise in incidence. In the absence of screening, attempts to reduce this cancer must focus on recognizing precursor lesions, namely, lichen sclerosus and VIN. The steep rise in HPV-repeated VIN will fall after the introduction of vaccination against HPV. In the meantime, those patients with VIN must be treated and then reviewed carefully and frequently. Lichen sclerosus has a 3% to 5% risk of progressing to vulvar cancer [297].

Vaginal cancer, 2% of all female genital malignancies, has a worse prognosis than cervical cancer.

SCC, the most common histologic subtype, may be associated partly with HPV. Most patients present with vaginal bleeding and discharge. Radiation or surgery are the main treatment modalities, but the physical and psychosexual morbidity can be significant [298]. Ovarian SCC is usually derived from a teratoma, a Brenner tumor, or endometriosis. Association with an HPV infection is rare. The development of bone metastases in association with an ovarian SCC is a rare finding, and it does not respond to treatment with a tyrosine kinase [299].

An isolated report of atypical squamous cells (ASC) on cervical cytology obtained at the initial prenatal visit does not warrant colposcopic evaluation during pregnancy, unless a repeat cytology suggests CIN. Repeat cytology and evaluation to exclude infections and inflammatory lesions is appropriate. However, if a subsequent cytology is abnormal, postpartum colposcopy and colposcopically directed biopsies seem appropriate, since the prevalence of HPV or CIN is 21% [300]. RRP is a benign yet aggressive neoplasm that produces considerable morbidity in children. Previous studies have linked RRP in children to mothers with genital tract HPV. Risk factors for vertical transmission have not been well identified. Controversy exists among obstetricians and otolaryngologists regarding the role of CS in preventing MTCT of HPV disease. The results of a national survey of otolaryngologists, the ACOG position statement, the relevant literature regarding the association between RRP and maternal HPV, and the proposed mechanisms for HPV transmission at birth make us postulate a very limited role for CS in preventing transmission of RRP, given our present knowledge of this disease [301]. It is unknown whether there is a disease correlate in children chronically infected with oncogenic HPV. Low-risk HPV genotypes 6 and 11 are the primary cause of condylomata acuminata, although in children non-genital genotypes are also found in a proportion, with the mode of transmission being either perinatal, horizontal, or sexual. The finding of asymptomatic HPV DNA in children, and correlation with live virus, infectivity, or disease is unclear. Long term follow-up for children with anogenital warts is recommended, although there are no longitudinal studies available to clarify whether they are at risk of developing carcinoma in young adulthood [302]. An understanding of the natural history of this common STI is necessary to allow diagnosis of clinically significant disease and judicious application of treatment modalities, especially in young adolescents [303].

Over the past decades, the ever-increasing volume of evidence implicating HPV types in genital neoplasia has stimulated much research interest into all aspects of the biology of this interesting group of viruses.

This research has led to the identification of a growing heterogeneity of HPV types. It is not surprising, therefore, that the clinical profile of disease associated with genital HPV types is much broader than previously recognized.

Knowledge of this clinical spectrum is mandatory to the understanding of the possible role of specific HPV types in human carcinogenesis [304-306]. HPV are associated with a spectrum of diseases, ranging from common warts to invasive carcinoma of the genital tract. The clinical manifestations of HPV infection depend on the viral subtype, the immune status of the patient, and environmental co-carcinogens. Infection with HPV is often asymptomatic, which makes viral detection challenging. Current therapies do not reliably eradicate HPV infection, and benign genital warts and genital tract intraepithelial neoplasia often recur after treatment [307].

The long, tedious search for the causes of and cure for cancer has not resulted in one astounding breakthrough discovery. Instead, researchers have slowly and painstakingly made small inroads into the understanding of the way cell growth goes awry and becomes malignant, destroying tissues and, if unchecked, spreading to other organs of the body and eventually causing death.

One of those inroads is the discovery that a cancer of the uterine cervix is almost certainly caused by a virus transmitted through sexual contact. Cancer of the cervix usually is preceded by a slowly progressive preinvasive lesion, dysplasia, which can be detected by a screening test, the Pap smear, and effectively treated with organ-preserving local therapy. Because dysplasia and early invasive cancer usually develop in young women, the need for conservative management is of utmost importance to preserve a woman's ability to have children.

The social and psychological impacts of a cancer occurring in young women are enormous and are further magnified by the fact that this cancer may be caused by a sexually transmitted virus. Sexual practice patterns, number of sexual partners, smoking, and other behavioral aspects contribute to the complexity of this disease. However, early detection of preinvasive and invasive cancer is possible with fairly simple and inexpensive means, and curative therapy is available. The disastrous impact of cervical cancer theoretically could be contained if patients at risk regularly participate in early detection programs.

Also, the disease could, to a large extent, be prevented altogether through healthful behavior and sexual practices. The social challenge is to provide this information to the public in a nonthreatening, nonmoralistic fashion.

We especially need to help young people to accept that sex within a caring, responsible relationship is a healthy human response and, at the same time, understand that there are dangers associated with transmittable diseases that can have profound effects on their ability to have children and on their lives [308]. There are no RCT to review regarding information for women about HPV but a number of well-conducted qualitative studies explore the issues that are faced both by the women undergoing cervical screening and their healthcare providers [309]. Cervical cancer patients are affected on a psychological, psychosocial, and sexual level, resulting in an overall decrease in QOL. Clinicians can better patients' QOL after an abnormal Pap test or diagnosis and treatment of cervical cancer. Fear, self-blame, distress, and anxiety about cervical cancer are common in women who receive abnormal Pap test results or positive HPV DNA tests. Such results impact body image, self-esteem, relationships with partners, and sexual and reproductive issues, while adding to an overall decrease of QOL in women with cervical cancer. In order to minimize the deleterious effects, the impact of cervical cancer and precancerous lesions on QOL should be managed as part of a complete healthcare plan. To improve QOL, cervical cancer patients should seek supportive counseling and education about self-care and adherence to treatment and follow-up plans, continue cervical cancer screening, and receive vaccination against prevalent oncogenic virus types [310]. Psychosexual vulnerability increases with number of recurrences of HPV infections. Depression, anxiety, and anger are the emotions most frequently reported. However, to date, there is no conclusive evidence of a specific correlation between HPV infection and a specific female sexual disorder. The relationship between HPV and vulvar vestibulitis/vulvodynia-related dyspareunia seems not to be direct. The evidence of psychosexual consequences of HPV-related genital warts and intraepithelial lesions is limited. Specific research on the sexual impact of genital warts and intraepithelial HPV-related lesion in women is urgently needed [311].

Only an effective cytological screening programme with effective follow-up arrangements will prevent the prospect of an "epidemic" of cervical and possibly of other squamous genital cancers. These should be priorities for future preventive medicine strategies [312]. The Pap smear is one of the most successful of the screening tools for cancer. However, refinements are continually being made in the terminology used to define the gradations of disease, in the classifications used to describe test results, and in the appropriate technique for performing the test [313]. Detection of high-risk HPV has a high potential value for secondary prevention of cervical cancer.

HPV testing can augment the sensitivity of conventional cytologic screening and can be used for triaging patients with a history of mild cytological abnormalities or low-grade CIN [314]. HPV typing provides the most rational basis for selecting women with L-SIL to be colposcoped and treated or given follow-up treatment with Pap smears. Management decisions may be based on an individual's risk factors such as age, compliance, past history of abnormal Pap smears, sexual habits, and access to adequate cytologic diagnosis [315].

The subjectivity of morphologic methods contributes to a "swamping" of colposcopic services, excessive costs, overdiagnosis, and overtreatment. HPV DNA testing provides the objectivity required to clarify difficult patient management issues, including follow-up, for low-grade cytologic abnormalities (ASC and L-SIL), noncorrelating (nonconfirmed) Pap smears, evaluation of nondiagnostic lower genital tract lesions, and cytology and histology laboratory quality assurance. Additionally, favorable preliminary data on HPV testing as a primary screen raise the exciting prospect of potentially lowering costs of cervical cancer screening programs, while further decreasing the incidence of cervical cancer [316].

The Pap smear has been the classic screening strategy for preventing cervical cancer for 50 years. The finding that infection with HPV is associated with an increased risk of cervical cancer has prompted the development of new strategies for cervical cancer screening and prevention [317]. Conventional viral detection assays, including serologic assays and growth in cell culture, are not available for the diagnosis and tracking of HPV infection. Pap tests are a valuable screening tool, but they miss a large proportion of HPV-infected persons. Accordingly, HPV DNA detection assays have become a key research tool in the detection of HPV infection, particularly in asymptomatic individuals. Several types of HPV DNA tests are now available, including Southern blots, dot blots, ISH, PCR, and solution hybridization (Hybrid Capture [HC] assay). Of these, the PCR assay is the most sensitive, whereas dot blots and solution hybridization are the least labor intensive. HPV DNA detection assays are not routinely used in screening patients, in part because the clinical relevance of asymptomatic infection is unclear. Nevertheless, these tests may be beneficial in confirming differential diagnoses and in providing prognostic information, particularly with respect to the HPV type involved [318]. In an effort to reduce the false-negative rate of cervical cytologic findings, several new technologies have recently evolved. Automated cytologic testing (PapNet, AutoPap 300 QC) proposes to rescreen negative conventional cytologic findings to identify smears likely to be false negative.

Fluid-based monolayers (ThinPrep, CytoRich) propose to reduce the false-negative rates by optimizing the collection and preparation of cells. HPV DNA testing by HC-2 (Digene Corporation, Gaithersburg, MD) has been proposed for a variety of screening and triage roles. Visual screening after application of acetic acid is done by cervicography by use of a photographic technique, whereas in speculoscopy the screening is done by direct visualization of the cervix by the primary care provider. Polarprobe uses biophysical parameters and a computer algorithm to give an instantaneous prediction of the likelihood of cervical disease [319]. In predicting the presence of high-grade or invasive disease in the cervix in women with Pap smears reported as ASC of undetermined significance (ASC-US) or L-SIL, the approach to management by cytologic screening and colposcopy, when indicated, appeared over the long term to be equal to HPV testing [320]. Testing for high-risk HPV types should become a standard of care for women because cervical cancer is an infectious disease.

Current care is based on cytologic screening and a pathologic staging of cellular tissue changes. Before these cellular modifications, there is a demonstrable pattern of HPV infection. Currently, adding HPV screening to the Pap smear identifies a population for closer follow-up studies [321]. HPV-DNA testing in association with the Pap smear performed either conventionally or, preferably, with the new liquid-based cytology is a valuable adjunct with high sensitivity and acceptable specificity rates in defining those patients most likely to demonstrate H-SIL at the time of colposcopy. At present, available evidence indicates that the best reason for performing HPV-DNA testing is the triage of selected patients with ASC-US and in specific settings with L-SIL [322].

Pap smear screening for cervical cancer has been a preventive health success. Although improved technology is increasing the accuracy of this technique, more women who have never been tested will need to undergo screening in order to further decrease the incidence of cervical cancer. Prevention of cervical cancer by detecting the disease process at an early and pre-malignant stage is practiced globally either through population-based screening programmes (PSP) or through non-organized ones. High-grade CIN detected by cervical cytological screening is extensively visualized by colposcopy and successively treated by, for instance, large loop electro-surgical excision of the transformation zone (LEETZ). Testing for the presence of high-risk HPV DNA should increase the ability to identify women who are truly at risk for cancer and true cancer precursors and to more efficiently plan further diagnostic evaluation [323, 324].

The ASCCP National Consensus Conference for the Management of Women with Cervical Cytological Abnormalities and Cervical Cancer Precursors was held on the National Institutes of Health campus in Bethesda, MD, September 6-8, 2001.

The conference was attended by 121 representatives from 29 national organizations interested in cervical cancer screening issues. For the first time, guidelines for the management of women with abnormal cervical cytology, developed from evidence-based literature, were presented to delegates from the majority of organizations with interest in cervical cancer screening, voted on, and revised when necessary to achieve a majority two-thirds approval. This development of consensus-approved guidelines is likely to be considered one of the most important milestones to date in the management of women with abnormal cervical cytology.

The timing of this Consensus Conference resulted from the convergence of many different factors, including new cytologic terminology developed at the Bethesda 2001 workshop and publication of the enrollment data from the National Cancer Institute (NCI)'s ASC-US)/L-SIL Triage Study, otherwise known as ALTS.

Additionally, new preliminary longitudinal ALTS data provided much of the information on the natural history of abnormal Pap tests and CIN, as well as data on the performance of both new liquid-based cytology and HPV DNA testing in the management of women following colposcopy. The result was a large database of new information that provided the foundation for the ASCCP Consensus Conference. The management of women with equivocal (ASC-US) and low-grade (L-SIL) cytologic abnormalities has been particularly problematic, because individually these women are at least risk for CIN 3 and cancer, yet their sheer numerical dominance ensures that they account for the majority of high-grade CIN detected in the US in the follow-up of abnormal cervical cytology.

Data from ALTS confirmed that women with ASC-US could be safely managed by any of the conventional approaches (repeat Pap test, immediate colposcopy, or HPV testing), but that the preferred management approach for women having an ASC-US report from liquid-based cytology was to assess the patient's risk by testing for HPV. Additionally, longitudinal ALTS data determined that repeat liquid-based cytology at 6 and 12 months and an HPV test at 12 months were nearly equivalent options in the follow-up of women referred for HPV-positive ASC or L-SIL, yet not found to have CIN 2+ at initial colposcopy. Therefore, all follow-up recommendations for women with CIN 1 or lower postcolposcopy findings include these two options [325].

The 2001 revisions in the Bethesda System reflect our improved understanding of the epidemiology and natural history of cervical epithelial abnormalities and cervical cancer. These revisions are designed to facilitate communication between the clinician and the laboratory and to improve the clinician's ability to accurately interpret the cytology report and plan initial management of any abnormalities [323].

The finding of atypical and low-grade cervical cytology on routine Pap test is considered problematic for gynecologists and pathologists. The interpretation and management of these cases can be difficult when Pap test results fall into the Bethesda 2001 categories of ASC, ASC-cannot rule out high-grade (ASC-H), atypical glandular cells (AGC), or L-SIL. Although liquid-based Pap tests may have resulted in some improvement in detection, a large amount of variability in cytologic interpretations continues to exist [326]. The options for management of CIN 1, 2, and 3 are ranked according to the strength of the recommendation and the quality of the evidence. Follow-up with repeat cytology at six and 12 months or DNA testing for high-risk types of HPV at 12 months is the preferred management approach for women with CIN 1 and satisfactory initial colposcopy.

If results from repeat cytology are reported as ASC-US or greater, or if HPV DNA testing is positive for oncogenic types of the virus, repeat colposcopy is preferred. When the initial colposcopy is unsatisfactory, a diagnostic excisional procedure is preferred. Follow-up without treatment is acceptable only in women who are pregnant and adolescents with CIN 1 who had unsatisfactory colposcopy. Biopsy-confirmed CIN 2 and 3 requires treatment except during pregnancy and in compliant adolescents with CIN 2 and negative endocervical curettage. When colposcopy is satisfactory, treatment includes ablative or excisional procedures. A diagnostic excisional procedure is recommended in women with biopsy-confirmed CIN 2 or 3 and unsatisfactory colposcopy [327].

The changes in cervical cytology characterization agreed on by the Bethesda committee meeting in 2001 created a category of atypical findings that has caused some management confusion.

By description, the characterization of cervical cytology as only atypical implies a less worrisome prognosis.

However, more than 40% of high-grade (CIN 2 or 3 or cancer) will be discovered within this category. The development and FDA approval of the HC-2 for detecting high-risk HPV subtypes and the subsequent level I evidence supporting use of this test in the triage of women with atypical cytology has revolutionized the management of this cytology.

With this success has come numerous additional uses for high-risk HPV testing in the treatment and follow-up of women with a variety of cytologic abnormalities [328].

Recent decades have witnessed a reduction in the incidence of cervical cancer in countries where screening programmes have achieved broad coverage. The recognized importance of high-risk HPV infection in the etiology of cervical cancer may introduce a role for HPV DNA testing in cervical screening programmes. Positive HPV DNA tests indicate women at risk of cervical cancer with greater sensitivity, but reduced specificity, compared with exfoliative cytology.

Combining HPV testing with cytology may be useful in the triage of minor cytological abnormalities into those requiring referral to colposcopy (HPV positive) compared with those who can be safely managed by cytological surveillance (HPV negative). With its high sensitivity and high-negative-predictive value, HPV testing may also be useful for predicting treatment failure, since residual disease is very unlikely in the event of a negative HPV test. Compared to cytology, the HC-2 and PCR are substantially more sensitive for prevalent CIN 2 or worse but significantly less specific. The combination of HC-2 and cytology has the highest sensitivity and lowest specificity. However, reduction of the incidence of or mortality from invasive cervical cancer among HPV screened subjects compared to cytologically screened subjects has not yet been demonstrated.

Ultimately, prevention is better than cure, and the advent of HPV prophylactic vaccines may obviate the need for population-based cervical screening programmes in the future.

A multivalent vaccine administered to adolescents prior to the onset of sexual activity and boosted at regular intervals throughout their sexually active life may provide protection against type-specific HPV infection, malignant precursors, and invasive cervical disease. Several large RCT have been conducted with promising results. For those generations of women already exposed to high-risk HPV infection, therapeutic vaccines may offer advantages over conventional treatment, although much work still needs to be done. Cervical screening in the post-vaccination era cannot be abolished but could be altered. Algorithms with the primary objective of hr-HPV testing followed by subjective cytology assessment in HPV-positive women could be a solution for both pre- and post-vaccination screening [324, 329, 330]. US-based guidelines recommended that screening should be initiated approximately 3 years after initiation of sexual intercourse, but no later than age 21 years and be continued at least until age 65 or 70.

Annual screening was recommended by the ACS and the ACOG, although in women aged ≥30 years with ≥3 negative Pap tests, screening may be conducted every 2 to 3 years. HPV testing has been approved by the US FDA and most US guidelines say that it is reasonable to consider HPV testing, in combination with triennial cytology screening. Pharmacoeconomic analyses indicate that combined cytology and HPV testing every three years in women aged ≥30 years is comparable in sensitivity to annual liquid-based cytology for the detection of cervical cancer precursors and is more cost-effective. Both surgical and nonsurgical therapies are commonly employed in patients with HPV lesions although recurrence is not uncommon. Treatment should be individualized based on the extent of disease and the needs of the patient. Current treatment of cervical cancer reflects the stage of the disease and should take into account patient- and tumor-related factors to ensure optimal patient outcomes [331].

The ACS, the ASCCP, and the ASCP have released revised consensus recommendations for cervical cancer screening. These new recommendations integrate molecular testing and include significant changes in screening, particularly in women from 30 to 65 years of age without complications who now may be screened every 5 years by co-testing with cervical cytology and high-risk HPV testing and women 21-29 years who may be screened with cervical cytology alone every 3 years. The revised recommendations include clarification on when to start and stop screening and management of women who have undergone hysterectomy. They also clarify the management of results of co-testing. The new recommendations achieve the same degree of protection against cervical cancer as previous recommendations. They require less screening and will be much more convenient for our patients. They are a further step away from the days of annual Pap tests, and the decreased requirements for cervical cancer screening pose an exciting opportunity for focusing on many other important health issues during the well woman visit [332]. Testing for HPV has been shown to be more sensitive than cervical cytology in detecting both high-grade and low-grade dysplasia. When screening for cervical cancer, unfortunately, the HPV test lacks specificity and has limited its usefulness as a primary screening modality for cervical cancer [333, 334].

Cervical cancer is the most common malignancy amongst females in developing countries, mainly due to a lack of precursor screening. This absence of screening is the result of inherent disadvantages of the Pap smear: high cost, low sensitivity, the need for a laboratory with high human expertise, and a complex screening program logistic system.

The prerequisites for screening in a developing country include a screening method that is affordable, which can be effectively applied once in a lifetime at the age of 30-35 years, provide an immediate result and thereby allowing for on-site treatment of positive cases. None of the current screening methods comply with these prerequisites. A screening program based on cytology analysis requires too much training, infrastructure, and repeated screening to be feasible. Visual inspection with acetic acid, often used throughout the world, is inexpensive and both sensitive and specific, but it lacks reproducibility. Although HPV testing is too expensive for widespread use, its negative predictive value and sensitivity make it a promising method of screening. More research is necessary into different combinations of tests, which improve sensitivity. On-site HPV identification, alone or in combination with other tests, is promising. Another promising development is immunization against HPV infection, either as a preventative measure or for stimulating immunity in infected women [335, 336]. Utilizing HPV vaccines as a primary mode of prevention may not be financially feasible and does not obviate the need for screening. Cervical cancer has been considered an AIDS-defining illness, with HPV and HIV often coexisting, and screening methods have been shown to be as reliable for women with HIV as those without. Ultimately, the most clinically effective and cost-effective methods for reducing cervical cancer incidence are those that limit the number of visits that women are required to attend. Providing immediate cryotherapy for those with a positive screen, whether by visual inspection or HPV testing, is promising to have quite an impact, although the type of program implemented will depend on the needs and expectations of each country [337].

The exact histologic diagnosis of CIN lesions is essential for a differentiated therapy. Data indicate that mild and moderate CIN lesions are detected more frequently by Pap smear and colposcopically directed punch biopsy than by cervical smears alone. Histological diagnosis and HPV-typing by ISH offers the possibility to establish a differentiated therapy, e.g., by way of close follow-up, local destruction, or cone biopsy. Main attention should be directed at early detection of dysplasia, at timely institution of follow-up programs, and a possibly conservative therapeutic management [338]. Target biopsy and transformation zone ablation on excision is the mainstay of management for cervical lesions that can be adequately visualized. For the physician who does not progress beyond whimsical estimates of lesion prominence (which cannot differentiate minor- from major-grade lesions), the colposcope will never be more than a simple aid to the collection of directed biopsy specimens.

Unfortunately, in situations in which the clinician's only option is passive response to the histopathology report, optimal management of the patient's disease will not occur. Indeed, the best prospect for diagnosing or prognosticating confusing disease patterns can sometimes be lost by blind precipitous intervention. Because the most prominent areas of colposcopic change do not necessarily coincide with the areas of greatest histologic abnormality, less experienced colposcopists may not be able to select the most abnormal sites for target biopsy. Peripheral areas of prominent aceto-whitening tend to be overinterpreted, and the subtle acetowhitening of high-grade CIN near the canal tends to be easily overlooked. This problem is best solved by using colposcopic criteria that are based on critical analysis, rather than "pattern recognition". It is easy to derive the four proven colposcopic criteria, and they can be quickly compiled into an index that helps the clinician recognize lesion severity while he or she is performing the colposcopy. Of course, using the Reid colposcopic index (RCI) to infer approximate histologic findings does not eliminate the importance of biopsy (Table 2). Skilled physicians will conscientiously follow the triage rules, including the need to collect carefully sited target biopsy specimens [339]. An awareness of the pitfalls associated with the various aspects of the colposcopic examination should minimize erroneous diagnosis and inappropriate treatment. The colposcopist, armed with current knowledge and guided by a diagnostic and therapeutic protocol, should be able to avoid them [340]. Colposcopic practice continues to evolve. As its need has expanded, so has the role of training, audit, and continuing medical education (CME). The recently published National Health Service (NHS) Cervical Screening Programme clinical guidelines document covers almost every aspect of clinical practice in an evidence-based directory. Excision of the transformation zone may be a very minor or major entity. The recent transformation zone classification system of the International Federation of Cervical Pathology and Colposcopy (IFCPC) attempts to clarify and standardize nomenclature so that therapy can be realistically compared. Colposcopic evaluation of the vagina and vulva is an important adjunct to cervical colposcopy because HPV disease can be multifocal and multicentric. Other reasons for vulvar and vaginal colposcopy include cytology unexplained by cervical findings, vaginal and vulvar symptoms, and diethylstilbestrol (DES) exposure. VIN and VaIN lesions are important cancer precursors to evaluate and treat. Many lesion types have a similar appearance, and biopsies should be used to elucidate the cause of the colposcopic findings. For the evaluation of borderline nuclear abnormal smear and for post-treatment surveillance, HPV is clinically useful and efficient.

Other biological tumor markers are likely to become clinically useful as their predictive profiles emerge [341, 342]. p16(INK4a) is a biomarker for transforming HPV infections that could act as an adjunct to current cytological and histological assessment of cervical smears and biopsies, allowing the identification of those women with ambiguous results that require referral to colposcopy and potentially treatment. Although there is good evidence that p 16(INK4a) immunostaining correlates with the severity of cytological/ histological abnormalities, the reproducibility is limited due to insufficiently standardized interpretation of the immunostaining.

Therefore, a consensus needs to be reached regarding the evaluation of p 16(INK4a) staining and the biomarker needs to be assessed in various clinical settings addressing specific clinical questions [343].

In conclusion, gynecologic cytopathology is a heavily regulated field, with Clinical Laboratory Improvement Amendments (CLIA) of 1988 mandating the collection of many quality metrics. There is a lack of consensus regarding methods to collect, monitor, and benchmark these data and how these data should be used in a quality assurance program. Furthermore, the introduction of HPV testing and proficiency testing has provided more data to monitor [344]. The number of Pap tests from high-risk patients should be maximized in prospective and retrospective rescreening. Unsatisfactory Pap tests should also be included. All readily identifiable high-risk HPV-positive cases with an interpretation of negative for intraepithelial lesion or malignancy should be prospectively rescreened. Cervical biopsy results with high-grade CIN or worse (CIN 2+) should trigger retrospective rescreening. Regular feedback should be provided to cytotechnologists and cytopathologists. Upgraded diagnoses from negative for intraepithelial lesion or malignancy to ASC-H should be monitored [345]. HPV testing is now routinely used to screen for cervical carcinoma and precursor lesions of the cervix (cotesting and reflex testing) and these results are considered in patient triage and management. It is not appropriate for laboratories to offer low-risk HPV testing for any clinical circumstance in gynecologic cytology. Laboratories should not order HPV testing to resolve diagnostic discrepancies. It is a valuable broad measure of laboratory quality to monitor the HPV-positive rates in Pap tests with ASC [346].

The WHO classification has clarified the typing of cervical tumors. The category of early stromal invasion has been eliminated from the International Federation of Gynecology and Obstetrics (FIGO) staging scheme of cervical carcinoma. Stage lAl is defined now as depth of invasion $\leq$3 mm, stage lA2 is

Table 2. Reid colposcopic index (RCI)*

Colposcopic signs	0	1	2
Color	• Low-intensity acetowhitening (not completely opaque) • Indistinct acetowhitening • Transparent or translucent acetowhitening • Acetowhitening beyond the margin of the transformation zone • Pure snow-white color with intense surface shine	Intermediate shade - grey/white color and shiny surface (most lesions should be scored in this category)	Dull, opaque, oyster white; grey
Lesion margin and surface configuration	• Microcondylomatous or micropapillary contour[1] • Flat lesions with indistinct margins • Feathered or finely scalloped margins • Angular, jagged lesions[3] • Satellite lesions beyond the margin of the transformation zone	Regular-shaped, symmetrical lesions with smooth, straight outlines	• Rolled, peeling edges[2] • Internal demarcations between areas of differing colposcopic appearance (a central area of high-grade change and peripheral area of low-grade change)
Vessels	• Fine/uniform-calibre vessels[4] (closely and uniformly placed) • Poorly formed patterns of fine punctation and/or mosaic • Vessels beyond the margin of the transformation zone • Fine vessels within microcondylomatous or micropapillary lesions[6]	Absent vessels	Well defined coarse punctation or mosaic, sharply demarcated[5] and randomly and widely placed
Iodine staining	• Positive iodine uptake giving mahogany-brown color • Negative uptake of insignificant lesion, i.e., yellow staining by a lesion scoring three points or less on the first three criteria • Areas beyond the margin of the transformation zone, conspicuous on colposcopy, evident as iodine-negative areas (such areas are frequently due to parakeratosis)[7]	Partial iodine uptake - variegated, speckled appearance	Negative iodine uptake of significant lesion, i.e., yellow staining by a lesion already scoring four points or more on the first three criteria

Colposcopic prediction of histologic diagnosis using the Reid Colposcopic Index (RCI)	
RCI (overall score)	Histology
0 - 2	Likely to be cervical intraepithelial neoplasia (CIN) 1
3 - 4	Overlapping lesion: likely to be CIN 1 or CIN 2
5 - 8	Likely to be CIN 2-3

*Colposcopic grading performed with 5% aqueous acetic acid and Lugol's iodine solution.
[1]Microexophytic surface contour indicative of colposcopically overt cancer is not included in this scheme.
[2]Epithelial edges tend to detach from underlying stroma and curl back on themselves. Note: Prominent low-grade lesions often are overinterpreted, while subtle avascular patches of high-grade squamous intraepithelial lesion (H-SIL) can easily be overlooked.
[3]Score zero even if part of the peripheral margin does have a straight course.
[4]At times, mosaic patterns containing central vessels are characteristic of low-grade histological abnormalities. These low-grade-lesion capillary patterns can be quite pronounced. Until the physician can differentiate fine vascular patterns from coarse, overdiagnosis is the rule.
[5]Branching atypical vessels indicative of colposcopically overt cancer are not included in this scheme.
[6]Generally, the more microcondylomatous the lesion, the lower the score. However, cancer also can present as a condyloma, although this is a rare occurrence.
[7]Parakeratosis: a superficial zone of cornified cells with retained nuclei.
Adapted from International Agency for Research on Cancer (IARC), 2013.

defined as depth of invasion between 3 and 5 mm in depth. The width should not exceed 7 mm. Persons with stage IA1 disease have a high cure rate with either simple hysterectomy or, where fertility preservation is an issue, by cone biopsy with clear margins. For patients with other stage I and stage IIA disease, radical surgery and radiation are equally effective treatments. These patients should be carefully selected to receive one treatment or the other but not both, as their combined use substantially increases the cost and morbidity of treatment. Women with more advanced, nonmetastatic disease should be treated with radiation. Recurrent cervical cancer confined to the pelvis should be treated with the modality not previously received.

Radiation is recommended to palliate symptoms in patients with metastatic disease. There is an active Cochrane Collaborative Review Group in Gynecological Cancer (Cochrane Gynecological Cancer Group, CGCG). As far as evidence for the effective management of cervical cancer is concerned, the strongest evidence would relate to the effectiveness of concurrent chemoradiation for treating locally advanced disease compared with radiation alone. Small cell carcinoma has been better delineated. The better understanding of pseudomalignant lesions, that is, deep cervical glands, various metaplasias, and inflammatory pseudo tumors, as well as some rare tumors, enables the surgical pathologist to make a more accurate diagnosis, resulting in better patient care [347-349].

Before the initiation of screening and treatment for cervical cancer precursors, approximately 3% to 4% of women were destined to eventually develop cervical cancer. During the last 60 years, the rate of cervical cancer incidence and mortality has decreased by more than 75% primarily because of the widespread availability of cervical cytologic screening and of treatment for documented cervical precancer. Successful screening of the entire population and appropriate treatment of lesions could theoretically reduce this risk to 1/10 of the risk of an unscreened population. The relatively recent understanding of the etiology of cervical cancer precursor lesions and of the immune response to them has given new direction to management options that incorporate healthy habits and dietary measures as part of traditional ablative or excisional treatment options. As we look to the future, we can expect that new markers that more specifically identify individuals at-risk for cervical precancer and cancer will be developed and take precedence in cervical screening. At the same time, treating the cause of these lesions, rather than the result, should provide less traumatic and more successful therapies. To this end, harnessing the immune system through immune response modifiers and HPV vaccines seems to be the solution, as do new chemopreventative approaches. Of all human cancers, only cervical cancer, once the second most common cancer among women, stands on the threshold of being virtually eliminated [350]. Estrogen interacts with HPV at a cellular level causing cell growth and inhibition of apoptosis. Indole derivatives, formed during digestion of cruciferous vegetables, have been shown to have chemopreventative properties inhibiting HPV transcription and influencing estrogen metabolism. Further clinical research is required to evaluate the chemopreventative properties of these agents [351].

The psychological stress of having genital warts is often greater than the morbidity of the disease, and therefore successful treatment is crucial.

Current treatments are patient-applied and provider-administered therapies. Immunomodulators have been used for some time in various medical specialities, but have only recently been used in gynecology. The first drug in this therapeutic class, imiquimod (Aldara, Meda AB, Solna, SW), has been shown to be effective in treating lesions induced by HPV such as genital warts or cervical and vulvar dysplasia, by stimulating the immune system of an infected individual. Thanks to its ease of use and its few side effects, imiquimod would appear to be, in the future, the treatment of choice for these types of viral infections, alone or in association with therapeutic vaccines or physical abative therapies as a prevention of relapses. Imiquimod 5% cream, a patient-applied therapy, is an efficacious treatment with a low recurrence rate, and has the potential to be an effective strategy for the management of genital warts [352, 353]. Alternative medical interventions, such as cidofovir, should be explored [354]. IFN have proved useful in the management of recalcitrant condylomata acuminata. Dosage schedules have been established that balance efficacy and systemic toxicity. Alone, however, IFN are not entirely effective in every patient. In combination with conventional medical and surgical modalities, they offer hope for the control of an often frustrating and potentially serious virus infection [355]. Because of their antiviral, antiproliferative, and immunoregulatory properties, IFN are potentially well suited for use in the management of benign HPV-related anogenital diseases. Parenteral and intralesional therapy of condylomata with various natural and recombinant IFN preparations has consistently resulted in beneficial response rates ranging between 40% and 60%, often in patients in whom other therapeutic measures have repeatedly failed. Adverse effects from IFN are dose dependent and generally tolerable at concentrations of IFN found to be effective in the treatment of condylomata, and they are not associated with any known long-term sequelae [356]. Studies have shown that therapy of condylomata acuminata with IFN is effective. The route of administration does not appear to influence the results: the intralesional, intramuscular, and subcutaneous routes were effective. Additional research is required to determine whether the natural IFN or recombinant product is superior. The appropriate administration schedule may also not have been attained [357]. Topical 5-FU is indicated for therapy-resistant condylomas and for extensive untreated vulvar condylomas. It may be the treatment of choice for vaginal condylomas. Applications of 5-FU once weekly to the vagina and twice weekly to the vulva for 10 weeks appear to be as effective as continued regimens but are better tolerated.

Perhaps the greatest value of 5-FU lies in the periodic application for prevention of recurrences of condylomas removed by surgical methods [358].

Management of cervical preneoplasia starts with an abnormal smear result. The use of the Bethesda System is recommended. The management of patients with low-grade abnormal smear results varies around the world. Patients with ASC on cytology are recommended to be subclassified into ASC-US and ASC-H groups.

While patients with ASC-US can be followed with cytology or colposcopy, the risk of having CIN is higher in patients with ASC-H. Such patients, as well as those with L-SIL on cytology, should be referred for colposcopy to ensure that diagnosis and treatment in CIN is detected. Patients with H-SIL should be referred promptly for colposcopic assessment. This should, usually at the same clinic visit, be followed by LLETZ. Although this is effective treatment, around 15% of patients will have persistent/recurrent disease on cytological follow-up. Patients with positive HPV DNA tests at follow-up seem to have a considerably higher risk of recurrent preneoplasia than those who have negative tests. Patients over 50 years of age have much higher recurrence risks than younger patients. These factors impact on second-line treatment and follow-up schedules.

An important benefit of conservative treatment for CIN with LLETZ is retention of fertility. LLETZ is associated with an increased risk of preterm PROM and preterm birth, but not with other adverse pregnancy outcome measures. Conservative excisional management of adenocarcinoma in situ (AIS) by LLETZ or cold knife cone biopsy is not reported to be as effective as that of CIN, with high risk of residual and recurrent disease at follow-up. Conversely, LLETZ may be acceptable treatment for micro-invasive SCC if the excision margins are free of disease and there is no evidence of lymphovascular space involvement (LVSI).

The ability to detect and treat premalignant lesions on the cervix reversed the natural history of cervical cancer. Methods of conservative treatment that evolved over decades have been proven safe and effective, allowing retention of fertility. Good clinical guidelines have been developed for most clinical scenarios while some uncertainties persist for other scenarios [359].

Current evidence supports the use of colposcopy for the detection of intraepithelial lesions as a second line tool. CIN treatment involves either excisional or destructive techniques, usually performed under local anesthesia. Although a debate exists about the most efficient approach, the currently available evidence reveals no differences in efficacy among the available conservative methods of treatment.

New evidence supports treatment by destructive rather than excisional techniques, at least for low-grade lesions in women wishing future childbearing, as they appear to have no apparent pregnancy-related morbidity. Treatment failures rates might increase in cases of involved excision margins, older age, or glandular involvement. There is no worldwide consensus on the optimal follow-up policy, interventions or frequency in surveillance after treatment. HPV DNA test combined with either colposcopy or cytology is a promising combination for the early detection of treatment failures due to residual disease. Existing guidelines should probably be updated incorporating the new information emerged from recently published work [360]. Surgical approaches using lasers and electricity are available to treat the clinical diseases and in turn provide good cosmetic and functional anatomy. The surgical method employed depends upon the anatomical and histological distribution of disease regardless of its site. Of the three areas (cervix, vagina, and vulva), CIN is the least difficult to cure. VIN is the most difficult, since recurrences can occur at any time and in some patients for many years [361].

There is widespread misconception that the unique physical properties of the carbon dioxide (CO_2) laser essentially guarantee favorable results. In reality, the margin between excellence and mediocrity is very narrow. Unless sophisticated strategies are employed to restrict lateral heat conduction during photovaporization, the laser will produce the same kind of conduction burn as a hot cautery [362].

In view of the precision, high success rate, and low risk of complications, CO_2 laser surgery appears to offer the best option in patients with extensive condylomas and those whose disease proves resistant to simpler therapies [363]. Cervical cryotherapy offers the advantages of inexpensive outpatient therapy that is well tolerated without anesthesia. Previous series have focused on women beyond adolescence and have concluded that the risks and complications are rare. The risk of infectious complication in the adolescent population prompted a recommendation for aggressive preventive measures, including documentation of recent negative cultures for Neisseria gonorrhoeae and Chlamydia. The use of prophylactic antibiotics should be investigated for adolescents undergoing cervical cryotherapy [364].

The most effective treatments for cervical carcinoma to date are surgery in the form of LLETZ for pre-invasive disease, LLETZ or simple hysterectomy with laparoscopic pelvic lymphadenectomy for FIGO Stages IA1 and IA2 microinvasive carcinomas, and Wertheim's hysterectomy or celio-Schauta for FIGO Stage IB disease along with concurrent chemoradiotherapy in patents with at least FIGO Stage IB disease.

However, radical trachelectomy, which involves a radical excision of the cervix with simultaneous laparoscopic or extraperitoneal lymphadenectomy, may be used selectively in patients with up to FIGO Stage IB1 cancers, as this may preserve fertility in younger women [365]. For patients wishing to preserve fertility conization is regarded as an adequate treatment in cervical cancer stage IA1 without LVSI. Reviewing case series with IA1 cervical cancers without LVSI, lymph node metastasis (LNM) is present in 0.5%. Occurrence of LNM in IA1 cervical cancers is very rare, but if early diagnosed curative treatment is possible [366].

There is an emerging interest concerning the role HPV DNA testing in women with an initial diagnosis of CIN, who receive conservative surgical treatment, and are followed with HPV DNA testing in addition to cytology, colposcopy, and/or biopsy. There is a marked heterogeneity in the design, population, intervention, and follow-up policy across different studies. The sensitivity of HPV DNA testing in detecting treatment failures was quite good in most studies, reaching 100% in four of them, whereas the specificity of the test differed across the studies, ranging from 44% to 95%. Among women in whom the treatment was considered to be successful, 84.2% had a negative postoperative HPV DNA test and 15.8% a positive one. The corresponding rates for cases with treatment failures were 17.2% and 82.8%, respectively. It seems that a positive HPV test, even in the presence of normal cytology, may pick up early and accurately a treatment failure. Cytology and colposcopy may still be needed in order to rule out false positive and false negative results. A systematic review of studies concerning HPV DNA testing in the follow-up period after conservative treatment for CIN indicates that a positive HPV test, even in the presence of normal cytology, may pick up early and accurately a treatment failure. Cytology and colposcopy may still be needed in order to rule out false positive and false negative results [367]. Recurrences of CIN as well as invasive cervical carcinoma have been reported to arise following ablative or excisional treatment for CIN. Cervical cytology, colposcopy, endocervical curettage, and HPV typing have been advocated for use as tools for follow-up. Involvement of the surgical margins and the presence of HPV-DNA are associated with higher risks of recurrence and should be taken into consideration. The psychological impact of undergoing colposcopy may affect compliance with follow-up visits and should be dealt with appropriately [368]. However, protracted attendance for cytological follow-up decreases with time and might put some women at risk of developing invasive disease. The analysis revealed that compliance with follow-up declines over time and reaches significance at the end of 24 months of surveillance.

Cytological surveillance puts women at risk as many show poor compliance and such women might have occult high grade abnormalities [369]. The prevention of morbidity and mortality from cervical cancer will hinge upon our understanding of the epidemiology, the molecular basis, and natural history of the disease and its associated precursors [370]. Clinicians should not only understand how to treat HPV-related diseases but offer strategies to prevent them. This understanding encompasses patient education and counseling regarding modifiable lifestyle factors and patient participation in organized secondary screening programs. Finally, for the first time in history, patients may be offered safe and effective vaccines that promise to have a dramatic impact on these conditions [371]. Following identification of the HPV as the infectious etiological agent and elucidation of the long natural history of cervical neoplasia, cervical cancer is now one of the most preventable of all cancers.

Qualitative work on attitudes towards cervical cancer prevention, education needs, the creation of an environment for informed choice and uptake are essential aspects of effective prevention programs. Cervical cancer poses a huge health burden in Africa. It is a disease that is eminently preventable given political will, the availability of affordable vaccines, appropriate cervical screening, and access to cheap, point-of-care HPV testing. There are a number of unanswered questions for the prevention of cervical cancer and a need for demonstration projects to address these and further develop prevention strategies [372, 373].

The interaction of HPV with the immune system has been studied, but the results are still inconclusive for several reasons. Until now, we have not been able to understand the mechanisms of immune system regulation in the uterine cervix. HPV infection does not unleash an inflammatory response, and consequently an efficient and specific immune response against the virus. Moreover, an understanding of HPV infection and local immune response is indispensable for the development of new bioactive drugs and therapies for patients with both non invasive and invasive tumors, mainly for patients that do not present regression with radiotherapy or chemotherapy or in whom the tumors are surgically unresectable [374]. Oncogenic HPV types infecting the anogenital tract have the potential to induce natural immunity, but at present we do not clearly understand the natural history of infection in humans and the mechanisms by which the virus can evade the host immune response. Natural acquired immune responses against HPV may be involved in the clearance of infection, but persistent infection with oncogenic virus types leads to the development of precancerous lesions and cancer.

B cell responses are important for viral neutralization, but antibody responses in patients with cervical cancer are poor [375]. The available data on whether natural HPV infection infers cross protection against other related strains from the same species are equivocal. There are data to indicate that following HPV infection, there appears to be a reduced risk of contracting the same strain of HPV. However, there is also evidence to indicate that natural infection with HPV does not confer group-specific immune protection or general protection from reinfection with genital HPV mucosal types [256]. Recombinant HPV major capsid proteins, which self-assemble into VLP, are produced in quantity, mimic the conformation of native virions, react with neutralizing antibodies, and are type-specific. HPV early viral peptides induce CTL responses that retard tumor progression and protect against tumor development after challenge in animal models. Recombinant HPV VLP are highly antigenic, protective in animal models, lack potentially carcinogenic viral DNA, and are, therefore, ideal components for a prophylactic vaccine against HPV infection. Immunization with HPV tumor peptides may be beneficial in tumor prevention, regression, and rejection. Vaccines against HPV infection can be important in reducing the incidence of cervical dysplasia and carcinoma worldwide, particularly in developing countries [376]. Crucial for these vaccination protocols to be successful is that they will result in a long-lasting ability to generate an immune response that will eliminate the virus. HPV transmission and subsequent infection is a local event in the lower female genital tract and therefore the efficacy of vaccines against this locally transmitted infection can be best assessed by parameters of local immunity [377]. Interplay between host immune system and expression of HPV early and late genes during infection has a central role in the surveillance of virus-induced neoplastic cervical lesions. Recently, new features of this interplay have been discovered. However, not enough is yet known of the relative roles of different E and L proteins, human lymphocyte antigens and specific co-factors in the natural history of these lesions in order to guarantee efficacy of preventive HPV vaccination [378]. Prophylactic strategies focus on the induction of effective humoral and cellular immune responses that are potentially protective against subsequent HPV infection. VLP have been synthesized to induce neutralizing antibody responses, and impressive immunoprophylactic effects have been demonstrated in both animals and humans. It is hoped that the development of successful HPV-specific vaccines will diminish the costs of existing cervical cancer screening programs and reduce the morbidity and mortality associated with the treatment of cervical neoplasias [379].

HPV vaccines results in clinical trials have been promising, but due to assortative transmission of the infection and multiple HPV types the effect of large-scale immunization on their spread will vary between different populations and by HPV type. Thus, it is difficult to predict the effect of vaccination on cancer incidence on the basis of efficacy trials only [380]. At present, several vaccines have been developed and tested in clinical trials. The vaccines are generally well tolerated and highly immunogenic. The current clinical data indicate that prophylactic vaccines are very effective against new persistent infections and the development of CIN. The protection is type specific. However, the follow-up of the vaccination trials is still short. The effect of HPV vaccines on future cancer incidence will only be known after decades of follow-up [381]. HPV vaccines are created from noninfectious VLP of the major capsid protein, L1, which closely mimic natural HPV virions. Proof-of-principle trials of monovalent vaccines that protect against high-risk HPV types such as HPV 16 or 18 have confirmed that intramuscular injection with VLP induces the production of HPV type-specific neutralizing antibodies. A bivalent vaccine incorporating oncogenic HPV types 16 and 18 was shown to be safe, well tolerated, and 100% efficacious in preventing persistent HPV infection. A quadrivalent vaccine that protects against genital wart-causing HPV types (HPV 6 and 11) and oncogenic HPV types (HPV 16 and 18) demonstrated 100% efficacy in preventing clinical disease. Because VLP vaccines are prophylactic, vaccination before exposure to HPV will result in the greatest public health benefit. Therefore, a successful vaccination program should target preadolescents and stress the importance of vaccination before sexual debut [382]. The first prophylactic HPV VLP vaccine against HPV types 6/11/16/18 (Gardasil, Merck and Co., Whitehouse Station, NJ) was licensed in 2006. The second prophylactic HPV vaccine (Cervarix, GlaxoSmithKline, Brentford, United Kingdom [UK]) is a recombinant cervical cancer vaccine which has been licensed in 2008. This vaccine is an AS04 adjuvanted bivalent L1 VLP vaccine against HPV types 16 and 18, which together account for approximately 70% of cervical cancers worldwide. An interim analysis of a large, multicenter, phase III trial being conducted by the Papilloma Trial against Cancer In young Adults (PATRICIA) Study Group to assess the efficacy of this vaccine was recently published. These vaccines are almost 100% effective in preventing infection and high-grade precancer associated with the HPV types included in the vaccine. The vaccines are well tolerated, safe, and highly immunogenic when given in three doses within 6 months. Efficacy of the vaccine against external vulvar and HPV-related vaginal lesions is also high.

Even though the vaccine is highly effective against high-grade cervical, vaginal, or vulvar precancers, this only applies to women unexposed to these HPV types and only to high-grade intraepithelial lesions caused by these HPV types. Therefore, it is important to understand that the population impact of the vaccines will be much lower than vaccinating naive populations.

Implementing HPV vaccine is a great opportunity but also a great challenge. However, mandatory HPV vaccination may raise many questions, and more answers are needed [383, 384]. Only the quadrivalent vaccine is designed to prevent condylomata acuminata and low-grade CIN caused by HPV 6 and HPV 11. It has been approved by the FDA for women aged 9 to 26 years against vulvar and vaginal cancer, and against cervical cancer and precancer. The adjuvant of the bivalent vaccine more significantly accelerates an immune reaction. Both vaccines demonstrate cross-protection, although against different HPV types. The bivalent vaccine is registered for above age 26 in Australia and Israel, and the quadrivalent vaccine in the Philippines and Ecuador. Time will verify claims and reveal differences. In the meantime, both vaccines are safe and effective for their approved indications and recommendations should be based on individual patient characteristics [385]. The yearly costs for treating precursors of these cancers exceed the cost of vaccinating all girls born in a given year. Thus, HPV vaccination is cost effective, even when a modified cancer screening program is retained [386]. The implementation of the HPV vaccine is a tremendous milestone in our effort toward preventing cervical cancers. However, screening programs will continue to serve as a critical component in prevention due to the limitations of the current vaccines.

The greatest impact in cervical cancer incidence worldwide requires improved health care access to underserved areas. Advances are needed to develop single-dose, heat-stable, needle-free, and affordable formulations of the HPV vaccine to overcome the socioeconomic barriers associated with this disease [387]. Eventual implementation of an HPV vaccination program raises several key issues, including universal vs. targeted vaccinations, the age and gender of vaccine recipients, the acceptability of this vaccine to HCW, adolescents, and parents, and the effect of this vaccine on cervical cancer screening. Preventative HPV vaccination programs should ideally be executed universally in both women and men with an emphasis on children and adolescents prior to their first sexual experience. Parent education on HPV disease and vaccine efficacy and safety will be critical to the acceptability of HPV vaccination for their children. HPV vaccination will not eliminate the need for Pap screening.

Further research will be needed to develop rational and cost-effective cervical surveillance programs for women protected by HPV vaccines [388]. Achieving long-term protection following vaccination is crucial to ensuring that high levels of immunity are maintained within a population while eliminating the need to introduce booster vaccinations. Based on an analysis of the HBV vaccine, several factors have been shown to contribute to long-term protection, namely: specific lymphoproliferation, the in vivo humoral response, and immune memory.

To ensure protection against persistent HPV infection and the subsequent development of cervical lesions, an effective HPV vaccine must be able to induce strong humoral immune responses. Mathematical modeling analyses based on a three-dose regimen of HPV type 16 prophylactic vaccine indicated that 99% of 16- to 23-year-old women would have almost life-long detectable anti-HPV-16 levels. Available data on the quadrivalent HPV vaccine demonstrated that long-term immune memory was induced, with anti-HPV geometric mean titers after 5 years remaining at or above those observed with natural infection. Vaccination also resulted in a substantial reduction in the combined incidence of HPV-6/11/16/18 related persistent infection or disease, and there were no cases of precancerous cervical dysplasia compared with six cases in women receiving placebo.

Similarly, the bivalent HPV vaccine has been shown to induce long-term immunity with >98% seropositivity maintained after 4.5 years of follow-up and geometric mean titres at this time point remaining substantially higher than those noted with naturally acquired infection. Countrywide registration regarding population and health events in a stable population of approximately 25 million makes the Nordic countries an ideal setting for the evaluation of long-term cervical cancer control. Population-based long-term efficacy trials conducted in these countries aim to investigate the long-term efficacy of HPV vaccination with regard to invasive cervical cancer [389]. Recent studies conducted with HPV vaccines show data on cross-protection against related HPV strains.

In vitro experiments with serum from recipients of the quadrivalent HPV vaccine (HPV-6/8/16/18) show neutralization of HPV 45 pseudovirions. Cross-protection following vaccination of women with three doses of bivalent HPV vaccine (HPV-16/18) demonstrated that, over a period of up to 4.5 years, long-term vaccine efficacy was observed for HPV-16 and -18, and vaccine efficacy was also observed against incident infection with HPV-31 and -45. These findings are supported by the results of a large study in women aged 15 to 25 years vaccinated with the adjuvant bivalent HPV vaccine (HPV-16/18).

Over a period of 6 months, cross-protection was observed against persistent infections with HPV-45, -31, and -52, and at 12 months, modest protection was demonstrated against persistent infections with 12 combined oncogenic HPV types [256]. Prior to licensure the vaccines were trialed in over 60,000 women and assessed as safe, within the statistical constraints of the trials to detect very rare events. Post-licensure surveillance is underway as vaccination programs are undertaken. International advisory bodies state that both HPV vaccines are safe, effective, and of great importance for women's health. Ongoing monitoring is required to maintain confidence in the safety of the vaccines [390]. In the recent period following the approval of the first vaccine targeted against HPV, it is imperative that we re-evaluate the past, present, and future of cervical cancer prevention. It is clear that the subject of vaccinating young women against a STI has incited a candid debate among all groups involved. Therefore, we must make the most appropriate and accurate information available to the public and medical communities. The development of vaccines targeted against oncogenic HPV types has made it possible to eliminate approximately 70% of all invasive cervical cancers in women worldwide. However, knowledge about HPV infection and cervical cancer, as well as the need to vaccinate against oncogenic HPV infection, is still lacking among women and physicians. This deficiency could be a key reason why some parents continue to have reservations about vaccinating their daughters. In order for HPV vaccination programs to be highly successful, multiple barriers must be overcome. Review of lessons learned to date has demonstrated that continued tailored and targeted educational and awareness initiatives are required for healthcare professionals, media, patients, and parents [391]. HPV vaccination of pre-pubescent girls will be effective for many girls. Vaccinating girls and women older than 12 years of age may accelerate the reduction in cervical cancer rates. Currently, HPV vaccines are effective for at least 5 years in the prevention of HPV 16 and 18 associated precancerous lesions, however, the duration of vaccine protection is unknown. The need for booster shots must therefore be addressed with patients as unknown. Continued cervical cancer screening is necessary regardless of vaccination. Vaccination alone will not eliminate cervical cancer [392].

Organized cervical screening programs have reduced the incidence and mortality of cervical cancer. However, in developing countries scarce resources, poverty, lack of infrastructure and disenfranchisement of women have been major hurdles in the effective implementation of routine screening programmes. As a result, 83% of cervical cancers still occur in the developing countries and account for 15% of all female cancers [393].

Primary HPV prevention may be the key to reducing incidence and burden of cervical cancer particularly in resource-poor countries. Vaccination programmes are already established in several developed regions, but several grey areas stand in the path of similar success in developing countries. The potential benefit of mass HPV vaccination appears enormous. However, the challenges of competing health demands, poverty, ignorance, religion, culture, weak health system, establishment of an effective intersectoral collaboration, and underfunding must be overcome to make maximal vaccine uptake a reality. Education and effective communication is crucial in achieving successful immunization programmes [394].

Limited sensitivity and unequal access to screening have resulted in an imbalance in distribution of the burden of cervical cancer between developed and developing countries, between metropolitan and rural areas in developed countries, and among women from different ethnic groups. In screened populations, there is a relative increase in incidence of cervical cancer in young and elderly women, and an increased proportion of adenocarcinoma. A high coverage of the target population has been achieved in HPV vaccination programs in many countries. After 3 years of mass vaccination of adolescent girls, surveillance data in Australia confirmed a significant reduction in high-grade abnormalities for girls aged 18 years and below. HPV vaccination is more feasible than cytology screening for universal implementation across geographic sectors and demographic groups within individual countries and over the world. The high vaccine efficacy should significantly reduce the total burden and unequal distribution of invasive cervical cancer, including adenocarcinoma hitherto observed. These epidemiological changes provoke consideration for appropriate modifications of the current screening program [395, 396].

Whilst prophylactic vaccination has proven very effective in terms of preventing cervical cancer precursor lesions, therapeutic strategies have presented far greater challenges [397].

Several lines of evidence suggest that cell-mediated immune responses are important in controlling both HPV infections and HPV-associated neoplasia. Since HPV E6 and E7 oncoproteins are expressed in these lesions and are necessary for the maintenance of the malignant phenotype, these proteins might be potential tumor-specific target antigens for immunotherapy of cervical cancer. The gold standard treatment for locally advanced cervical cancer is primary radiation therapy combined with chemotherapy. A potential drawback of this potentially curative treatment is a profound and long lasting negative effect on the immune system.

Treatment-induced immunosuppression combined with tumor-induced subversion of the immune system may therefore impose severe limitations on the efficacy of conventional vaccination strategies in late stage cervical cancer patients. The recognition of dendritic cells (DC) as powerful antigen-presenting cells capable of inducing primary T cell responses in vitro and in vivo, has recently generated widespread interest in DC-based immunotherapy of several human malignancies.

Various therapeutic HPV vaccines are being developed and implemented in human clinical trials, in particular the use of autologous DC pulsed with full-length HPV 16 or 18 E7 oncoproteins as a novel strategy to induce HPV E7-specific and tumor-specific T cell responses in cervical cancer patients following conventional treatment [398,399]. To treat and eradicate pre-existing HPV infections and associated lesions which remain prevalent worldwide, effective therapeutic HPV vaccines are needed. DNA vaccination has emerged as a particularly promising form of therapeutic HPV vaccines due to its safety, stability, and ability to induce antigen-specific immunity.

Improving the potency of therapeutic HPV vaccines can be reached through modification of DC by:

1) increasing the number of antigen-expressing/antigen-loaded DC;
2) improving HPV antigen expression, processing, and presentation in DC; and
3) enhancing DC and T cell interaction.

Continued improvement in therapeutic HPV DNA vaccines may ultimately lead to an effective DNA vaccine for the treatment of HPV-associated malignancies [400].

Therefore, immunotherapy has been proposed as a potential treatment to be used in conjunction with surgery, or independently, as treatment for CIN. Currently, immunotherapy includes the application of recombinant viral proteins, vaccines, or antibody- and DC-based therapies [401].

Unfortunately these, in principal successful, therapeutic approaches also fail to induce clinical responses in a substantial number of cases. The potential mechanisms involved in the escape of HPV-induced lesions from the immune system indicate gaps in our knowledge. There are a number of pre-existing conditions that determine the patients' responsiveness to immunotherapy. An immunotherapeutic strategy in which different aspects of immune failure are attacked by complementary approaches, will improve the clinical response rate [402-424].

Hepatitis Viruses

Currently, six distinct types of Hepatitis Virus have been identified: A, B, C, D, E, and G. HAV infection does not cause a chronic carrier state, and perinatal transmission is extremely uncommon. Hepatitis B can be transmitted perinatally, but immunization of the newborn with hepatitis B Ig and hepatitis B vaccine markedly reduces the risk of neonatal infection (Figure 3). Hepatitis D Virus (HDV) is dependent on coinfection with the HBV for replication. Immunoprophylaxis against hepatitis B also is effective against hepatitis D. HCV is primarily transmitted by the parenteral route and is particularly likely to cause chronic liver disease. Perinatal transmission of hepatitis C principally occurs in women who have high titers of HCV-RNA or who are coinfected with HIV. At this time, no immunoprophylaxis for hepatitis C is available. Hepatitis G Virus (HGV), a recently described organism, is related to hepatitis

C. Its clinical significance remains undetermined. Hepatitis E Virus (HEV) is transmitted in a manner similar to hepatitis A.

Perinatal transmission is unusual, but maternal disease is often severe [425]. Pregnancy associated with chronic hepatitis B is a common and important problem with unique challenges. Pregnant women with chronic hepatitis B are different from the general population, and their special problems need to be considered, such as the effect of HBV infection on the mother and fetus, the effect of pregnancy on replication of the HBV, whether mothers should take HBV antiviral therapy during pregnancy, the effect of these treatments on the mother and fetus, how to carry out immunization of neonates, whether it can induce hepatitis activity after delivery, and other serious issues.

At present, there are about 350 million individuals with HBV infection worldwide, of which 50% were infected during the perinatal or neonatal period, especially in HBV-endemic countries. Currently, the rate of HBV infection in the child-bearing age group is still at a high level, and the infection rate is as high as 8.16%. Effective prevention of MTCT is an important means of reducing the global burden of chronic HBV infection. Even after adopting the combined immunization measures, there are still 5-10% of babies born with HBV infection in HBeAg positive pregnant women. As HBV perinatal transmission is the main cause of chronic HBV infection, we must consider how to prevent this transmission to reduce the burden of HBV infection. In this population of chronic HBV infected women of childbearing age, specific detection, intervention, and follow-up measures are particularly worthy of attention and discussion [426].

Although it is the most common cause of jaundice during pregnancy, viral hepatitis does not generally increase the risk of pregnancy complications, nor is it teratogenic. Vertical transmission of some types of viral hepatitis does occur, however [427]. Breastfeeding after proper immunoprophylaxis does not contribute to MTCT transmission of HBV [428].

Although liver dysfunction is infrequently seen in pregnancy, it can result in severe maternal and fetal compromise. An unrecognized case of acute fatty liver may result in both maternal and fetal death. Failure to screen for hepatitis B can result in a newborn who will be a hepatitis carrier for life. Because of such consequences, the obstetrician must remain vigilant for signs of liver dysfunction and must understand the pathophysiology of these disorders [429]. Surgeons engaged in the practice of obstetrics and gynecology should have a clear understanding of the hepatitis B surface antigen (HBsAg, once called "Australia antigen") serologic test.

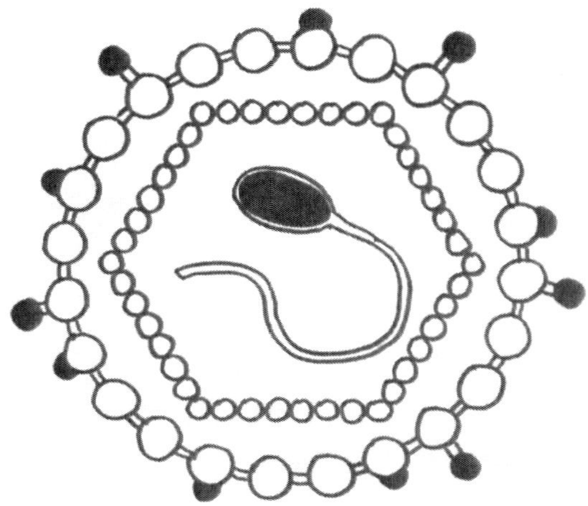

Modified from hepatitis-b-am-besten-testen-de.

Figure 3. Hepatitis B Virus (HBV).

When positive, it serves as a marker either for the carrier state or for subclinical to overt hepatitis B (once called "serum hepatitis"). Patients or health personnel with a positive test are potentially infectious and appropriate precautions should be taken. Surgeons are at increased risk for hepatitis B and, when acutely exposed and not vaccinated, should receive standard serum Ig, or perhaps high-titer hepatitis B Ig.

Infants born to mothers with a positive test may become HBsAg positive and develop chronic hepatitis [430]. Thus, routine serologic testing of all pregnant women is necessary to identify those HBSAg-positive women capable of transmitting the HBV to their infants.

All the other obstetric surveys support the need to screen obstetric patients and to provide immunoprophylaxis or vaccination to the infants at risk of perinatal infection. This policy is necessary to prevent perinatal transmission of HBV and is cost-effective [431]. Measurement of serum alphafetoprotein (AFP) might be a useful additional index of infectivity and prognosis in HBsAg-positive subjects and in the light of the association between chronic HBV infection, hepatocellular carcinoma, and raised AFP in non-European populations, consideration should be given to regular monitoring of AFP levels in HBsAg-positive subjects [432]. Infant hepatitis B infection increases risk of chronic infection, cirrhosis, or liver cancer (hepatocellular carcinoma) in adult. Perinatal transmission is a common route of infection. No RCT that assessed the effects of hepatitis B vaccine during pregnancy for preventing infant infection have been found. However, the need for well-designed RCT for the effect of hepatitis B vaccine during pregnancy on the incidence of infant infection and adverse effects has been identified [433]. Current pediatric vaccination schedules in the US are based on age. In contrast, adults are vaccinated against most infectious diseases, including hepatitis A and B, only when they are identified as at high risk or after a known exposure. There are multiple risk factors for hepatitis A and B of which clinicians often are not aware.

Consequently, many persons at high risk are never vaccinated. Universal vaccination against hepatitis A and B is recommended for adults to halt transmission of the virus and prevent long-term sequelae. Women and their offspring are an especially important population to consider in efforts to reduce the incidence of hepatitis. The following recommendations for expanding the use of hepatitis vaccines in obstetrics and gynecology are made: all older adolescents and adults should be vaccinated regardless of risk factors, and greater efforts should be made to educate physicians about the need to vaccinate their patients against hepatitis [434].

Hepatitis C is the most common chronic bloodborne infection in the US (Figure 4). Chronic infection with HCV is a major cause of liver disease-related death and is also the most frequent indication for liver transplantation in US. Infected individuals can remain asymptomatic for 20 years or more, but they remain at risk for progressive liver disease. They also represent a potential source of infection for others.

For reducing the future disease burden due to HCV, obstetrician/gynecologists and primary HCW should be aware of the factors that promote HCV transmission, how to provide counseling and testing, and when specialist referral is needed [435]. Because of the risk of perinatal transmission and possible sexual transmission, it is important for obstetrician-gynecologists to keep abreast of the rapidly expanding literature on hepatitis C. Acute hepatitis C represents about 5% of all reported cases of hepatitis. Approximately 50% of acute infections progress to chronic liver disease. Risk factors for infection include intravenous drug use (21-42% of cases), previous blood transfusion (6-17%), and multiple sexual partners (6%), while 40-50% of cases have no

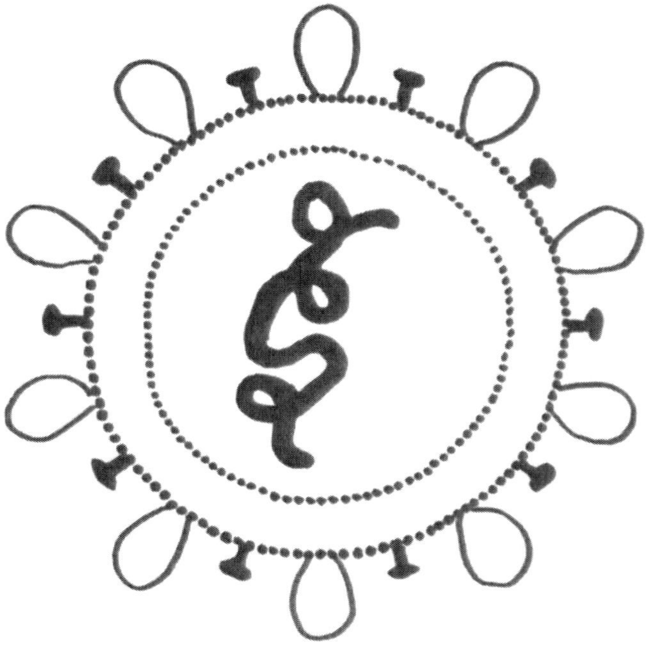

Modified from springerimages.com.

Figure 4. Hepatitis C Virus (HCV).

identified risk factors. The seroprevalence of anti-hepatitis C antibody is 70.8% in intravenous drug users, 11.6% in patients with HIV, 8.8% in prostitutes, 1.2% in hospital personnel, and 0.5-1.4% in volunteer blood donors. The risk of transmission to the neonate depends on the trimester at exposure. No perinatal transmission has been shown after acute maternal infection in the second trimester. Based on the few reported cases, chronic maternal infection or acute infection in the third trimester may result in neonatal infection rates of 45-87.5%.

Universal screening is probably not cost-effective because the prevalence is low and over 70% of screening tests can be falsely positive using the currently approved assay. Selective screening of high-risk patients is recommended [436]. In epidemiologic studies done primarily in Europe and in the US, antibody to hepatitis C has been present in approximately 1% to 4% of pregnant women. Although close to 50% of infected women have no known risk factors for infection, routine screening of pregnant women is not currently recommended. HCV may be transmitted to the newborn at a rate of approximately 5%: it is not clear whether this occurs in utero, intrapartum, or both [437]. Factors positively associated with maternal seropositivity include maternal age (between 25 to 29 years), prior history of delivering a stillborn infant, and seropositivity for syphilis during the index pregnancy [438]. The diagnosis of vertical transmission is reliably established by a positive serum HCV RNA on two occasions 3 to 4 months apart after the infant is at least 2 months old and/or by the detection of anti-HCV antibodies after the infant is 18 months old. Vertical transmission in HCV RNA-negative pregnant women is approximately 1% to 3% versus approximately 4% to 6% in HCV RNA-positive women. From the standpoint of vertical transmission, no critical HCV RNA titer has been established.

A high maternal HCV viral load and coinfection with HIV has been shown to increase the risk of vertical transmission of HCV, but HAART may decrease the risk significantly. In HIV-negative women, route of delivery does not influence vertical transmission and there is no evidence that a CS prevents transmission. In HCV/HIV-coinfected women, decisions regarding mode of delivery should be based on HIV status. There is no association between vertical transmission of HCV and gestational age at delivery or the presence of chorioamnionitis. The use of a scalp electrode has been associated with vertical transmission and this practice is discouraged. Data are conflicting regarding duration of ruptured membranes and the risk of vertical transmission of hepatitis C. When the duration of membrane rupture exceeds 6 hours, the risk may be increased. There is no evidence demonstrating an increased risk of HCV transmission in HIV-negative women who breast feed. In HCV/HIV-coinfected women, breastfeeding is discouraged in women who have consistent access to safe infant formula [439]. Given the relatively low seroprevalence of HCV and the fact that risk factors for HCV infection remain largely unknown, more studies are needed to identify high-risk populations likely to benefit from HCV screening and treatment programmes. There is currently no treatment for HCV infection that is approved for use in pregnancy or for use in the neonate.

IFN-alpha is used for the treatment of myeloproliferative diseases and chronic viral illnesses. Because the agent has antiproliferative activity, its effects on a fetus are a concern. An inadvertent administration of IFN-alpha during pregnancy may occur, but in that case IFN-alpha may not induce congenital malformations. These findings may encourage such women to continue pregnancy [440, 441].

HUMAN HERPESVIRUSES

The HHV infections (HSV, VZV, Epstein-Barr Virus [EBV], and CMV) create many dilemmas when encountered during pregnancy [442]. Viruses of the HHV family can have profound effects on pregnancy. Primary maternal infection with CMV and varicella during pregnancy has been associated with fetal abnormalities and neonatal disease. Public awareness of the role of CMV in the etiology of developmental disorders and chronic disabilities needs to increase. With time, we may see new interventions for treatment of infected pregnant women and prevention of long-term effects. Attention must be focused on development of a safe and effective vaccine. With the introduction of an efficacious varicella vaccine, the rate of varicella in pregnancy is expected to decrease dramatically. Physicians caring for women have the opportunity to prevent the complications of varicella by identifying and vaccinating susceptible women [443].

HSV infection is prevalent worldwide (Figure 5). Herpes labialis, caused predominantly by HSV-1, and herpes vulvovaginitis, caused predominantly by HSV-2, may result in significant morbidity and mortality for infected neonates exposed during delivery.

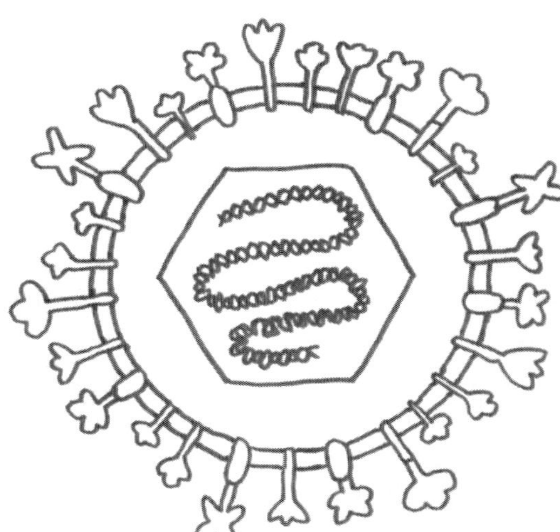

Modified from bio.davidson.edu.

Figure 5. Herpes Simplex Virus (HSV).

The diagnosis of HSV infection is made by serological testing, viral culture, or PCR. Women with primary herpes vulvovaginitis exhibit a painful vesicular rash which is self-limited but may be followed by multiple recurrences. Women at greatest risk to transmit HSV to their neonates are those who experience their first episode of HSV during the latter stage of pregnancy. If infected, their neonates may have localized skin, eye, and mucosal lesions, invasive CNS infection, or disseminated disease. Because of the potentially devastating outcome for a baby infected with HSV, pregnant women with active HSV lesions at delivery should be offered a CS. Still, many neonates who are infected with HSV are born to women with asymptomatic HSV shedding. Therefore, prevention of HSV during pregnancy is exceedingly important [444].

In contrast to the frequent occurrence of localized HSV infections during pregnancy, disseminated disease has rarely been reported. In the third trimester of pregnancy, HSV can occasionally disseminate in immunocompetent women. A clinical syndrome of unexplained fever, pneumonia, anicteric hepatitis, leukopenia, and disseminated intravascular coagulation (DIC) without mucocutaneous lesions should prompt investigation and possible treatment for disseminated HSV infection [445]. Disseminated HSV infection during pregnancy is a life-threatening condition that has a typical presentation, which includes a nonspecific viral prodrome. During pregnancy, fever and anicteric hepatitis unresponsive to empiric antibiotics should prompt an evaluation for disseminated HSV infection.

Pharyngitis or skin lesions with a positive HSV culture are common, specific signs associated with dissemination [446]. Fulminant hepatic dysfunction in the third trimester of pregnancy accompanied by fever may result from disseminated HSV. Mucocutaneous lesions are present in only half of cases, therefore, suspicion for diagnosis of this disease is low. Twenty-five percent of cases are not diagnosed until autopsy. Maternal and perinatal mortality are high, approaching 39% for both mother and fetus [447].

Hepatitis is a rare but serious complication of a HSV infection. Pregnancy is a risk factor and has been associated with a high maternal and fetal mortality rate. Early recognition with initiation of antiviral therapy appears to be most important in maximizing survival [448]. Using three criteria:

1) herpetic infection and altered organogenesis of inflammatory etiology that antedates dissolution of the fetal membranes;
2) documented herpetic infection present at birth and within 24 hours of rupture of the fetal membranes; and

3) evidence of viral herpetic placentitis the induction of which antedates rupture of the membranes, cases of congenital transplacental HSV infection have been identified.

Disease occurring early in gestation produces a cluster of congenital malformations that is clinically indistinguishable from that produced by the CMV. Disease manifesting after the shortest recognized incubation period for the induction of the disease in experimental animals does not necessarily preclude transplacental acquisition. Various factors mask the perception of congenital transplacental HSV infection as a valid disease entity [449]. Genital herpes is feared in particular during birth, when the virus can infect the baby during its passage through the birth canal, and lead to the death of the neonate or lasting severe morbidity. Neonatal HSV infection can have severe consequences. Skin, eye, and mouth infection is rarely fatal, but disseminated or CNS disease has a mortality rate of 80% in the absence of therapy, and most surviving infants have neurological sequelae, such as CP and developmental delay. Much more frequent, however, is recurrent herpes genitalis that can occur up into old age, and which is usually nothing worse than a nuisance. Owing to the wide spectrum of possible symptoms and their intensity, it is not infrequently recognized either very late in its evolution, or not at all. Varicella in pregnancy is also particularly feared, since it can (rarely) lead to congenital damage or, in the case of maternal peripartal varicella, to severe infection in the neonate [450]. Both HSV type 1 and HSV type 2 can cause genital herpes. Because the infection is chronic, genital herpes has become the most common STD among women. The prevalence of the HSV-2 antibody among women in the US is 26%, although genital herpes has been diagnosed in only a small proportion (10-25%) of individuals with HSV-2 antibodies. HSV type 1 is becoming a more frequent cause of genital herpes, especially among young women. Overall, HSV-1 seroprevalence in the US is estimated at 67%, although serologic data do not provide information about site of infection.

Therefore, the use of condoms is recommended to lessen the likelihood of disease transmission. Recent advances in diagnostic methods and therapeutic options are likely to change the management of genital herpes [451]. The appropriate obstetric management of women with a history of genital herpes remains controversial. Past management protocols have stressed frequent third trimester viral cultures in an attempt to identify those at risk for asymptomatic viral shedding at delivery. CS was recommended if asymptomatic shedding was suspected. Subsequent research has shown that surveillance schema aimed at identifying asymptomatic shedding in term gestations will fail to identify antepartum the majority of cases of neonatal herpes. Furthermore, weekly surveillance cultures have failed to predict intrapartum viral shedding accurately. The current literature supports mode of delivery decisions based on clinical history and careful intrapartum examination. The development of rapid diagnostic tests for intrapartum diagnoses of viral shedding as well as the prophylactic use of antiviral agents have influenced the recommendations [452]. Recent guidelines suggest a rationale for the management of women at risk for genital HSV. Nevertheless, as the newer immunologic and serologic techniques became clinically reliable and allowed a correct and rapid diagnosis of HSV infection, identification of the infected woman in labor must be made using detailed clinical history, physical examination, and viral culture [453]. Decision analysis techniques have been used to compare three strategies for antepartum screening for HSV in women with no history of infection:

1) universal screening;
2) targeted screening in women estimated to be at high risk for infection; and
3) current care (no screening).

For the screening strategies, screening has been considered at 35 weeks of gestation, with prophylactic antiviral therapy for seropositive women. For all women, CS has been assumed in the setting of symptomatic infection at delivery. Universal maternal screening reduced the total number of deaths and severe sequelae secondary to neonatal HSV. Universal screening required treatment of 3849 women to prevent one case of neonatal death or disease with severe sequelae from HSV. Targeted screening of high-risk women treatment of 2277 women to prevent one death or case of severe disease. Universal screening reduced the rate of neonatal HSV attributable to recurrent HSV by 79.3%. CS was reduced with both screening strategies. One-way sensitivity analyses have been used to evaluate the robustness of this model.

Maternal screening reduced the number of cases of neonatal HSV. Screening also reduced the rate of CS. However, employing universal screening will likely result in a significant expenditure of medical resources because the number needed to treat to avert a single case of neonatal herpes is high [454]. Although PCR can detect HSV in the cerebrospinal fluid (CSF), HSV encephalitis remains a significant cause of neurologic impairment in pregnant women. Assessment of fetal contamination also remains a problem. As soon as encephalitis in pregnancy is suspected, a combination of ACV and penicillin is recommended because the potential benefits far outweigh the risks. Using the HSV PCR, HSV infection in the fetus can be diagnosed [455]. Diagnosis of genital herpes relies on laboratory confirmation with culture or PCR assay of genital lesions and type-specific glycoprotein G-based serologic testing. Despite advances in the diagnosis and treatment of neonatal herpes, little change in the incidence or serious sequelae from this infection has occurred. As such, prevention of the initial neonatal infection is critically important. Obstetricians are in a unique position to prevent vertical HSV transmission by identifying women with genital lesions at the time of labor for CS, prescribing antiviral suppressive therapy as appropriate, and avoiding unnecessary invasive intrapartum procedures in women with genital herpes. Enhanced prevention strategies include identification of women at risk for HSV acquisition during pregnancy by testing women and possibly their partners for HSV antibodies and providing counseling to prevent transmission to women in late pregnancy [456]. All HCW who manage patients with genital herpes need to know the limitations of serologic testing. Current information suggests that serologic commercial testing that is most commonly available cannot discriminate between infections caused by HSV type 1 and type 2. Laboratory methods still rely on culturing HSV in living cells in vitro. However, the availability of monoclonal antibodies allows for rapid assays for the confirmation of cultured HSV. In addition, assays have been developed and tested, suggesting that perhaps antigen-detection systems may be available that could replace culturing the virus in living cells. New information on neonatal herpes points out the predictors of morbidity and mortality in newborns who contract herpes within the first few weeks of life. Information concerning asymptomatic shedding in labor will provide the clinician with a better understanding of this disease entity in the pregnant woman. Several studies have confirmed that HSV infection is a risk factor for developing HIV infection. A new study clearly shows that treatment using daily ACV therapy over a prolonged period of time can control and may modify HHV infection [457].

Numerous and varied antiviral compounds have been approved by the FDA to treat genital HSV infections. The treatment of these conditions has been advanced over the past three decades by the introduction of guanosine nucleoside antivirals such as ACV (Zovirax, Glaxo Wellcome, London, UK), valacyclovir (Valtrex, Glaxo Wellcome, London, UK), the highly bioavailable prodrug of the antivirals, and famciclovir (Famvir, SmithKline Beecham, Brentford, UK). They all have the same mechanism of action. ACV, valacyclovir, and famciclovir have been approved for the treatment of primary and recurrent disease. All three agents can be used for daily administration for the suppression of recurrent disease. Appropriate use of these antiviral compounds in the nonpregnant and pregnant woman can significantly alter the disease and influence transmission rates to sexual partners and the newborn along with decreasing the morbidity and mortality associated with HSV infections [48, 49]. Suppressive treatment is suggested for patients who have:

1) at least 6 recurrences per year;
2) significant complications, but fewer than 6 recurrences per year;
3) their quality of life significantly affected;
4) social and sexual dysfunction; and
5) to lower the risk of transmission to a sexual partner or fetus/neonate [458].

The data demonstrate that valacyclovir is more effective than placebo and as effective as other antivirals in the episodic and suppressive treatment of recurrent genital herpes. Valacyclovir is the only antiviral shown to be effective with a short (3-day) course in the episodic treatment of recurrent genital herpes, as well as with once-daily dosing for daily suppressive therapy. In VZV infection, valacyclovir is as effective as famciclovir and more effective than either placebo or acyclovir at facilitating cutaneous healing and healing of zoster-associated pain and post-herpetic neuralgia. Valacyclovir is well tolerated, with convenient dosing frequencies for the treatment of genital herpes or herpes zoster, it also has the option for use as a short course therapy in the episodic treatment of recurrent genital herpes, all of which are important benefits in the management of these conditions. The use of the antiviral valacyclovir, coupled with condoms and safer sex counseling, is recommended for individuals with proven genital herpes. Routine or targeted HSV screening is not indicated [459]. Although there are as yet no established indications for ACV use in pregnancy, the most reasonable uses are for maternal infections such as disseminated HSV, varicella pneumonia, and severe primary genital herpes. Other potential, but more problematic, uses during pregnancy are for uncomplicated primary genital herpes infections, maternal varicella, and for prophylaxis against the recurrence of genital herpes near term [460]. Continuous oral therapy with ACV (200 mg four times a day or 400 mg twice daily) has been shown to be safe and effective in reducing recurrence of genital herpes by 74-93%. Continuing therapy appears to be safe, even when used for up to 4 years. When an episode of genital herpes is diagnosed in term pregnancy, CS should be considered, even if intrauterine infection is possible until the rupture of membranes [461]. Use of ACV in infants, even in those that are premature, is very well tolerated, with a wide margin of safety. In addition, the pharmacokinetics studies, as well as the animal studies, suggest that maternal use of ACV may actually provide a prophylactic and therapeutic benefit to an infant who is exposed to HSV. The information provided indicated that ACV suppression actually decreases asymptomatic shedding, along with decreasing clinical recurrences. Because asymptomatic shedding seems to be similar in pregnant and nonpregnant patients, it would be reasonable to assume that asymptomatic shedding also would be decreased at delivery in pregnant women with HSV infection. This supposition is supported by the data from the RCT and cohort studies that demonstrated a lower than expected asymptomatic shedding rate. Women who experience their first genital herpes outbreak while they are pregnant seem to benefit from ACV suppression, with both a decrease in the risk of clinical recurrences at delivery and a decreased need for CS. This is well documented by a RCT and other cohort studies. ACV's efficacy in patients who have a history of genital herpes infections antedating their pregnancy is less clear. The data appear to indicate a clinically important decrease in the likelihood of symptomatic reactivations at the time of delivery, although the sample sizes in the randomized studies have been too small to draw a statistically significant conclusion one way or the other. Unfortunately, a definitive trial for this group of women may never be done. Assuming a 13% recurrence risk at the time of delivery and a 50% decrease in recurrences with the use of ACV, 652 women would have to complete the study to achieve a power of 80%. With valacyclovir and famciclovir now available, it is unlikely that any further work will be done with ACV. Information from the valacyclovir trials, however, may reach statistical significance because of changes in the study design that will allow smaller sample sizes to reach adequate power. The antiviral agent famciclovir has been shown to shorten the course and decrease the severity of episodes of recurrent genital herpes. In addition, famciclovir has been shown to be effective in suppressing recurrent genital herpes.

Famciclovir treatment holds promise because of its longer intracellular half-life, but until concerns about potential mutagenicity are resolved and more information on its efficacy for suppressive therapy becomes available, it should not be considered for maternal suppressive therapy. ACV appears to be effective, at least in some cohorts, and is probably safe for the fetus [462, 463]. ACV therapy can improve the outcome of neonatal herpes, but is often delayed due to the early non-specific symptoms of the disease. Even with early therapy, some infants develop disseminated infection or CNS complications. The virus is usually vertically transmitted to the neonate from an infected mother during delivery. As such, the optimal strategy for reducing the morbidity of neonatal herpes is to prevent the neonate from acquiring HSV infection at delivery. The highest risk of neonatal infection occurs when the mother sheds HSV at labor, which happens more frequently in women who acquire genital herpes in the third trimester. Therefore, one approach for reducing maternal-fetal transmissions is to prevent HSV acquisition in late pregnancy. Definitive classification of genital HSV infection during pregnancy as either primary, non-primary first episode, or recurrent can be accomplished only when clinical evaluation is accompanied by laboratory testing, including the use of IgG-specific serological tests. The serological status of the mother's sexual partner should be considered when determining her risk of infection. The use of weekly viral cultures in pregnant women with confirmed genital herpes is not warranted, as they do not predict an infant's risk of acquisition of HSV at delivery and are not cost-effective. High-risk susceptible women should be counseled about abstinence and reducing oral-genital contact near term. Observational studies suggest that CS can reduce transmission of neonatal herpes, and is warranted for women who shed HSV at delivery, although different countries vary in their approach to CS and so universal recommendations are not available. If maternal antiviral therapy is considered, the potential benefits of treatment should be balanced against potential adverse outcomes for mother and fetus, although it may be warranted when the mother has severe or life-threatening disease. Studies on the use of antiviral prophylaxis in women with known recurrences at labor are ongoing. Invasive fetal monitoring can increase the risk of neonatal herpes, and should only be used in HSV-2 seropositive women for defined obstetrical indications [464]. There is insufficient evidence to determine if antiviral prophylaxis reduces the incidence of neonatal herpes. Antenatal antiviral prophylaxis reduces viral shedding and recurrences at delivery and reduces the need for CS for genital herpes. Limited information exists regarding the neonatal safety of prophylaxis.

The risks, benefits, and alternatives to antenatal prophylaxis should be discussed with women who have a history and prophylaxis initiated for women who desire intervention [465].

In conclusion, herpes genitalis has become one of the most common STD and has reached epidemic proportions. It presents a grave risk to immunocompromised patients and to newborns. The advent of effective therapy with ACV has dramatically modified the morbidity and mortality of disseminated HHV infection and has helped in the therapy of primary and recurrent herpes genitalis. Current work has indicated that the disease can be transmitted by asymptomatic patients who are shedding the virus in the absence of visible lesions, which presents a diagnostic and therapeutic problem, especially significant for the pregnant patient, because infection of the neonate leads to serious consequences. Close follow-up of the pregnant woman with genital herpes therefore is imperative to minimize the risk to the newborn [466]. One of the most deleterious consequences of maternal infection with HSV is neonatal herpes, which results in death or significant neurodevelopmental impairment in the majority of infected babies. The ability to minimize the risk of HSV transmission has improved in tandem with advances in understanding of the mechanisms and epidemiology of acquisition of neonatal HSV. In particular, antiviral pharmacotherapy is now recognized as an important option both for reducing the risk of transmission of HSV from a seropositive to a seronegative partner and, potentially, for modifying several risk factors for transmission of the virus from a HSV-infected mother to the neonate. HSV infection during pregnancy can also impact the psychologic health of the mother [467].

In fact, although not life threatening, the physical symptoms of the disease, and the ensuing psychosocial complications, can be overwhelming to patients. The life cycle of the HSV is complex, comprising multiple stages. Following infection, the virus establishes life-long latency in its host and can reactivate at any time as a recurrent infection. Successful management of genital HSV infections involves patient education and psychological support, as well as antiviral agents [463]. Physicians must understand that the psychologic impact of genital HSV infections frequently is more disabling than the physical manifestations. Sensitivity, compassion, and support are necessary from members of the medical community, and psychologic counseling may help patients cope with HSV and all its implications.

Similarly, physicians must downplay the hysteria that has been associated with HHV infections, emerging as a result of intense media coverage in the 1970s and 1980s.

Minimizing the number of cases of neonatal herpes through identification of infected women during parturition continues to be important [453]. Substantial advances have been made in our understanding of HSV and genital herpes. The molecular biology of viral structure and function and the pathogenesis of infection have been elucidated to a large degree, and epidemiologic investigations, based on reliable type-specific assays, have been done. Diagnostic techniques have been refined, and the value of therapy has been defined. Currently, management strategies for pregnant women and their neonates are based on data rather than hypothesis, and rational counseling is feasible. The next major advance in the field would be the availability of a safe and effective vaccine, the development and investigation of which is being pursued vigorously. At this time, no vaccines have been demonstrated to be safe and effective, therefore, prevention is of the utmost importance [468-472].

VZV infection ("shingles") can be serious for pregnant women and their babies, although it is rare (Figure 6). The implications of primary VZV infection vary with the gestational age at infection.

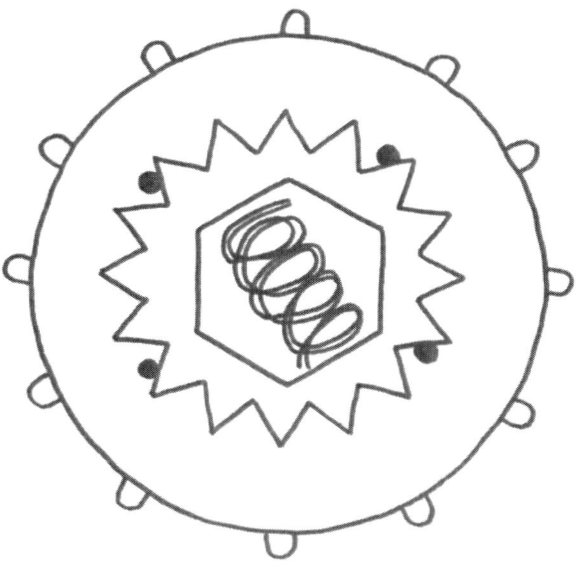

Modified from pediatrics.aappublications.org.

Figure 6. Varicella Zoster Virus (VZV).

For the mother, the risk of severe illness is greatest after mid-pregnancy, when she is relatively immunocompromised. For the fetus, the risk of congenital infection is greatest when maternal infection occurs in the first or second trimester. Maternal infection is preventable by preconception vaccination [473]. Obstetric populations born in tropical or subtropical regions are likely to be seronegative for VZV. Obstetric populations containing a large proportion of women born in tropical or subtropical regions will benefit greatly from being screened for varicella immunity. Physicians should therefore know the geographic origin of the community they serve and should consider testing varicella immunity in their obstetric patients born in tropical or subtropical regions. To ensure that passive immunization is received when indicated, physicians should obtain serostatus without relying on patients' recollection of their exposure to VZV [474].

Genital ulcerations can be the initial manifestation of EBV in adolescents who are neither sexually active nor immunocompromised (Figure 7) [475]. Burkitt lymphoma during pregnancy is a rare event, and outcomes have been poor.

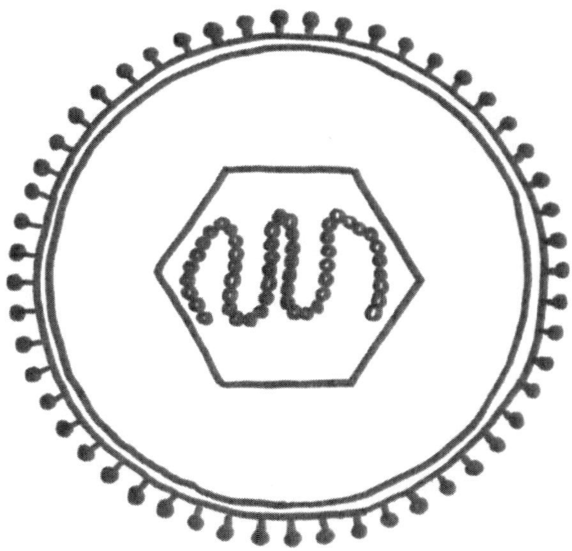

Modified from hindawi.com.

Figure 7. Epstein-Barr Virus (EBV).

However, few patients were treated by current standards, with nearly half receiving single-agent cyclophosphamide or no chemotherapy. When Burkitt lymphoma is encountered in pregnancy, immediate cytotoxic combination chemotherapy is indicated [476].

CMV is one of the most common causes of congenital infections in developed countries with reported incidences varying between 0.15% and 2.0% (Figure 8).

The effects of congenital CMV infection may vary from a congenital syndrome to an asymptomatic course. Infants that are asymptomatic at birth may still present handicaps at a later age. Congenital CMV infection is an important cause of hearing impairment, mental retardation, and CP. It is generally accepted that symptoms of congenitally infected children are more severe after primary infection than after recurrent infection.

The outcome of recurrent maternal CMV infection may be severe and congenital CMV infection should be considered in cases of pregnancy loss and necrotizing enterocolitis (NEC) with recurrent maternal CMV infection [477].

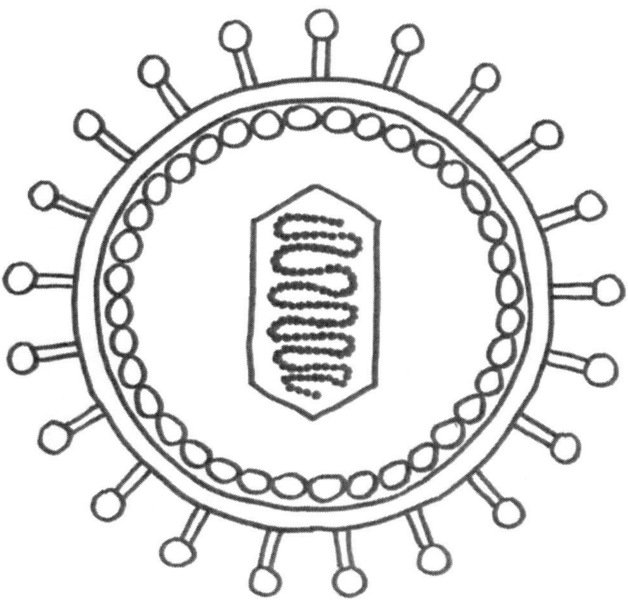

Modified from mbioblog.asm.org.

Figure 8. Cytomegalovirus (CMV).

It is suggested that CMV enteritis is added to the spectrum of clinical manifestations of postnatal CMV infection. Signs suggestive of NEC with atypical features should prompt investigations for CMV infection [478]. The annual cost of treating CMV infection complications in the US is two billion US dollars.

Many issues regarding CMV infection such as routine screening, antenatal diagnosis, and vaccination during pregnancy are unsettled and disputed. At present, it appears that there is no indication for routine prenatal screening, while other issues, such as the most accurate method for antenatal diagnosis and the indications for pregnancy termination are, as yet, unsettled [479]. The high incidence and the serious morbidity associated with congenital CMV infection emphasise the need for effective interventions to prevent the antenatal transmission of CMV infection. To date, no RCT are available that examine antenatal interventions for preventing MTCT of CMV during pregnancy and adverse outcomes in the congenitally infected infant. Further research is needed to assess the efficacy of interventions aimed at preventing MTCT of CMV during pregnancy including a long-term follow-up of exposed infants and a cost effective analysis [480]. Recent findings include an enhanced understanding of the epidemiology, pathogenesis, and treatment of CMV infections, a knowledge of high-risk women particularly those with chronic exposure to a young child in the home, the availability of accurate methods for the serologic diagnosis of a primary CMV infection using either single or serial blood samples, accurate methods for the diagnosis of fetal infection via amniotic fluid, sensitive fetal and placental indicators for neonatal outcomes, and the availability of potentially effective interventions such as hygienic intervention and CMV hyperimmune globulin. These findings suggest that serologic testing for CMV during pregnancy may be appropriate either using one-time testing or serial serologic testing throughout the first two trimesters of pregnancy and that education of pregnant women about CMV is necessary so that they can assess their risk and make informed choices about serologic screening [481]. Principal sources of infection during pregnancy are young children and intimate contacts. Prevention of maternal and congenital CMV infection depends on counseling women regarding the sources of infection and hygienic measures that might prevent infection. There is currently insufficient evidence to support use of antiviral treatment or passive immunization for postexposure prophylaxis of pregnant women or as a maternal treatment aimed at preventing fetal infection. Vaccines for CMV are under development but it will be a number of years before one is licensed [482].

Preeclampsia/eclampsia remains an important cause of maternal and perinatal morbidity and mortality. Its origins lie in a mismatch between fetoplacental demands and the ability of the uteroplacental arteries to supply those demands, a situation that also arises in normotensive IUGR (the fetal syndrome of preeclampsia in isolation).

The evidence surrounds a potential trigger for the differential response, namely infection. This builds on the inflammatory model of preeclampsia for which there is increasing support. The evidence for an infectious trigger is principally indirect, linking the similarities between acute atherosis in preeclampsia and atherosclerosis, the increased likelihood of developing CVD later in life following a preeclampsia pregnancy, and the association between chronic infection and atherogenesis [483].

Like atherosclerosis, there is a potential link between CMV infection and preeclampsia. CMV infection seems to affect the occurrence of preeclampsia. Evaluation of the relation between CMV infection and preeclampsia may provide mechanistic insights into preeclampsia-related inflammation [484]. The British Andrology Society (BAS) guidelines for the screening of semen donors have undergone a recent review, and following consultation with members of the Society and with experts in the allied professions, revised guidelines have been issued.

Major changes include the introduction of an upper age limit for semen donors (<40 years old) and the general exclusion of men who are seropositive for CMV as donors. The BAS recommends the screening of prospective semen donors for chromosomal abnormalities and for cystic fibrosis carrier status. Following the report of cross-contamination of human cells with HBV within a liquid nitrogen storage vessel, the BAS recommends that steps be taken to ensure the safe cryopreservation of donor gametes [485]. The recommendation is based on the results of recent studies that identified a high percentage of symptomatic congenital CMV infections in newborns of women with CMV seropositivity pre-existing to pregnancy and on the fact that CMV can be detected in semen of CMV seropositive men.

These are not new data. CMV seropositive women can infect their fetuses with their own latent CMV strain that can reactivate, or with an exogenous strain that can be transmitted to them by a sexual partner, but also by contacts, for example with an excreting child.

The efficiency of these various ways of transmission to the fetus and the factors that could influence this transmission are for the moment completely unknown. An infectious virus is recovered by culture in the semen of <5% of CMV seropositive men.

Exclusion of a large population of donors on the sole criteria of a positive CMV serology introduces the general message that this part of the male population is also not suitable as possible partners in couples who have no fertility problems [486-490].

HUMAN PARVOVIRUS

Human Parvovirus B19 is a common infection in children occurring in winter and spring months that can affect pregnant women and their unborn fetuses (Figure 9). Adverse fetal sequelae may include anemia and myocarditis. Fortunately, several noninvasive testing schemes are available to assess the fetus, and invasive testing is reserved for fetuses with marked anemia [489]. Histologic and DNA hybridization studies suggest Parvovirus infection ("fifth disease") as a cause for nonimmune hydrops fetalis (NIHF) and fetal death.

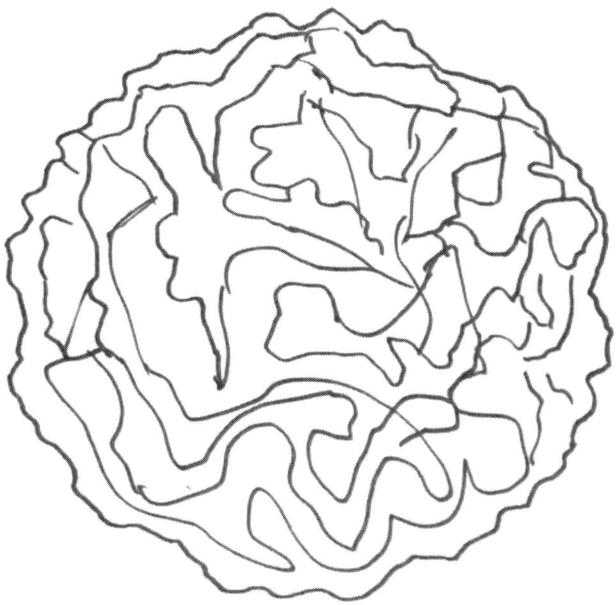

Modified from virology.wisc.edu.

Figure 9. Human Parvovirus (B19).

Women at high risk for exposure (school teachers) should have screening for Parvovirus IgG-specific antibodies: if these are absent, they should avoid close contact with schoolchildren. Pregnant women with evidence of recent infection should have a level II ultrasound. Because no vaccine is currently available, routine screening cannot be recommended [492]. From the point of view of obstetrics and pediatrics, the importance of B19 infection lies in the potential for intraueterine infection following maternal B19 infection. Ongoing prospective studies of B19 infection in pregnant women indicate a risk of adverse pregnancy outcomes considerably lower than previous estimates from retrospective studies and case reports. The occurrence, however, of severe

NIHF or stillbirths or both in even a small percentage of progeny of B19-infected pregnant women is a concern. It thus behooves physicians caring for pregnant women and their offspring to be thoroughly familiar with B19 and issues related to B19 infection in pregnancy [493]. Postexposure passive immunization is not currently recommended. Once there is maternal infection, maternal disease is usually self-limited, but the effects to the fetus can be devastating.

Even so, additional studies of the risks and benefits of intrauterine therapy such as transfusion and digitalization are necessary before definitive recommendations can be made. Cases where congenital viral infection is suspected should be handled in an appropriate manner and should include serology on mother and infant (both acute and convalescent), viral cultures, and ophthalmologic evaluation. HCW must be aware that the infant and its body fluids and organs may be infective to susceptible nursery and laboratory personnel [494].

Recent improvements in diagnosing Parvovirus infections by sensitive molecular biology techniques now allow for a new insight into its pathogenic rule, immunology, and the varied clinical manifestations. The estimated overall risk of fetal loss after maternal exposure is about 6.5%, which is much less than previously thought. Inasmuch as complete spontaneous reversal of fetal hydrops has been commonly described, controversy exists regarding the management of the fetus with clinical signs of infection by Parvovirus B19. According to the experience that has accumulated, it seems that only cases with severe fetal anemia or signs of fetal compromise should be managed by intrauterine transfusion. This procedure, however, is not without risk. Although an association between fetal viral infection and structural abnormalities has been described, it has not been proved yet. However, infection by Parvovirus B19 has been recently proposed as a causative factor for congenital red blood cell aplasia due to bone marrow suppression [495].

The critical period during which maternal Parvovirus B19 infection leads to NIHF correlates with the hepatic period of hematopoietic activity. These findings suggest that Parvovirus B19 may have an affinity for erythroid lineage cells at the hepatic stage of hematopoiesis, which may strongly influence the clinical features of feto-maternal B19 infection [496].

Adverse outcome of pregnancy can occur after symptomatic and asymptomatic maternal infection. Only rare cases of congenital malformations and fetal disease in live-born infants have been associated with intrauterine B19 virus infection. Laboratory results obtained from paired maternal and fetal cord blood samples indicate that a reliable diagnosis of fetal B19 virus infection should be based on detection of Parvovirus B19 DNA [497]. Parvovirus B19 infection during pregnancy causes up to 27% cases of NIHF in anatomically normal fetuses.

The virus is believed to cause arrest of maturation of red blood cell precursors at the late normoblast stage and also causes a decrease in the number of platelets. Fetal anemia is presently thought to be responsible for the development of skin edema and effusions. Myocarditis leading to heart failure may contribute to the development of fetal hydrops. The most promising diagnostic techniques are PCR of amniotic fluid or fetal blood and electron microscopy.

There are some reports of fetal abnormalities occurring (probably coincidentally) in cases of Parvovirus infection, but the majority of postmortem findings are infection-related, in particular myocarditis and hepatic abnormalities. There is no treatment, but preventive measures can be used to decrease perinatal mortality.

Although management guidelines cannot be derived due to the variable degree of hydrops, the present data suggest a benefit of transfusion therapy over conservative management in infected fetuses. The only study which was corrected for severity of hydrops using ultrasound criteria showed a clear benefit of intrauterine transfusion [498].

Thus, if the fetus exhibits hydrops in the latter part of pregnancy, the main treatment options include either correcting the associated anemia with intrauterine blood transfusion or birth with extrauterine management. Although the serious problems associated with this virus during pregnancy are uncommon, they can be fatal.

In view of this, a pregnant woman who is antibody negative should try to avoid contact with large groups of young children in order to decrease contact with potential vectors [499-501].

Rubella Virus

Rubella and rubeola are common viral exanthems that may affect women of reproductive age (Figure 10). Effective vaccination programs have greatly decreased their incidence.

Although rubella is a relatively innocuous illness for the nonpregnant patient, transplacental fetal infection with rubella can result in significant and crippling fetal malformations and handicap. Because some women of reproductive age are not appropriately immunized, rubella is still a threat.

The practitioner needs to be vigilant in assuring vaccination of susceptible individuals when seen for routine health maintenance. Additionally, at times the obstetrician will be challenged with the evaluation and care of a susceptible pregnant patient who is exposed to rubella.

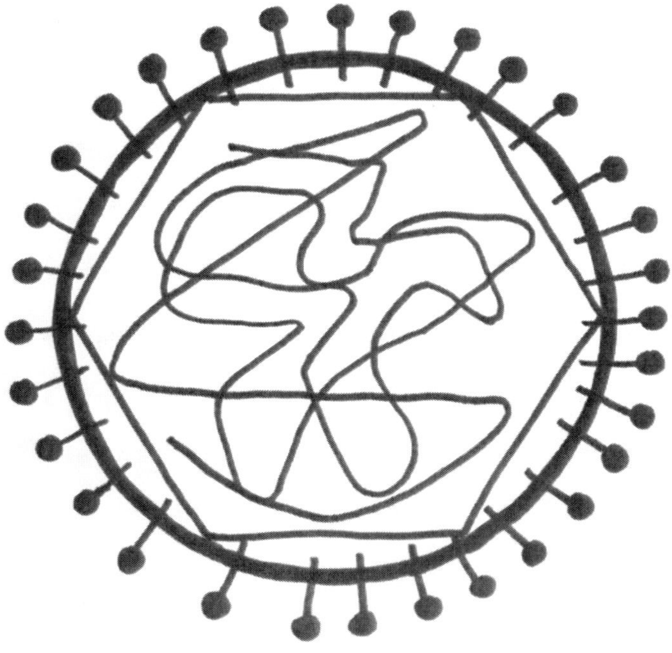

Modified from pathmicro.med.sc.edu.

Figure 10. Rubella Virus.

In contrast, rubeola ("measles") infection during pregnancy has not been associated with congenital malformations.

Affected mothers, however, experience a higher incidence of spontaneous abortions and premature delivery and are themselves at risk for serious complications such as pneumonia and encephalitis [502]. Rubella Virus is the first virus demonstrated as a teratogen. There is a high risk to develop congenital rubella syndrome (CRS) if the infection occurs in the first part of pregnancy, particularly in women without specific immunological protection. Specific therapies to prevent CRS are not available.

Many developed countries have specific vaccination programs and maternal rubella is rare. However, in developing countries or where campaigns of rubella surveillance and preconceptional vaccination are inadequate, there are still cases of CRS registered despite primary possibilities of prevention. Maternal infection is not indicative of vertical transmission in 100% of cases, and damage does not necessarily occur in all cases of fetal infection. This is the reason why an adequate prenatal counseling is mandatory, particularly in cases of proven maternal infection.

Advanced prenatal diagnostic techniques, invasive or not, should be offered to the women especially in order to distinguish the cases without fetal damage. Prevention of voluntary interruption of pregnancy (VIP) for the latter or in case of maternal false IgM rubella antibody positivity or IgM "chronic carrier" patients is mandatory. World wide, the aim is to perform an adequate primary prevention through vaccination of childbearing age women without specific immunological protection [503].

Nationally, nearly one of every five practicing obstetricians may not have documented rubella immunity, and the majority of office-based practices have no system for assuring such immunity. Rubella immunity should extend beyond the hospital setting, with consideration for requiring rubella immunity as a condition for employment. Methods for effective implementation and documentation of current guidelines need to be addressed, particularly in the office setting [504].

HUMAN T-LYMPHOTROPIC VIRUS

Worldwide, 20-30 million people are estimated to be infected with HTLV (Figure 11). HTLV-1 is endemic in Western Africa and Southern Japan, whereas HTLV-2 is considered to be spread among native American people. Transmission may occur by sexual intercourse or cellular blood products. Although materno-fetal transmission is debated, transmission through maternal breast milk has been confirmed.

An HTLV-infection can lead to adult T-cell leukemia (ATL) or cumulative opportunistic and neurological disorders that can occur with varying degrees of severity. Diagnosis can be done by antibody detection via the use of ELISA and Western blot analysis as well as PCR diagnosis. Due to inadequate treatment options and the lack of an effective vaccination, prevention is currently only possible by restricting transmission, including the usage of condoms during sexual intercourse or avoiding breastfeeding in

HTLV-seropositive mothers. If, due to socio-economic reasons, breastfeeding cannot be avoided, short-term breastfeeding for a maximum of up to 6 months is suggested [505]. In the past two decades, a large initiative has been put forth to understand the biological and pathogenic properties of the HTLV-1: this has ultimately led to the development of various experimental vaccination and therapeutic strategies to combat HTLV-1 infection. These strategies include peptide, recombinant protein, DNA, and viral vectors. These strategies also include the development of envelope glycoprotein derived B-cell epitopes for the induction of neutralizing antibodies, as well as a strategy to generate a multivalent CTL response against the HTLV-1 Tax antigen [506].

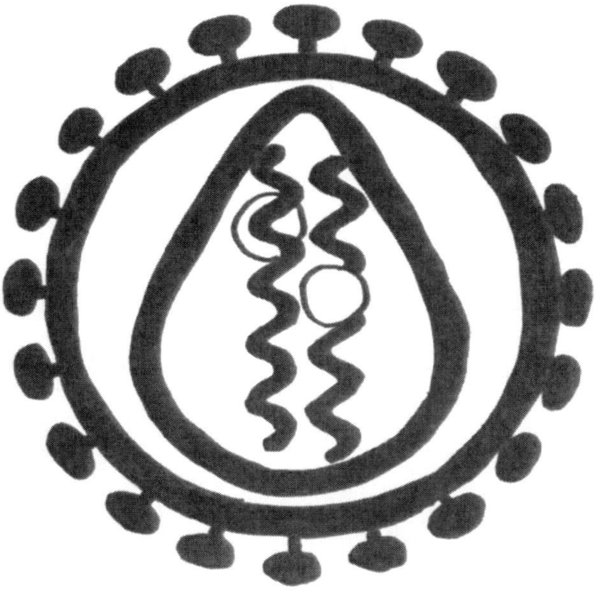

Modified from my-personaltrainer.it.

Figure 11. Human T-Lymphotropic Virus (HTLV).

Other Viruses

Emerging infections, many zoonotic, are caused by a variety of pathogens with global distribution. Previously rare pathogens have emerged: global travel facilitates their rapid spread. Human encroachment on remote areas has brought contact with zoonotic diseases never before characterized. Although systematic study of rare outbreaks can be challenging, knowledge of emerging pathogens and their effects on women (Lymphocytic Choriomeningitis Virus [LCMV], West Nile Virus [WNV], Severe Acute Respiratory Syndrome Coronavirus [SARS-CV], Avian Influenza A Virus, viral hemorrhagic fevers, etc.) is accumulating [507].

Recently, there has been an increased concern over viral respiratory infections and their potential for a pandemic. This concern makes it important to review the most current guidelines for the management of viral respiratory diseases in pregnancy. Pregnant women have an increased susceptibility to viral respiratory diseases. The most common respiratory virus to infect pregnant women is influenza (Figure 12).

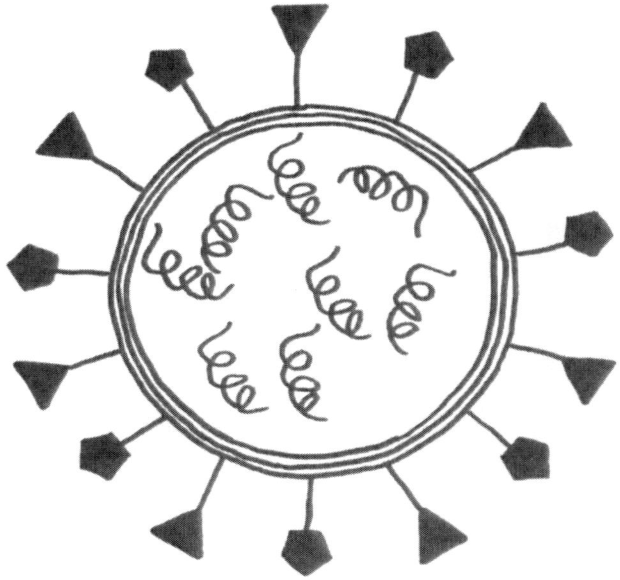

Modified from sciencebuz.com.

Figure 12. Influenza Virus.

Influenza is a significant cause of morbidity and mortality from febrile respiratory illness worldwide. Influenza in pregnant women has historically been associated with a higher rate of morbidity and mortality.

All women who intend to become pregnant or are pregnant should receive the influenza vaccine. If a pregnant woman develops influenza, she should be treated with supportive care. Antiviral medications should be reserved for cases where the benefits outweigh the risks. Avian Influenza Virus (H5N1) is a new emerging virus usually contracted from direct contact with diseased birds.

There is no commercially available vaccine at this time to prevent infection. Pregnant women should be treated aggressively with supportive care and antiviral medications, as the significant risk of maternal mortality outweighs the potential fetal risks [508]. Human infection with the novel H1N1 Influenza Virus, initially popularly termed "swine flu", was first reported in April 2009 and has since prompted the WHO to raise its pandemic alert to the highest level. During pregnancy, both mother and baby are at increased risk when infected with either pandemic or seasonal influenza. Because of concerns about the severity of the disease during pregnancy, the CDC has implemented enhanced surveillance for infection with this novel virus in pregnant women and has placed them in a group that merits priority vaccine administration.

The benefit of treatment with the antiviral medication oseltamivir outweighs its theoretical risk, as pregnant women are at increased risk of severe complications from H1N1 virus infection. In addition to confirmed H1N1 cases, the associated symptoms, particularly fever, merit immediate attention. Moreover, precautions must be taken by both patients and health care professionals when confirmed or suspected H1N1-infected pregnant women present to labor and delivery, or the doctor's office. After delivery, pregnant women infected with H1N1 may breastfeed but must follow specific guidelines. Although the current strain of H1N1 virus has fairly mild sequelae, the virus may mutate over the summer months and so there can be a possible second wave of more severe illness moving into fall and winter [509, 510]. Reproductive endocrinologists often have the opportunity to evaluate patients before conception and are able to counsel them before they become part of this high-risk obstetrics group. The CDC, ACOG, and American Society of Reproductive Medicine (ASRM) have universal agreement in recommending vaccination for all pregnant women and all women attempting conception. Patients should be counseled regarding the vaccine and consider delaying conception until the immunization has been received [511].

Both the rate of vaccination of pregnant women against influenza and the rate of a documented discussion regarding vaccination increased after implementation of the best-practice alert. It is recommended that users of electronic medical records add a best-practice alert to improve influenza vaccination rates [512-517].

Pneumonia is the sixth leading cause of death in the US, and is the number one cause of death from an infectious disease (Figure 13). Although pregnant women do not get pneumonia more often than nonpregnant women, it can result in greater morbidity and mortality because of the physiologic adaptations of pregnancy. Pregnant patients who have either of these conditions require a higher level of surveillance and intervention [518]. Although the advent of broad-spectrum antibiotics has markedly improved the maternal outcomes of pneumonia complicating pregnancy, pneumonia remains a significant condition that may complicate pregnancy. The clinical course of bacterial pneumonia seems to be minimally altered by pregnancy, whereas viral pneumonia carries a significantly worse prognosis when encountered during gestation.

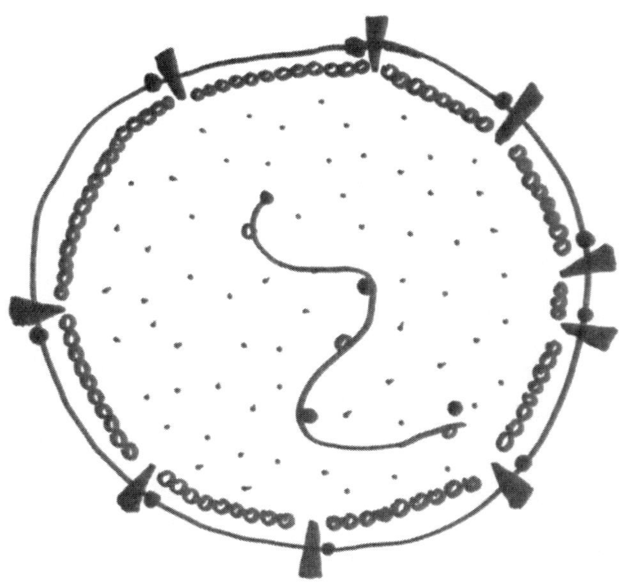

Modified from enfermerosmicrobiologicos.blogspot.com.

Figure 13. Pneumovirus.

Prompt diagnosis, the initiation of respiratory support, and appropriate antimicrobial/antiviral therapy are key components of therapy for women in whom pregnancy is complicated by pneumonia. Because preterm labor frequently accompanies pneumonia, women should be monitored closely for the occult onset of preterm labor and appropriate interventions initiated if indicated. Perhaps even more important than interventions to treat acute pneumonia are efforts directed at active immunization or prophylactic therapy to prevent the development of pneumonia in select patient populations. The combination of these efforts is essential to optimize medical care for pregnant women [519]. Three recent high-profile infectious disease threats have affected the US: SARS, WNV, and LCMV. The three emerging infectious diseases pose very different threats: SARS is a newly identified pathogen that caused an international pandemic, the WNV investigation involved an old pathogen that was identified in a new location, and LCMV has particular relevance to obstetrics, as it is likely an under-recognized abortifacient and fetal teratogen. All three outbreaks highlight the importance of obstetrician-gynecologists keeping current with new information as it emerges. Pregnant women diagnosed clinically with SARS should be treated empirically, as a serologic diagnosis can take weeks to confirm (Figure 14).

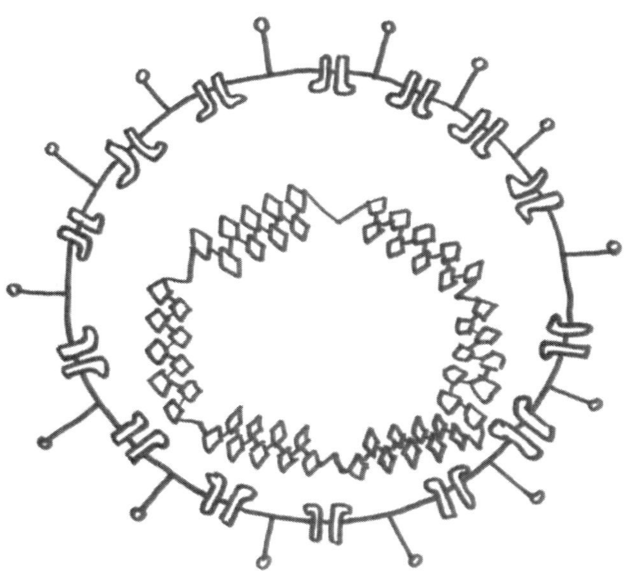

Modified from globalinfocenter.blogspot.com.

Figure 14. Severe Acute Respiratory Syndrome (SARS) Virus.

The treatment of pregnant women with SARS should be without ribavirin [520]. WNV, a relatively new infectious agent to North America, can cause significant morbidity including severe meningoencephalopathy and death (Figure 15). Infection by this virus during pregnancy has been previously reported in only two cases, one of which may have resulted in adverse neonatal neurologic sequelae. WNV infection during pregnancy does not uniformly result in maternal-fetal transmission. Further research is necessary in order to counsel parents appropriately about potential adverse fetal effects [521]. A report in May 2005 from the CDC describing a cluster of LCMV infections among 4 solid organ recipients has increased awareness of and clinical interest in this pathogen (Figure 16). Human infection with LCMV results from direct or indirect contact with rodents. There have been 54 cases of congenital LCMV reported since 1955, with 34 of the cases diagnosed since 1993. Chorioretinitis and hydrocephalus are the predominant characteristics among children diagnosed with congenital LCMV infection. Obstetricians should educate their pregnant patients about the risks of exposure to laboratory, pet, and wild rodents [522].

HCW must be prepared for the threat of bioterrorism. So, primary HCW, obstetricians in particular, shoul be educated in the prevention, diagnosis, and treatment of smallpox (Figure 17).

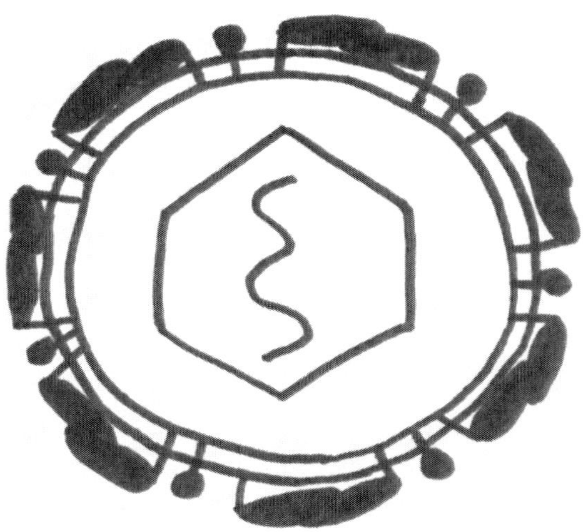

Modified from fairfoxcounty.gov.

Figure 15. West Nile Virus (WNV).

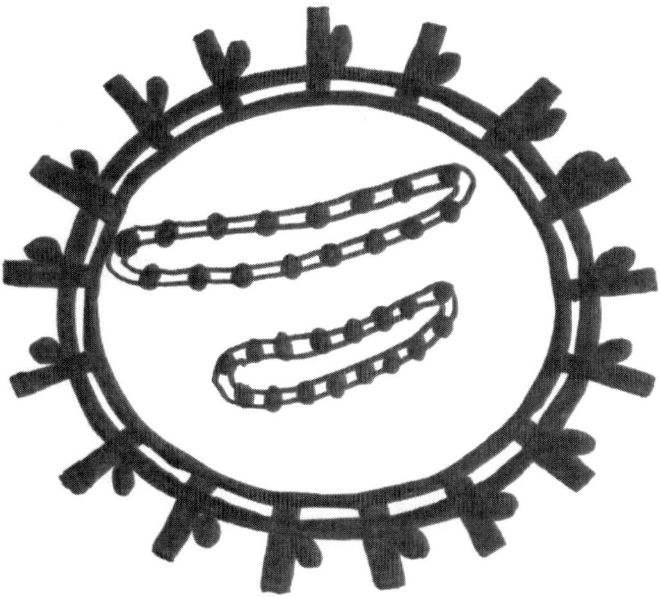

Modified from virology.net.

Figure 16. Lymphocytic Choriomeningitis Virus (LCMV).

Smallpox poses a particularly serious threat because of its high case-fatality rate in unvaccinated populations (no one younger than 25 years has been vaccinated, and older persons have little remaining residual immunity). Routine nonemergency smallpox vaccination is restricted to laboratory staff working with smallpox-related viruses. Under these circumstances, contraindications to vaccination are pregnancy, immunodeficiency, exfoliative skin conditions (eczema), and allergy to vaccine components.

In case of an intentional release of the Smallpox Virus, those directly exposed and their close contacts must be vaccinated and isolated. Under such emergency circumstances, pregnant women exposed to the Variola Virus should be vaccinated because of the lethality of the disease during pregnancy. Currently, there is a limited supply of vaccine available [523]. Early in June 2003, the CDC announced yet another unique infectious disease outbreak, the first evidence of community-acquired monkeypox in the US (Figure 18).

Modified from scq.ubc.ca.

Figure 17. Smallpox Virus.

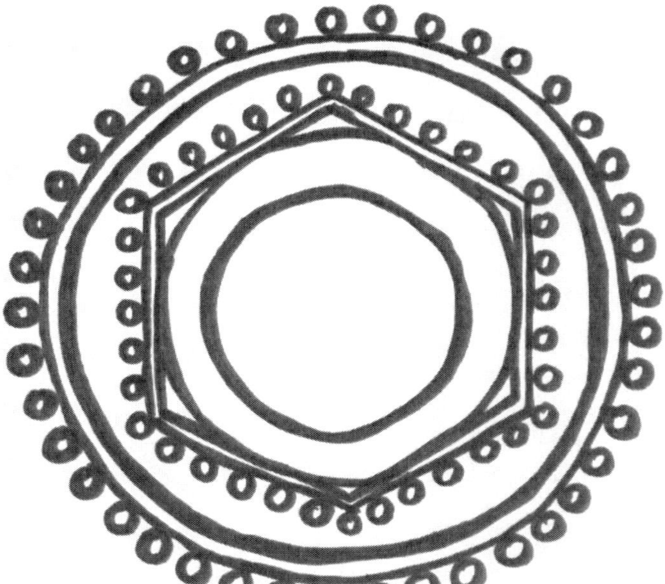

Modified from pics5.this-pic.com.

Figure 18. Monkeypox Virus.

When emerging infectious diseases are reported in the US, particularly when these reports receive widespread media attention, obstetrician-gynecologists may be called upon to rapidly respond to queries from their patients and to address certain infectious disease risks within their clinical practices. In addition, obstetrician-gynecologists may have specific concerns about the implications for an infectious disease outbreak, such as monkeypox, for pregnant women. Therefore, it is important that obstetrician-gynecologists know how to gather up-to-date and accurate information about infectious disease outbreaks and that they be familiar with the public health response system for responding to such outbreaks [524].

The cluster of neural tube defects (NTD) appears to be due to Dengue Virus infection (Figure 19) [525]. Dengue is a major public health problem in several countries. Few reports document presentations and outcomes of dengue during pregnancy. In many endemic countries, as the average age of getting dengue infections is shifting upwards, dengue in pregnancy is likely to be encountered more frequently.

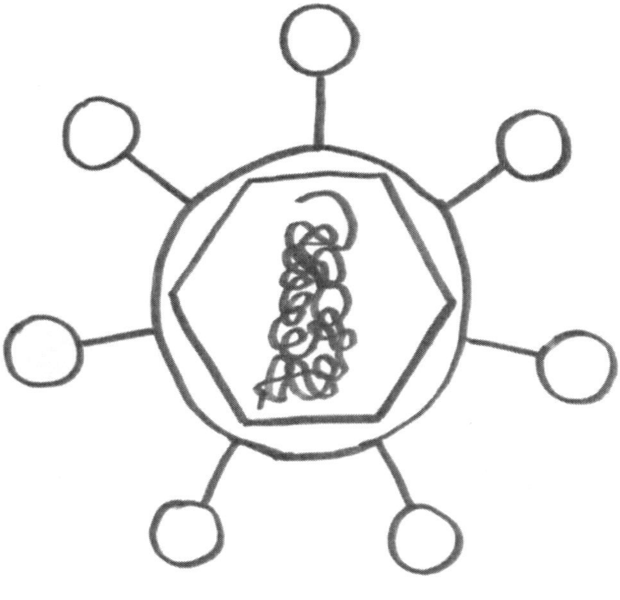

Modified from nature.com.

Figure 19. Dengue Virus.

Patterns of dengue in patients from different regions are needed if we are to draft evidence based management guidelines. Awareness of clinical and laboratory manifestations of dengue in pregnancy should allow its early recognition and institution of appropriate treatment. Reports on dengue in pregnancy from different regions should allow more evidence-based guidelines to be formulated for optimum evaluation and care of such patients [526].

Molluscum contagiosum is a common condition that often occurs in children, sexually active young adults, and immunocompromised patients (Figure 20). Generally, molluscum contagiosum lesions are self-limited. They often resolve spontaneously [527].

CONCLUSION

At the beginning of the millennium, it is important that experts and official organizations direct their strategic plans towards the improvement of reproductive sexual health. Adolescents represent the major target of these plans in an effort to improve their sexual behavior.

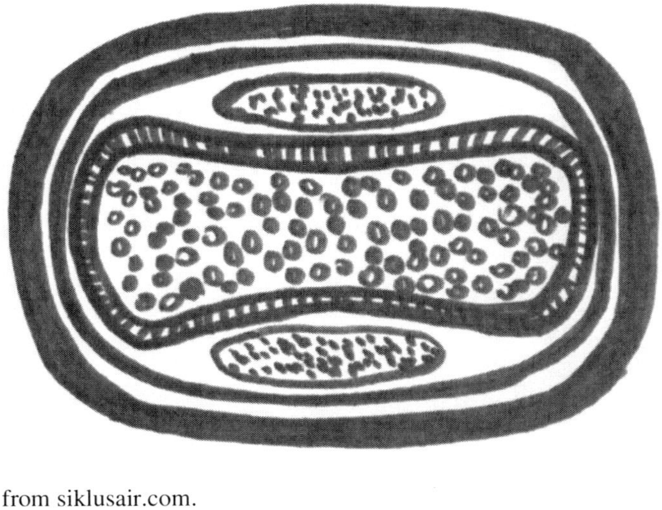

Modified from siklusair.com.

Figure 20. Molluscum Contagiosum Virus (MCV).

STD must be reduced since their prevalence is very high in certain Eastern European countries. These plans should be considered together with the development of new fertility control methods which provide at the same time bactericidal and antiviral properties. Education, provided especially through the media, should be considered a tool for the improvement of the present situation [528]. STD in women are of great concern to all HCW since many of them are preventable and/or treatable conditions which, if left untreated, could have serious sequelae such as PID, infertility, cervical cancer, systemic disease, etc. They may also become a major public health problem when dealing with diseases such as hepatitis, etc., or in people with HIV [529]. RCT provide evidence that female condoms confer as much protection from STI as male condoms. Observational studies suggest that the diaphragm protects against STI pathogens. Several microbicide effectiveness studies are under way and new directions, such as adaptation of therapeutic agents as preventive products, are being examined. Substantial attention is now given to product formulation and novel delivery strategies. Combining microbicide products with different mechanisms of action as well as combining chemical and physical barriers will be necessary to maximize prevention effectiveness. Increased investment in the development and identification of female controlled barrier methods offers promise that additional products will be available in the years ahead. Generalizing trial results to a community setting, promoting products that may be less effective than male condoms, and bringing an effective product to scale introduce public health challenges that warrant attention. The need for female controlled barrier methods that provide women with the opportunity to take an active role in reducing their STI/HIV risk are urgently needed and constitute an essential tool to prevent continued spread of these infections [530].

The AIDS epidemic weighs heavily on the already burdened health care delivery systems of developing countries especially in central Africa. AIDS not only incurs high morbidity and mortality but has a severe impact on productivity, economic infrastructures, and development in those countries which need them the most. HIV is mainly spread through heterosexual intercourse in central Africa. Vertical transmission of HIV and breastfeeding are other means. The key vehicle of HIV transmission in the US is still homosexual intercourse. STD facilitate HIV transmission via intercourse. Research shows that subsequent infection by other STD hastens the development of AIDS in HIV-infected people. Some evidence indicates that pregnancy increases the risk of developing AIDS in a woman who is positive for HIV.

The main means to prevent HIV transmission is the condom. Yet, in Rwanda, only 7% of women had ever used condoms despite the high rate (32%) of HIV-positive serology. The University of Zimbabwe Medical School believes adolescents are the most appropriate starting point for AIDS prevention since they tend to experiment with sexual behaviors. Its youth counseling program involves education and prevention messages within and outside educational settings through youth meeting places, youth workers, and other mass media. It hosts workshops at meeting places which use the problem solving approach to risk-reduction behavior. The program invites schools, churches, and other educational settings to form anti-AIDS clubs. It advocates use of drama and music to promote AIDS awareness. The program has also branched out into community counseling where it works to eliminate the stigma and guilt associated with talking about sexual transmission of AIDS. Governments must learn who the STD and HIV transmission high-risk groups are and then target them with information, education, and communication AIDS prevention programs [531]. The use of ZDV for the prevention of MTCT of HIV, as well as continuing advances in our understanding of the determinants of that transmission, and of potential new avenues of intervention augur ever more efficient perinatal prevention strategies in the near future. At least four factors will be critical in determining what the evolving role of prenatal testing in an era of ever more successful interventions will be: clinical, legal, ethical and economic. Each of these are parochial, i.e., they will feature in eradication strategies in different ways in different geographical, economic, and cultural settings. An understanding of these factors will help to suggest what course testing policy should take and to determine the role clinicians must play if any testing policy is to succeed in contributing to the end of pediatric HIV disease [532]. Cervical cancer is the second most common cancer in women worldwide. There are about 60,000 newly detected cases and 30,000 deaths annually in Europe, with the highest incidence reported from Eastern Europe countries. According to data from the National Public Health Institute (NPIH), it is the eighth most common malignancy in women. A large study carried out in 1995 by the IARC, which included cervical cancer material collected from 22 countries all over the world, revealed HPV genome in 99.7% of cases. Efficient methods of cervical cancer detection and screening methods for identification of precancerous lesions (conventional Pap smear) are available. Cervical cancer prevention programs should include education (of health care providers and women), stressing the benefits of screening, the age of the peak cervical cancer incidence, and the signs and symptoms of precancerous lesions and invasive disease.

The aim of screening actions is to detect precancerous lesions that may lead to cancer if left untreated. Screening can only be effective if there is a well-organized system of follow-up, diagnosis, and treatment. Cervical cytology, or Pap testing, has for decades been a cornerstone of cervical cancer screening.

According to recent guidelines issued by the WHO Regional Office for Europe, the primary task of the public health system is the introduction of secondary prevention through properly organized screening programs. Launching the national immunization program is only possible in the countries with well-organized secondary prevention programs and in those that can afford it [533]. With the introduction of cervical screening programs, the incidence and mortality of cervical cancer has been drastically reduced.

Techniques such as the traditional Pap test and the newer liquid-based cytology allow for the early detection of cervical abnormalities prior to the development of invasive cervical cancer. As oncogenic HPV infection is necessary for cervical cancer, HPV-DNA testing has also been proposed as a routine screening method for the general population. Screening limitations, such as adherence, test sensitivity and specificity, access, and cost-effectiveness are reflected in current screening guidelines. The development of prophylactic cervical cancer vaccines is a major milestone in cervical cancer prevention. These vaccines protect against the initial infection of certain oncogenic HPV types, and therefore prevent the development of cervical dysplasia, precancerous lesions, and cervical cancer. Considering routine cervical cancer vaccination in adolescent girls, screening guidelines must adapt in order to retain efficient and cost-effective prevention measures. Although the true epidemiological and economic impact of cervical cancer vaccines cannot be immediately realized, mathematical models predict various scenarios in which vaccination, in addition to cervical screening, will be cost-effective and further reduce cervical cancer disease [534]. Many vaccine platforms for both prevention of HPV infection and treatment of associated disease have been developed. VLP constructs containing HPV capsid proteins have been shown to protect against HPV infection. Novel peptide or protein constructs containing modified E6 or E7 proteins, novel adjuvants, fusion proteins such as IgG-heavy chain E7, or heat shock proteins (HSP) have been made as therapeutic modalities. In addition, many new recombinant vaccine vectors such as Vaccinia, Listeria species, Adenovirus, Semliki Forest vectors, and others have been developed as carriers of immunotherapeutic agents. Recently, chimeric VLP vaccines have been developed to treat existing HPV-induced neoplasms.

Immunotherapy protocols using a variety of recombinant vectors and modified HPV proteins induce in-vitro T cell responses and may lead to tumor regression. Vaccine-induced in-vitro immune reactivity and clinical vaccine effects are often not well associated. Further analysis of ongoing human immunotherapy trials is awaited [535].

The world government community made a commitment in 1994 to make reproductive health care universally available no later than the year 2015. The commitment has been confirmed by a special session of the UN General Assembly in July 1999. The commitment has to be backed-up by resources, and the health profession has to provide the know-how. In this global environment, it is likely that novel disease threats will continue to emerge. Social action will also be needed. Progress has been made, but challenges remain [536].

REFERENCES

[1] Larsen, B. Host defence mechanisms in obstetrics and gynaecology. *Clin. Obstet. Gynaecol.*, 1983 10, 37-64.

[2] Nasu, K., Narahara, H. Pattern recognition *Mediators Inflamm.,* 2010 2010, 976024.

[3] Koga, K., Mor, G. Expression and function of toll-like receptors at the maternal-fetal interface. *Reprod. Sci.*, 2008 15, 231-242.

[4] Baecher-Lind, L. E., Miller, W. C., Wilcox, A. J. Infectious disease and reproductive health: a review. *Obstet. Gynecol. Surv.*, 2010 65, 53-65.

[5] Huddleston, H., Schust, D. J. Immune interactions at the maternal-fetal interface: a focus on antigen presentation. *Am. J. Reprod. Immunol.*, 2004 51, 283-289.

[6] Rote, N. S., Chakrabarti, S., Stetzer, B. P. The role of human endogenous retroviruses in trophoblast differentiation and placental development. *Placenta*, 2004 25, 673-683.

[7] Mor, G., Cardenas, I. The immune system in pregnancy: a unique complexity. *Am. J. Reprod. Immunol.*, 2010 63, 425-433.

[8] Brabin, L. Interactions of the female hormonal environment, susceptibility to viral infections, and disease progression. *AIDS Patient Care STDS*, 2002 16, 211-221.

[9] Bergström, S. Genital infections and reproductive health: infertility and morbidity of mother and child in developing countries. *Scand. J. Infect. Dis.* Suppl., 1990 69, 99-105.

[10] ACOG Committee on Practice Bulletins – Gynecology. ACOG Practice Bulletin. Clinical management guidelines for obstetrician-gynecologists, Number 72, May 2006: Vaginitis. *Obstet. Gynecol.*, 2006 107, 1195-1206.

[11] Faro, S. New considerations in treatment of urinary tract infections in adults. *Urology*, 1992 39, 1-11.

[12] Donders, G. G. Management of genital infections in pregnant women. *Curr. Opin. Infect. Dis.*, 2006 19, 55-61.

[13] Haun, L., Kwan, N., Hollier, L. M. Viral infections in pregnancy. *Minerva Ginecol.*, 2007 59, 159-174.

[14] Ghidini, A., Lynch, L. Prenatal diagnosis and significance of fetal infections. *West. J. Med.*, 1993 159, 366-373.

[15] Durand-Réville, M., Bongain, A., Gillet, J. Y. Update on maternal-fetal infections by hepatitis C, HIV and cytomegalovirus. *J. Gynecol. Obstet. Biol. Reprod.* (Paris), 2000 29, 306-308.

[16] Newton, E. R. Diagnosis of perinatal TORCH infections. *Clin. Obstet. Gynecol.*, 1999 42, 59-70.

[17] Al-Adnani, M., Sebire, N. J. The role of perinatal pathological examination in subclinical infection in obstetrics. *Best Pract. Res. Clin. Obstet. Gynaecol.*, 2007 21, 505-521.

[18] Ault, K. A., Faro, S. Viruses, bacteria, and protozoans in pregnancy: a sample of each. *Clin. Obstet. Gynecol.*, 1993 36, 878-885.

[19] Guerina, N. G. Management strategies for infectious diseases in pregnancy. *Semin. Perinatol.*, 1994 18, 305-320.

[20] Puro, V., Scognamiglio, P., Ippolito, G. HIV, HBV, or HDV transmission from infected health care workers to patients. *Med. Lav.*, 2003 94, 556-568.

[21] Ross, R. S. Nosocomial transmission of viruses to pregnant women by infected medical personnel. *Bundesgesundheitsblatt Gesundheitsforschung Gesundheitsschutz*, 2007 50, 1399-1403.

[22] Danzmann, L., Gastmeier, P., Schwab, F., Vonberg, R. P. Health care workers causing large nosocomial outbreaks: a systematic review. *BMC Infect. Dis.*, 2013 13, 98.

[23] Davis, M. S. Occupational hazards of operating: opportunities for improvement. *Infect. Control Hosp. Epidemiol.*, 1996 17, 691-693.

[24] Gelber, S. E., Ratner, A. J. Hospital-acquired viral pathogens in the neonatal intensive care unit. *Semin. Perinatol.*, 2002 26, 346-356.

[25] Anderson, B. L., Cu-Uvin, S. Clinical parameters essential to methodology and interpretation of mucosal responses. *Am. J. Reprod. Immunol.*, 2011 65, 352-360.

[26] Leroy, S. Infectious risk of endovaginal and transrectal ultrasonography: systematic review and meta-analysis. *J. Hosp. Infect.*, 2013 83, 99-106.

[27] Henderson, J. L., Weiner, C. P. Congenital infection. *Curr. Opin. Obstet. Gynecol.*, 1995 7, 130-134.

[28] Weiner, C. P. The elusive search for fetal infection. Changing the gold standards. *Obstet. Gynecol. Clin. North Am.*, 1997 24, 19-32.

[29] Gibbs, R. S. The origins of stillbirth: infectious diseases. *Semin. Perinatol.*, 2002 26, 75-78.

[30] Goldenberg, R. L., Thompson, C. The infectious origins of stillbirth. *Am. J. Obstet. Gynecol.*, 2003 189, 861-873.

[31] Wolfberg, A. J., Dammann, O., Gressens, P. Anti-inflammatory and immunomodulatory strategies to protect the perinatal brain. *Semin. Fetal Neonatal Med.*, 2007 12, 296-302.

[32] Gibson, C. S., MacLennan, A. H., Goldwater, P. N., Dekker, G. A. Antenatal causes of cerebral palsy: associations between inherited thrombophilias, viral and bacterial infection, and inherited susceptibility to infection. *Obstet. Gynecol. Surv.*, 2003 58, 209-220.

[33] Jacobsson, B., Hagberg, G. Antenatal risk factors for cerebral palsy. *Best Pract. Res. Clin. Obstet. Gynaecol.*, 2004 18, 425-436.

[34] Alanen, A. Polymerase chain reaction in the detection of microbes in amniotic fluid. *Ann. Med.*, 1998 30, 288-295.

[35] Bailão, L. A., Osborne, N. G., Rizzi, M. C., Bonilla-Musoles, F., Duarte, G., Bailão, T. C. Ultrasound markers of fetal infection part 1: viral infections. *Ultrasound Q.*, 2005 21, 295-308.

[36] Degani, S. Sonographic findings in fetal viral infections: a systematic review. *Obstet. Gynecol. Surv.*, 2006 61, 329-336.

[37] Weiner, C. P., Grose, C. F., Naides, S. J. Diagnosis of fetal infection in the patient with an ultrasonographically detected abnormality but a negative clinical history. *Am. J. Obstet. Gynecol.*, 1993 168, 6-11.

[38] Gonçalves, L. F., Chaiworapongsa, T., Romero, R. Intrauterine infection and prematurity. *Ment. Retard. Dev. Disabil. Res. Rev.*, 2002 8, 3-13.

[39] Hagberg, H., Peebles, D., Mallard, C. Models of white matter injury: comparison of infectious, hypoxic-ischemic, and excitotoxic insults. *Ment. Retard. Dev. Disabil. Res. Rev.*, 2002 8, 30-38.

[40] Feldman, D. M., Timms, D., Borgida, A. F. Toxoplasmosis, parvovirus, and cytomegalovirus in pregnancy. *Clin. Lab. Med.*, 2010 30, 709-720.

[41] Vrachnis, N., Vitoratos, N., Iliodromiti, Z., Sifakis, S., Deligeoroglou, E., Creatsas, G. Intrauterine inflammation and preterm delivery. *Ann. N. Y. Acad. Sci.*, 2010 1205, 118-122.
[42] Coccia, M. E., Cammilli, F., Ginocchioni, L., Rizzello, F. Role of infection in in vitro fertilization treatment. *Ann. N. Y. Acad. Sci.*, 2004 1034, 219-235.
[43] Keck, C., Gerber-Schäfer, C., Clad, A., Wilhelm, C., Breckwoldt, M. Seminal tract infections: impact on male fertility and treatment options. *Hum. Reprod. Update*, 1998 4, 891-903.
[44] Savasi, V., Ferrazzi, E., Fiore, S. Reproductive assistance for infected couples with bloodborne viruses. *Placenta*, 2008 29 Suppl. B, 160-165.
[45] Englert, Y., Lesage, B., Van Vooren, J. P., Liesnard, C., Place, I., Vannin, A. S., Emiliani, S., Delbaere, A. Medically assisted reproduction in the presence of chronic viral diseases. *Hum. Reprod. Update*, 2004 10, 149-162.
[46] Tulsiani, D. R., Abou-Haila, A. Is sperm capacitation analogous to early phases of Ca^{2+}-triggered membrane fusion in somatic cells and viruses? *Bioessays*, 2004 26, 281-290.
[47] Bronson, R. Biology of the male reproductive tract: its cellular and morphological considerations. *Am. J. Reprod. Immunol.*, 2011 65, 212-219.
[48] Baker, D. A. Antiviral therapy for genital herpes in nonpregnant and pregnant women. *Int. J. Fertil. Womens Med.*, 1998 43, 243-248.
[49] Baker, D. A. The use of antiviral medications in the treatment of herpes simplex virus infections of women. *Int. J. Fertil. Womens Med.*, 1999 44, 227-233.
[50] Money, D. M. Antiviral and antiretroviral use in pregnancy. *Obstet. Gynecol. Clin. North Am.*, 2003 30, 731-749.
[51] Watts, D. H. Antiviral agents. *Obstet. Gynecol. Clin. North Am.*, 1992 19, 563-585.
[52] Von Rheinbaben, F. Virucidal disinfection in gynecology. *Zentralbl Gynakol*, 1992 114, 265-269.
[53] Hubka, T. A., Wisner, K. P., Advisory Committee on Immunization Practices (ACIP) of the Centers for Disease Control and Prevention. Vaccinations recommended during pregnancy and breastfeeding. *J. Am. Osteopath. Assoc.*, 2011 111, S23-S30.
[54] Gall, S. A. Maternal immunization. *Obstet. Gynecol. Clin. North Am.*, 2003 30, 623-636.

[55] Gonik, B. Passive immunization: the forgotten arm of immunologically based strategies for disease containment. *Am. J. Obstet. Gynecol.*, 2011 205, 444.e1-6.

[56] Naz, R. K. Female genital tract immunity: distinct immunological challenges for vaccine development. *J. Reprod. Immunol.*, 2012 93, 1-8.

[57] Fortner, K. B., Kuller, J. A., Rhee, E. J., Edwards, K. M. Influenza and tetanus, diphtheria, and acellular pertussis vaccinations during pregnancy. *Obstet. Gynecol. Surv.*, 2012 67 251-257.

[58] Fox, K. A., Theiler, R. Vaccination in pregnancy. *Curr. Pharm. Biotechnol.*, 2011 12, 789-796.

[59] McGregor, J. A., French, J. I., Spencer, N. E. Prevention of sexually transmitted diseases in women. *Obstet. Gynecol. Clin. North Am.*, 1989 16, 679-702.

[60] Mårdh, P. A. Aetiology, diagnosis and therapy of sexually transmitted and allied infections – Reflections on novel observations and current trends. *Eur. J. Contracept. Reprod. Health Care*, 2006 11, 169-174.

[61] Paavonen, J., Stamm, W. E. Sexually transmitted diseases. Lower genital tract infections in women. *Infect. Dis. Clin. North Am.*, 1987 1, 179-198.

[62] McGregor, J. A., French, J. I., Spencer, N. E. Prevention of sexually transmitted diseases in women. *J. Reprod. Med.*, 1988 33, 109-118.

[63] Spence, M. R. Epidemiology of sexually transmitted diseases. *Obstet. Gynecol. Clin. North Am.*, 1989 16, 453-466.

[64] Sulak, P. J. Sexually transmitted diseases. *Semin. Reprod. Med.*, 2003 21, 399-413.

[65] Hollier, L. M., Workowski, K. Treatment of sexually transmitted infections in women. *Infect. Dis. Clin. North Am.*, 2008 22, 665-691.

[66] Doherty, I. A., Padian, N. S., Marlow, C., Aral, S. O. Determinants and consequences of sexual networks as they affect the spread of sexually transmitted infections. *J. Infect. Dis.*, 2005 191 Suppl. 1, S42-S54.

[67] Peaceman, A. M., Gonik, B. Sexually transmitted viral disease in women. *Postgrad. Med.*, 1991 89, 133-140.

[68] Baker, D. A. Diagnosis and treatment of viral STDs in women. *Int. J. Fertil. Womens Med.*, 1997 42, 107-114.

[69] Hoyme, U. B. Sexually transmitted diseases in adult, non-pregnant women. *Curr. Opin. Obstet. Gynecol.*, 1993 5, 521-526.

[70] Persson, E. Family planning and prevention strategies for sexually transmitted diseases. *Adv. Contracept.*, 1991 7, 181-186.

[71] McGregor, J. A., Hammill, H. A. Contraception and sexually transmitted diseases: interactions and opportunities. *Am. J. Obstet. Gynecol.*, 1993 168, 2033-2041.

[72] Berer, M. Dual protection: more needed than practised or understood. *Reprod. Health Matters*, 2006 14, 162-170.

[73] Stuart, G. S., Castaño, P. M. Sexually transmitted infections and contraceptives: selective issues. *Obstet. Gynecol. Clin. North Am.*, 2003 30, 795-808.

[74] Stone, K. M. Avoiding sexually transmitted diseases. *Obstet. Gynecol. Clin. North Am.*, 1990 17, 789-799.

[75] Hassan, E., Creatsas, G., Gravanis, A., Georgoulias, V., Psychoyos, A. Anti-STD vaginal contraceptive sponges. *Ann. N. Y. Acad. Sci.*, 1997 816, 451-456.

[76] Hatcher, R. A., Warner, D. L. New condoms for men and women, diaphragms, cervical caps, and spermicides: overcoming barriers to barriers and spermicides. *Curr. Opin. Obstet. Gynecol.,* 1992 4, 513-521.

[77] Kirkman, R., Chantler, E. Contraception and the prevention of sexually transmitted diseases. *Br. Med. Bull.*, 1993 49, 171-181.

[78] Creatsas, G. Sexually transmitted diseases and oral contraceptive use during adolescence. *Ann. N. Y. Acad. Sci.*, 1997 816, 404-410.

[79] Creatsas, G. Contraception and sexually transmitted diseases. *Eur. J. Contracept. Reprod. Health Care*, 1997 2, 259-262.

[80] Beksinska, M. E., Smit, J. A., Mantell, J. E. Progress and challenges to male and female condom use in South Africa. *Sex. Health*, 2012 9, 51-58.

[81] Genuis, S. J., Genuis, S. K. Orgasm without organisms: science or propaganda? *Clin. Pediatr.* (Phila.), 1996 35, 10-17.

[82] Lurie, S. Does intercourse during menses increase the risk for sexually transmitted disease? *Arch. Gynecol. Obstet.*, 2010 282, 627-630.

[83] Creatsas, G. K. Sexuality: sexual activity and contraception during adolescence. *Curr. Opin. Obstet. Gynecol.*, 1993 5, 774-783.

[84] Vermillion, S. T., Holmes, M. M., Soper, D. E. Adolescents and sexually transmissible diseases. *Obstet. Gynecol. Clin. North Am.*, 2000 27, 163-179.

[85] Hassan, E. A., Creatsas, G. C. Adolescent sexuality: a developmental milestone or risk-taking behavior? The role of health care in the prevention of sexually transmitted diseases. *J. Pediatr. Adolesc. Gynecol.*, 2000 13, 119-124.

[86] Welner, S. L. Sexually transmitted infections in women with disabilities: diagnosis, treatment, and prevention: a review. *Sex. Transm. Dis.*, 2000 27, 272-277.

[87] Holmes, M. Sexually transmitted infections in female rape victims. *AIDS Patient Care STDS*, 1999 13, 703-708.

[88] Kaye, D. K. Gender inequality and domestic violence: implications for human immunodeficiency virus (HIV) prevention. *Afr. Health Sci.*, 2004 4, 67-70.

[89] Weström, L. V. Sexually transmitted diseases and infertility. *Sex. Transm. Dis.*, 1994 21, S32-S37.

[90] Watts, D. H., Eschenbach, D. A. Sexually transmitted diseases in pregnancy. *Infect. Dis. Clin. North Am.*, 1987 1, 253-275.

[91] Jackson, S. L., Soper, D. E. Sexually transmitted diseases in pregnancy. *Obstet. Gynecol. Clin. North Am.*, 1997 24, 631-644.

[92] Roberts, R., Dinsmore, W. Sexually transmitted diseases in pregnancy. *Br. J. Hosp. Med.*, 1992 47, 674-679.

[93] Wendel, G. D Jr. Sexually transmitted diseases in pregnancy. *Semin. Perinatol.*, 1990 14, 171-178.

[94] Minkoff, H. L. Preventing fetal damage from sexually transmitted diseases. *Clin. Obstet. Gynecol.*, 1991 34, 336-344.

[95] Goldenberg, R. L., Andrews, W. W., Yuan, A. C., MacKay, H. T., St Louis, M. E. Sexually transmitted diseases and adverse outcomes of pregnancy. *Clin. Perinatol.*, 1997 24, 23-41.

[96] Martens, M. G. Office diagnosis of sexually transmitted diseases. *Obstet. Gynecol. Clin. North Am.*, 1989 16, 659-677.

[97] Shih, S. L., Graseck, A. S., Secura, G. M., Peipert, J. F. Screening for sexually transmitted infections at home or in the clinic? *Curr. Opin. Infect. Dis.*, 2011 24, 78-84.

[98] Hollier, L. M., Workowski, K. Treatment of sexually transmitted diseases in women. *Obstet. Gynecol. Clin. North Am.*, 2003 30, 751-775.

[99] Amaral, E. Current approach to STD management in women. *Int. J. Gynaecol. Obstet.*, 1998 63 Suppl. 1, S183-S189.

[100] Brabin, L. Clinical management and prevention of sexually transmitted diseases: a review focusing on women. *Acta Trop.*, 2000 75, 53-70.

[101] Hollier, L. M., Workowski, K. Treatment of sexually transmitted infections in pregnancy. *Clin. Perinatol.*, 2005 32, 629-656.

[102] Genuis, S. J., Genuis, S. K. Managing the sexually transmitted disease pandemic: a time for reevaluation. *Am. J. Obstet. Gynecol.*, 2004 191, 1103-1112.

[103] Genuis, S. J., Genuis, S. K. Primary prevention of sexually transmitted disease: applying the ABC strategy. *Postgrad. Med. J.*, 2005 81, 299-301.

[104] Minkin, M. J. Sexually transmitted infections and the aging female: placing risks in perspective. *Maturitas*, 2010 67, 114-116.

[105] Wenstrom, K. D., Gall, S. A. HIV infection in women. *Obstet. Gynecol. Clin. North Am.*, 1989 16, 627-643.

[106] Lazenby, G. B. Opportunistic infections in women with HIV AIDS. *Clin. Obstet. Gynecol.*, 2012 55, 927-937.

[107] Viscarello, R. R. AIDS. Natural history and prognosis. *Obstet. Gynecol. Clin. North Am.*, 1990 17, 545-555.

[108] Osborne, N. G. AIDS and the obstetrician-gynecologist. *J. Natl. Med. Assoc.*, 1987 79, 1057-1067.

[109] Potts, M. Acquired immunodeficiency syndrome (AIDS): a commentary on the international aspects of the disease. *Int. J. Gynaecol. Obstet.*, 1988 26, 1-3.

[110] Hickl, E. J., Koch, M. G. The AIDS epidemic and its importance in obstetrics and gynecology. *Geburtshilfe Frauenheilkd*, 1989 49, 313-327.

[111] Minkoff, H. L. Care of pregnant women infected with human immunodeficiency virus. *JAMA*, 1987 258, 2714-2717.

[112] Fleming, A. F. AIDS in Africa. *Baillieres Clin. Haematol.*, 1990 3, 177-205.

[113] Chersich, M. F., Rees, H. V. Vulnerability of women in southern Africa to infection with HIV: biological determinants and priority health sector interventions. *AIDS*, 2008 22 Suppl. 4, S27-S40.

[114] Van der Spuy, Z. M. HIV and reproductive health: a South African experience. *Reprod. Biomed. Online*, 2009 18 Suppl. 2, 3-10.

[115] Scorgie, F., Chersich, M. F., Ntaganira, I., Gerbase, A., Lule, F., Lo, Y. R. Socio-demographic characteristics and behavioral risk factors of female sex workers in sub-saharan Africa: a systematic review. *AIDS Behav.*, 2012 16, 920-933.

[116] Allen, M. H. Primary care of women infected with the human immunodeficiency virus. *Obstet. Gynecol. Clin. North Am.*, 1990 17, 557-569.

[117] Minkoff, H. L., DeHovitz, J. A. Care of women infected with the human immunodeficiency virus. *JAMA*, 1991 266, 2253-2258.

[118] Allen, M. H., Marte, C. HIV infection in women: presentations and protocols. *Hosp. Pract.* (Off Ed.), 1992 27, 155-162.

[119] Shah, P. N., Smith, J. R., Kitchen, V. S., Barton, S. E. HIV infection and the gynaecologist. *Br. J. Obstet. Gynaecol.*, 1994 101, 187-189.
[120] Conde, D. M., Silva, E. T., Amaral, W. N., Finotti, M. F., Ferreira, R. G., Costa-Paiva, L., Pinto-Neto, A. M. HIV, reproductive aging, and health implications in women: a literature review. *Menopause*, 2009 16, 199-213.
[121] Cejtin, H. E. Gynecologic issues in the HIV-infected woman. *Infect. Dis. Clin. North Am.*, 2008 22, 709-739.
[122] Agboghoroma, C. O. Gynaecological and reproductive health issues in HIV-positive women. *West Afr. J. Med.*, 2010 29, 135-142.
[123] ACOG Committee on Practice Bulletins – Gynecology. ACOG Practice Bulletin No. 117: Gynecologic care for women with human immunodeficiency virus. *Obstet. Gynecol.*, 2010 116, 1492-1509.
[124] Korn, A. P., Landers, D. V. Gynecologic disease in women infected with human immunodeficiency virus type 1. *J. Acquir. Immune Defic. Syndr. Hum. Retrovirol.,* 1995 9, 361-370.
[125] Carosi, G., Nasta, P., Fiore, S., Matteelli, A., Cauda, R., Ferrazzi, E., Tamburrini, E., Savasi, V., Bini, T., Ravizza, M., Bucceri, A., Vichi, F., Murri, R., Mazzotta, F., d'Arminio Monforte, A., Italian Working Group for the Women with HIV Management Guidelines. Women facing HIV. Key question on women with HIV infection: Italian consensus workshop. *Infection*, 2009 37, 168-178.
[126] Helfgott, A. TORCH testing in HIV-infected women. *Clin. Obstet. Gynecol.*, 1999 42, 149-162.
[127] Thurman, A. R., Doncel, G. F. Herpes simplex virus and HIV: genital infection synergy and novel approaches to dual prevention. *Int. J. STD AIDS*, 2012 23, 613-619.
[128] Ferrero, S., Bertoldi, S., Lungaro, P., Nicoletti, A., Gotta, C., Bentivoglio, G. HIV-HCV co-infection during pregnancy. *Minerva Ginecol.*, 2005 57, 627-635.
[129] Sebitloane, M. H. HIV and gynaecological infections. *Best Pract. Res. Clin. Obstet. Gynaecol.*, 2005 19, 231-241.
[130] Ray, A., Ray, S., George, A. T., Swaminathan, N. Interventions for prevention and treatment of vulvovaginal candidiasis in women with HIV infection. *Cochrane Database Syst. Rev.*, 2011 8, CD008739.
[131] Schust, D. J., Ibana, J. A., Buckner, L. R., Ficarra, M., Sugimoto, J., Amedee, A. M., Quayle, A. J. Potential mechanisms for increased HIV-1 transmission across the endocervical epithelium during C. trachomatis infection. *Curr. HIV Res.*, 2012 10, 218-227.

[132] Korn, A. P. Pelvic inflammatory disease in women infected with HIV. *AIDS Patient Care STDS*, 1998 12, 431-434.

[133] Rojansky, N., Anteby, S. O. Gynecological neoplasias in the patient with HIV infection. *Obstet. Gynecol. Surv.*, 1996 51, 679-683.

[134] Abercrombie, P. D., Korn, A. P. Lower genital tract neoplasia in women with HIV infection. *Oncology* (Williston Park), 1998 12, 1735-1739.

[135] Spitzer, M. Lower genital tract intraepithelial neoplasia in HIV-infected women: guidelines for evaluation and management. *Obstet. Gynecol. Surv.*, 1999 54, 131-137.

[136] Stier, E. Cervical neoplasia and the HIV-infected patient. *Hematol. Oncol. Clin. North Am.*, 2003 17, 873-887.

[137] Chirenje, Z. M. HIV and cancer of the cervix. *Best Pract. Res. Clin. Obstet. Gynaecol.*, 2005 19, 269-276.

[138] Tebeu, P. M., Major, A. L., Mhawech, P., Rapiti, E. The recurrence of cervical intraepithelial neoplasia in HIV-positive women: a review of the literature. *Int. J. STD AIDS*, 2006 17, 507-511.

[139] De Vuyst, H., Lillo, F., Broutet, N., Smith, J. S. HIV, human papillomavirus, and cervical neoplasia and cancer in the era of highly active antiretroviral therapy. *Eur. J. Cancer Prev.*, 2008 17, 545-554.

[140] McKenzie, N. D., Kobetz, E. N., Hnatyszyn, J., Twiggs, L. B., Lucci, J. A. 3rd. Women with HIV are more commonly infected with non-16 and -18 high-risk HPV types. *Gynecol. Oncol.*, 2010 116, 572-577.

[141] Kojic, E. M., Cu-Uvin, S. Update: human papillomavirus infection remains highly prevalent and persistent among HIV-infected individuals. *Curr. Opin. Oncol.*, 2007 19, 464-469.

[142] Del Mistro, A., Chieco Bianchi, L. HPV-related neoplasias in HIV-infected individuals. *Eur. J. Cancer*, 2001 37, 1227-1235.

[143] Stier, E. A., Baranoski, A. S. Human papillomavirus-related diseases in HIV-infected individuals. *Curr. Opin. Oncol.*, 2008 20, 541-546.

[144] Abercrombie, P. D., Korn, A. P. Vulvar intraepithelial neoplasia in women with HIV. *AIDS Patient Care STDS*, 1998 12, 251-254.

[145] Brown, J. E., Sunborg, M. J., Kost, E., Cosin, J. A., Winter, W. E. 3rd. Vulvar cancer in human immunodeficiency virus-seropositive premenopausal women: a case series and review of the literature. *J. Low Genit. Tract. Dis.*, 2005 9, 7-10.

[146] Elit, L., Voruganti, S., Simunovic, M. Invasive vulvar cancer in a woman with human immunodeficiency virus: case report and review of the literature. *Gynecol. Oncol.*, 2005 98, 151-154.

[147] Macasaet, M. A., Duerr, A., Thelmo, W., Vernon, S. D., Unger, E. R. Kaposi sarcoma presenting as a vulvar mass. *Obstet. Gynecol.*, 1995 86, 695-697.

[148] Butler, S. A., Iles, R. K. Ectopic human chorionic gonadotropin beta secretion by epithelial tumors and human chorionic gonadotropin beta-induced apoptosis in Kaposi's sarcoma: is there a connection? *Clin. Cancer Res.*, 2003 9, 4666-4673.

[149] Ojwang, S. B., Otieno, M. R., Khan, K. S. Human immunodeficiency virus in gestational trophoblastic neoplasias – Is it a poor prognostic risk factor. *East Afr. Med. J.*, 1992 69, 647-648.

[150] Cejtin, H. E. Gynecologic issues in the HIV-infected woman. *Obstet. Gynecol. Clin. North Am.,* 2003 30, 711-729.

[151] Conde, D. M., Pinto-Neto, A. M., Costa-Paiva, L. Age at menopause of HIV-infected women: a review. *Gynecol. Endocrinol.*, 2008 24, 84-86.

[152] Fan, M. D., Maslow, B. S., Santoro, N., Schoenbaum, E. HIV and the menopause. *Menopause Int.*, 2008 14, 163-168.

[153] Santoro, N., Fan, M., Maslow, B., Schoenbaum, E. Women and HIV infection: the makings of a midlife crisis. *Maturitas*, 2009 64, 160-164.

[154] Anderson, J. R. Adolescents and human immunodeficiency virus infection. *Curr. Opin. Obstet. Gynecol.*, 1992 4, 849-854.

[155] Henry-Reid, L. M., Martinez, J. Care of the adolescent with HIV. *Clin. Obstet. Gynecol.*, 2008 51, 319-328.

[156] Cohan, D. Perinatal HIV: special considerations. *Top HIV Med.*, 2003 11, 200-213.

[157] Mola, G. HIV infections in obstetrics and gynaecology. *P N G Med. J.*, 1996 39, 190-195.

[158] Doncel, G. F. Exploiting common targets in human fertilization and HIV infection: development of novel contraceptive microbicides. *Hum. Reprod. Update*, 2006 12, 103-117.

[159] Korn, A. P., Abercrombie, P. D. Gynecology and family planning care for the woman infected with HIV. *Obstet. Gynecol. Clin. North Am.*, 1997 24, 855-872.

[160] Agboghoroma, C. O. Contraception in the context of HIV/AIDS: a review. *Afr. J. Reprod. Health*, 2011 15, 15-23.

[161] Heikinheimo, O., Lähteenmäki, P. Contraception and HIV infection in women. *Hum. Reprod. Update*, 2009 15, 165-176.

[162] Cejtin, H. E., Jacobson, L., Springer, G., Watts, D. H., Levine, A., Greenblatt, R., Anastos, K., Minkoff, H. L., Massad, L. S., Schmidt, J.

B. Effect of hormonal contraceptive use on plasma HIV-1-RNA levels among HIV-infected women. *AIDS*, 2003 17, 1702-1704.

[163] Stringer, E., Antonsen, E. Hormonal contraception and HIV disease progression. *Clin. Infect. Dis.*, 2008 47, 945-951.

[164] Robinson, J. A., Jamshidi, R., Burke, A. E. Contraception for the HIV-positive woman: a review of interactions between hormonal contraception and antiretroviral therapy. *Infect. Dis. Obstet. Gynecol.*, 2012 2012, 890160.

[165] Castaño, P. M. Use of intrauterine devices and systems by HIV-infected women. *Contraception*, 2007 75, S51-S54.

[166] Henrion, R., Mandelbrot, L., Firtion, G., Crémieux, N., Henrion-Géant, E. HIV seropositivity and desire for children. *Contracept. Fertil. Sex.*, 1993 21, 217-221.

[167] Politch, J. A., Mayer, K. H., Abbott, A. F., Anderson, D. J. The effects of disease progression and zidovudine therapy on semen quality in human immunodeficiency virus type 1 seropositive men. *Fertil. Steril.*, 1994 61, 922-928.

[168] Pudney, J., Nguyen, H., Xu, C., Anderson, D. J. Microscopic evidence against HIV-1 infection of germ cells or attachment to sperm. *J. Reprod. Immunol.*, 1998 41, 105-125.

[169] Pudney, J., Nguyen, H., Xu, C., Anderson, D. J. Microscopic evidence against HIV-1 infection of germ cells or attachment to sperm. *J. Reprod. Immunol.*, 1999 44, 57-77.

[170] Quayle, A. J., Xu, C., Tucker, L., Anderson, D. J. The case against an association between HIV-1 and sperm: molecular evidence. *J. Reprod. Immunol.*, 1998 41, 127-136.

[171] Chu, M. C., Pena, J. E., Thornton, M. H. 2nd; Sauer, M. V. Assessing the treatment efficacy of IVF with intracytoplasmic sperm injection in human immunodeficiency virus-1 (HIV-1) serodiscordant couples. *Reprod. Biomed. Online*, 2005 10, 130-134.

[172] Sauer, M. V. Sperm washing techniques address the fertility needs of HIV-seropositive men: a clinical review. *Reprod. Biomed. Online*, 2005 10, 135-140.

[173] Agboghoroma, C. O., Giwa-Osagie, O. F. Management of infertility in HIV infected couples: a review. *Afr. J. Reprod. Health*, 2012 16, 13-20.

[174] Sauer, M. V. American physicians remain slow to embrace the reproductive needs of human immunodeficiency virus-infected patients. *Fertil. Steril.*, 2006 85, 295-297.

[175] Mmeje, O., Cohen, C. R., Cohan, D. Evaluating safer conception options for HIV-serodiscordant couples (HIV-infected female/HIV-uninfected male): a closer look at vaginal insemination. *Infect. Dis. Obstet. Gynecol.*, 2012 2012, 587651.

[176] Feinkind, L., Minkoff, H. L. HIV in pregnancy. *Clin. Perinatol.*, 1988 15, 189-202.

[177] Dinsmoor, M. J. HIV infection and pregnancy. *Med. Clin. North Am.*, 1989 73, 701-711.

[178] Coyne, B. A., Landers, D. V. The immunology of HIV disease and pregnancy and possible interactions. *Obstet. Gynecol. Clin. North Am.*, 1990 17, 595-606.

[179] Valente, P., Main, E. K. Role of the placenta in perinatal transmission of HIV. *Obstet. Gynecol. Clin. North Am.*, 1990 17, 607-616.

[180] MacGregor, S. N. Human immunodeficiency virus infection in pregnancy. *Clin. Perinatol.*, 1991 18, 33-50.

[181] Sperling, R S. Human immunodeficiency virus and the acquired immunodeficiency syndrome in obstetrics. *Curr. Opin. Obstet. Gynecol.*, 1991 3, 692-697.

[182] Sperling, R. S., Stratton, P. Treatment options for human immunodeficiency virus-infected pregnant women. Obstetric-Gynecologic Working Group of the AIDS Clinical Trials Group of the National Institute of Allergy and Infectious Diseases. *Obstet. Gynecol.*, 1992 79, 443-448.

[183] Johnstone, F. D. Management of pregnancy in women with HIV infection. *Br. J. Hosp. Med.*, 1992 48, 664-665.

[184] Dinsmoor, M. J. HIV infection and pregnancy. *Clin. Perinatol.*, 1994 21, 85-94.

[185] Zorrilla, C. D. Obstetric factors and mother-to-infant transmission of HIV-1. *Infect. Dis. Clin. North Am.*, 1997 11, 109-118.

[186] Lindsay, M. K., Nesheim, S. R. Human immunodeficiency virus infection in pregnant women and their newborns. *Clin. Perinatol.*, 1997 24, 161-180.

[187] Minkoff, H. L. Human immunodeficiency virus infection in pregnancy. *Semin. Perinatol.*, 1998 22, 293-308.

[188] Groginsky, E., Bowdler, N., Yankowitz, J. Update on vertical HIV transmission. *J. Reprod. Med.*, 1998 43, 637-646.

[189] Phuapradit, W. Timing and mechanism of perinatal human immunodeficiency virus-1 infection. *Aust. N. Z. J. Obstet. Gynaecol.*, 1998 38, 293-297.

[190] Zorrilla, C. D. Mother-to-child HIV-1 transmission: state of the art and implications for public policy. *P. R. Health Sci. J.*, 2000 19, 29-34.
[191] Krist, A. H. Obstetric care in patients with HIV disease. *Am. Fam. Physician*, 2001 63, 107-116.
[192] Lindsay, M. K. Prevention of perinatal HIV infection: cause for optimism. *AIDS Clin. Care*, 1999 11, 95-9.
[193] Goldenberg, R. L., Stringer, J. S., Sinkala, M., Vermund, S. H. Perinatal HIV transmission: developing country considerations. *J. Matern. Fetal Neonatal. Med.*, 2002 12, 149-158.
[194] Minkoff, H. Human immunodeficiency virus infection in pregnancy. *Obstet. Gynecol.*, 2003 101, 797-810.
[195] Moodley, J., Moodley, D. Management of human immunodeficiency virus infection in pregnancy. *Best Pract. Res. Clin. Obstet. Gynaecol.*, 2005 19, 169-183.
[196] Anderson, B. L., Cu-Uvin, S. Pregnancy and optimal care of HIV-infected patients. *Clin. Infect. Dis.*, 2009 48, 449-455.
[197] Morfaw, F. L., Thabane, L., Mbuagbaw, L C., Nana, P. N. Male participation in prevention programmes of mother to child transmission of HIV: a protocol for a systematic review to identify barriers, facilitators and reported interventions. *Syst. Rev.*, 2012 1, 13.
[198] Vallone, C., Rigon, G., Lucantoni, V., Putignani, L., Signore, F. Pregnancy in HIV-positive patients: effects on vaginal flora. *Infect. Dis. Obstet. Gynecol.*, 2012 2012, 287849.
[199] Minkoff, H., Mofenson, L. M. The role of obstetric interventions in the prevention of pediatric human immunodeficiency virus infection. *Am. J. Obstet. Gynecol.*, 1994 171, 1167-1175.
[200] Sison, A. V., Campos, J. M. Laboratory methods for early detection of human immunodeficiency virus type 1 in newborns and infants. *Clin. Microbiol. Rev.*, 1992 5, 238-247.
[201] Young, S. L., Mbuya, M. N., Chantry, C. J., Geubbels, E. P., Israel-Ballard, K., Cohan, D., Vosti, S. A., Latham, M. C. Current knowledge and future research on infant feeding in the context of HIV: basic, clinical, behavioral, and programmatic perspectives. *Adv. Nutr.*, 2011 2, 225-243.
[202] Clark, J., Lampe, M. A., Jamieson, D. J. Testing women for human immunodeficiency virus infection: who, when, and how? *Clin. Obstet. Gynecol.*, 2008 51, 507-517.
[203] Merhi, Z., Minkoff, H. Rapid HIV screening for women in labor. *Expert Rev. Mol. Diagn.*, 2005 5, 673-679.

[204] Moodley, J., Wennberg, J. L. HIV in pregnancy. *Curr. Opin. Obstet. Gynecol.*, 2005 17, 117-121.

[205] Giles, M. HIV and pregnancy: screening and management update. *Curr. Opin. Obstet. Gynecol.*, 2009 21, 131-135.

[206] Parisaei, M., Hemelaar, J., Govind, A. HIV in pregnancy: a case of Pneumocystis (carinii) jiroveci pneumonia. *Arch. Gynecol. Obstet.*, 2010 281, 1-3.

[207] Kästner, R., Härtl, K., Knobbe, A., Grubert, T. A., Stauber, M. Specific concepts of care for pregnant women with drug addiction or HIV infection. *Zentralbl Gynakol*, 2001 123, 48-50.

[208] Jones, T. B. Psychosocial dimensions of HIV infection in pregnancy. *Clin. Obstet. Gynecol.*, 2008 51, 456-466.

[209] Psaros, C., Geller, P. A., Aaron, E. The importance of identifying and treating depression in HIV infected, pregnant women: a review. *J. Psychosom. Obstet. Gynaecol.*, 2009 30, 275-281.

[210] Baker, D. A. Management of the female HIV-infected patient. *AIDS Res. Hum. Retroviruses*, 1994 10, 935-938.

[211] Drake, K., Youchah, J., Damus, K. Human immunodeficiency virus disease in pregnancy. *J. Assoc. Acad. Minor Phys.*, 1995 6, 105-111.

[212] De Santis, M., Noia, G., Caruso, A., Mancuso, S. Guidelines for the use of zidovudine in pregnant women with HIV infection. *Drugs*, 1995 50, 43-47.

[213] Rouse, D. J., Owen, J., Goldenberg, R. L., Vermund, S. H. Zidovudine for the prevention of vertical HIV transmission: a decision analytic approach. *J. Acquir. Immune Defic. Syndr. Hum. Retrovirol.*, 1995 9, 401-407.

[214] Minkoff, H., Augenbraun, M. Antiretroviral therapy for pregnant women. *Am. J. Obstet. Gynecol.*, 1997 176, 478-489.

[215] Dattel, B. J. Antiretroviral therapy during pregnancy. Beyond AZT (ZDV). *Obstet. Gynecol. Clin. North Am.*, 1997 24, 645-657.

[216] Sperling, R. Zidovudine. *Infect. Dis. Obstet. Gynecol.*, 1998 6, 197-203.

[217] Zorrilla, C. D. Antiretroviral combination therapy in HIV-1 infected women and men: are their responses different? *Int. J. Fertil. Womens Med.*, 2000 45, 195-199.

[218] Stek, A. M. Antiretroviral medications during pregnancy for therapy or prophylaxis. *Curr. HIV/AIDS Rep.*, 2009 6, 68-76.

[219] Delke, I. Special considerations for the HIV-infected patient with preterm labor. *Clin. Perinatol.*, 2003 30, 855-874.

[220] Bera, E., Mia, R. Safety of nevirapine in HIV-infected pregnant women initiating antiretroviral therapy at higher CD4 counts: a systematic review and meta-analysis. *S. Afr. Med. J.*, 2012 102, 855-859.

[221] Chirenje, Z. M., Marrazzo, J., Parikh, U. M. Antiretroviral-based HIV prevention strategies for women. *Expert Rev. Anti Infect. Ther.*, 2010 8, 1177-1186.

[222] Okwundu, C. I., Okoromah, C. A. Antiretroviral pre-exposure prophylaxis (PrEP) for preventing HIV in high-risk individuals. *Cochrane Database Syst. Rev.*, 2009 1, CD007189.

[223] Short, R. V. New ways of preventing HIV infection: thinking simply, simply thinking. *Philos. Trans. R. Soc. Lond. B Biol. Sci.,* 2006 361, 811-820.

[224] Hillier, S. L., Moench, T., Shattock, R., Black, R., Reichelderfer, P., Veronese, F. In vitro and in vivo: the story of nonoxynol 9. *J. Acquir. Immune Defic. Syndr.*, 2005 39, 1-8.

[225] Harper, C. C., Holt, K., Nhemachena, T., Chipato, T., Ramjee, G., Stratton, L., Blum, M., McCulloch, C. E., Mgweba, S., Blanchard, K. Willingness of clinicians to integrate microbicides into HIV prevention practices in southern Africa. *AIDS Behav.*, 2012 16, 1821-1829.

[226] Dezzutti, C. S., Hladik, F. Use of human mucosal tissue to study HIV-1 pathogenesis and evaluate HIV-1 prevention modalities. *Curr. HIV/ AIDS Rep.*, 2013 10, 12-20.

[227] Fichorova, R. N. Guiding the vaginal microbicide trials with biomarkers of inflammation. *J. Acquir. Immune Defic. Syndr.*, 2004 37 Suppl. 3, S 184-S193.

[228] Xu, X., Patel, D. A., Dalton, V. K., Pearlman, M. D., Johnson, T. R. Can routine neonatal circumcision help prevent human immunodeficiency virus transmission in the United States? *Am. J. Mens Health*, 2009 3, 79-84.

[229] Friend, D. R. Drug delivery in multiple indication (multipurpose) prevention technologies: systems to prevent HIV-1 transmission and unintended pregnancies or HSV-2 transmission. *Expert Opin. Drug Deliv.*, 2012 9, 417-427.

[230] Crombleholme, W. R. HIV infection. Managing exposure risks for the obstetrician/gynecologist. *Obstet. Gynecol. Clin. North Am.*, 1990 17, 627-636.

[231] Hirsch, H. A. Prevention of HIV infections in surgical gynecology and obstetrics. *Geburtshilfe Frauenheilkd*, 1990 50, 665-669.

[232] Hemsell, D. L. HIV and blood-borne diseases in relation to gynecologic surgery. *Curr. Opin. Obstet. Gynecol.*, 1993 5, 340-345.

[233] Safer needles work, but not penetrating market. *AIDS Alert*, 1997 12, 27-30.

[234] Levison, J. The ostrich syndrome: obstetrician gynecologists and human immunodeficiency virus exposure. *Obstet. Gynecol.*, 2008 111, 183-186.

[235] Cook, R J., Dickens, B. M. Patient care and the health-impaired practitioner. *Int. J. Gynaecol. Obstet.*, 2002 78, 171-177.

[236] Nolan, K. Human immunodeficiency virus infection, women, and pregnancy. Ethical issues. *Obstet. Gynecol. Clin. North Am.*, 1990 17, 651-668.

[237] Oldenettel, D., Dye, T. D., Artal, R. Prenatal HIV screening in pregnant women: a medical-legal review. *Birth*, 1997 24, 165-172.

[238] American College of Obstetrics and Gynecology. ACOG Committee Opinion No. 389, December 2007. Human immunodeficiency virus. *Obstet. Gynecol.*, 2007 110, 1473-1478.

[239] Thurman, A. R., Doncel, G. F. Innate immunity and inflammatory response to Trichomonas vaginalis and bacterial vaginosis: relationship to HIV acquisition. *Am. J. Reprod. Immunol.*, 2011 65, 89-98.

[240] Doncel, G. F., Joseph, T., Thurman, A. R. Role of semen in HIV-1 transmission: inhibitor or facilitator? *Am. J. Reprod. Immunol.*, 2011 65, 292-301.

[241] Doncel, G. F., Clark, M. R. Preclinical evaluation of anti-HIV microbicide products: New models and biomarkers. *Antiviral Res.*, 2010 88 Suppl. 1, S10-S18.

[242] Hladik, F., Doncel, G. F. Preventing mucosal HIV transmission with topical microbicides: challenges and opportunities. *Antiviral Res.*, 2010 88 Suppl. 1, S3-S9.

[243] Friend, D. R., Doncel, G. F. Combining prevention of HIV-1, other sexually transmitted infections and unintended pregnancies: Development of dual-protection technologies. *Antiviral Res.*, 2010 88 Suppl. 1, S47-S54.

[244] Moodley, J., Pattinson, R. C., Baxter, C., Sibeko, S., Abdool Karim, Q. Strengthening HIV services for pregnant women: an opportunity to reduce maternal mortality rates in Southern Africa/sub-Saharan Africa. *BJOG*, 2011 118, 219-225.

[245] Anderson, D., Politch, J. A., Pudney, J. HIV infection and immune defense of the penis. *Am. J. Reprod. Immunol.*, 2011 65, 220-229.

[246] Kushnir, V. A., Lewis, W. Human immunodeficiency virus/acquired immunodeficiency syndrome and infertility: emerging problems in the era of highly active antiretrovirals. *Fertil. Steril.*, 2011 96, 546-553.
[247] Onyangunga, O. A., Moodley, J. Managing pregnancy with HIV, HELLP syndrome and low platelets. *Best Pract. Res. Clin. Obstet. Gynaecol.*, 2012 26, 133-147.
[248] Hemelaar, J. The origin and diversity of the HIV-1 pandemic. *Trends Mol. Med.*, 2012 18, 182-192.
[249] Cejtin, H. E. Care of the human immunodeficiency virus-infected menopausal woman. *Am. J. Obstet. Gynecol.*, 2012 207, 87-93.
[250] Willers, D. M., Kizer, N., Schon, S., Keegan, M. B. Discussion: "Abnormal anal cytology in HIV-infected women" by Baranoski et al. *Am. J. Obstet. Gynecol.*, 2012 207, e1-3.
[251] Venkatesh, K. K., Cu-Uvin, S. Assessing the relationship between cervical ectopy and HIV susceptibility: implications for HIV prevention in women. *Am. J. Reprod. Immunol.*, 2013 69 Suppl. 1, 68-73.
[252] Diouf, K., Nour, N. Female genital cutting and HIV transmission: is there an association? *Am. J. Reprod. Immunol.*, 2013 69 Suppl. 1, 45-50.
[253] Denny, L. A., Franceschi, S., de Sanjosé, S., Heard, I., Moscicki, A. B, Palefsky, J. Human papillomavirus, human immunodeficiency virus and immunosuppression. *Vaccine*, 2012 30 Suppl. 5, F168-F174.
[254] Spitzer, M., Krumholz, B. A. Human papillomavirus-related diseases in the female patient. *Urol. Clin. North Am.*, 1992 19, 71-82.
[255] Paavonen, J. Human papillomavirus infection and the development of cervical cancer and related genital neoplasias. *Int. J. Infect. Dis.*, 2007 11 Suppl. 2, S3-S9.
[256] Ault, K. A. Human papillomavirus vaccines and the potential for cross-protection between related HPV types. *Gynecol. Oncol.*, 2007 107, S31-S33.
[257] Hines, J. F., Jenson, A. B., Barnes, W. A. Human papillomaviruses: their clinical significance in the management of cervical carcinoma. *Oncology* (Williston Park), 1995 9, 279-285.
[258] Lancaster, W. D., Jenson, A. B. Natural history of human papillomavirus infection of the anogenital tract. *Cancer Metastasis Rev.*, 1987 6, 653-664.
[259] American College of Obstetricians and Gynecologists. ACOG Practice Bulletin. Clinical Management Guidelines for Obstetrician-Gynecologists. Number 61, April 2005. Human papillomavirus. *Obstet. Gynecol.,* 2005 105, 905-918.

[260] Committee on Practice Bulletins – Gynecology. ACOG Practice Bulletin Number 131: Screening for cervical cancer. *Obstet. Gynecol.*, 2012 120, 1222-1238.

[261] Cox, J. T. Epidemiology and natural history of HPV. *J. Fam. Pract.*, 2006 Suppl., 3-9.

[262] Myers, E. R., McCrory, D. C., Nanda, K., Bastian, L., Matchar, D. B. Mathematical model for the natural history of human papillomavirus infection and cervical carcinogenesis. *Am. J. Epidemiol.*, 2000 151, 1158-1171.

[263] Anorlu, R. I. Cervical cancer: the sub-Saharan African perspective. *Reprod. Health Matters*, 2008 16, 41-49.

[264] Seoud, M. Burden of human papillomavirus-related cervical disease in the extended middle East and north Africa-a comprehensive literature review. *J. Low Genit. Tract. Dis.*, 2012 16, 106-120.

[265] Matsukura, T., Sugase, M. Pitfalls in the epidemiologic classification of human papillomavirus types associated with cervical cancer using polymerase chain reaction: driver and passenger. *Int. J. Gynecol. Cancer*, 2008 18, 1042-1050.

[266] Cox, J. T. Epidemiology of cervical intraepithelial neoplasia: the role of human papillomavirus. *Baillieres Clin. Obstet. Gynaecol.*, 1995 9, 1-37.

[267] Ault, K. A. Epidemiology and natural history of human papillomavirus infections in the female genital tract. *Infect. Dis. Obstet. Gynecol.*, 2006 2006 Suppl., 40470.

[268] Gadducci, A., Barsotti, C., Cosio, S., Domenici, L., Riccardo Genazzani, A. Smoking habit, immune suppression, oral contraceptive use, and hormone replacement therapy use and cervical carcinogenesis: a review of the literature. *Gynecol. Endocrinol.*, 2011 27, 597-604.

[269] Reid, R. Human papillomaviral infection. The key to rational triage of cervical neoplasia. *Obstet. Gynecol. Clin. North Am.*, 1987 14, 407-429.

[270] Ambros, R. A., Kurman, R. J. Current concepts in the relationship of human papillomavirus infection to the pathogenesis and classification of precancerous squamous lesions of the uterine cervix. *Semin. Diagn. Pathol.*, 1990 7, 158-172.

[271] Schneider, A., Koutsky, L. A. Natural history and epidemiological features of genital HPV infection. *IARC Sci. Publ.*, 1992 119, 25-52.

[272] Huh, W. K. Human papillomavirus infection: a concise review of natural history. *Obstet. Gynecol.*, 2009 114, 139-143.

[273] Reid, R. The management of genital condylomas, intraepithelial neoplasia, and vulvodynia. *Obstet. Gynecol. Clin. North Am.*, 1996 23, 917-991.
[274] Bornstein, J., Rahat, M. A., Abramovici, H. Etiology of cervical cancer: current concepts. *Obstet. Gynecol. Surv.*, 1995 50, 146-154.
[275] Heilmann, V., Kreienberg, R. Molecular biology of cervical cancer and its precursors. *Curr. Womens Health Rep.*, 2002 2, 27-33.
[276] Furumoto, H., Irahara, M. Human papilloma virus (HPV) and cervical cancer. *J. Med. Invest.*, 2002 49, 124-133.
[277] Motoyama, S., Ladines-Llave, C. A., Luis Villanueva, S., Maruo, T. The role of human papilloma virus in the molecular biology of cervical carcinogenesis. *Kobe. J. Med. Sci.*, 2004 50, 9-19.
[278] Moodley, M. Update on pathophysiologic mechanisms of human papillomavirus. *Curr. Opin. Obstet. Gynecol.*, 2005 17, 61-64.
[279] Yim, E. K., Park, J. S. Role of proteomics in translational research in cervical cancer. *Expert Rev. Proteomics*, 2006 3, 21-36.
[280] Lu, Q., Ma, D., Zhao, S. DNA methylation changes in cervical cancers. *Methods Mol. Biol.*, 2012 863, 155-176.
[281] Cai, Q., Lv, L., Shao, Q., Li, X., Dian, A. Human papillomavirus early proteins and apoptosis. *Arch. Gynecol. Obstet.*, 2013 287, 541-548.
[282] Gissmann, L. Immunologic responses to human papillomavirus infection. *Obstet. Gynecol. Clin. North Am.*, 1996 23, 625-639.
[283] Sheu, B. C., Chang, W. C., Lin, H. H., Chow, S. N., Huang, S. C. Immune concept of human papillomaviruses and related antigens in local cancer milieu of human cervical neoplasia. *J. Obstet. Gynaecol. Res.*, 2007 33, 103-113.
[284] Sasagawa, T., Takagi, H., Makinoda, S. Immune responses against human papillomavirus (HPV) infection and evasion of host defense in cervical cancer. *J. Infect. Chemother.*, 2012 18, 807-815.
[285] Sillman, F. H., Sedlis, A. Anogenital papillomavirus infection and neoplasia in immunodeficient women. *Obstet. Gynecol. Clin. North Am.*, 1987 14, 537-558.
[286] Sillman, F. H., Sentovich, S., Shaffer, D. Ano-genital neoplasia in renal transplant patients. *Ann. Transplant.*, 1997 2, 59-66.
[287] Moodley, M., Moodley, J., Chetty, R., Herrington, C. S. The role of steroid contraceptive hormones in the pathogenesis of invasive cervical cancer: a review. *Int. J. Gynecol. Cancer*, 2003 13, 103-110.
[288] Moodley, J. Combined oral contraceptives and cervical cancer. *Curr. Opin. Obstet. Gynecol.*, 2004 16, 27-29.

[289] Richart, R. M., Masood, S., Syrjänen, K. J., Vassilakos, P., Kaufman, R. H., Meisels, A., Olszewski, W. T., Sakamoto, A., Stoler, M. H., Vooijs, G. P., Wilbur, D. C. Human papillomavirus. International Academy of Cytology Task Force summary. Diagnostic Cytology Towards the 21st Century: An International Expert Conference and Tutorial. *Acta Cytol.*, 1998 42, 50-58.

[290] Leroy, J. L., Vinatier, D., Collier, F., Thomas, P. Diagnosis of vulvar intraepithelial neoplasias (VIN). *Gynecol. Obstet. Fertil.*, 2008 36, 190-199.

[291] Joura, E. A. Epidemiology, diagnosis and treatment of vulvar intraepithelial neoplasia. *Curr. Opin. Obstet. Gynecol.*, 2002 14, 39-43.

[292] Daayana, S., Winters, U., Stern, P. L., Kitchener, H. C. Clinical and immunological response to photodynamic therapy in the treatment of vulval intraepithelial neoplasia. *Photochem. Photobiol. Sci.*, 2011 10, 802-809.

[293] Kurman, R. J., Trimble, C. L., Shah, K. V. Human papillomavirus and the pathogenesis of vulvar carcinoma. *Curr. Opin. Obstet. Gynecol.*, 1992 4, 582-585.

[294] Ansink, A. C., Heintz, A. P. Epidemiology and etiology of squamous cell carcinoma of the vulva. *Eur. J. Obstet. Gynecol. Reprod. Biol.*, 1993 48, 111-115.

[295] Monk, B. J., Burger, R. A., Lin, F., Parham, G., Vasilev, S. A., Wilczynski, S. P. Prognostic significance of human papillomavirus DNA in vulvar carcinoma. *Obstet. Gynecol.*, 1995 85, 709-715.

[296] Rosenthal, A. N., Hopster, D., Ryan, A., Jacobs, I. J. Immunohistochemical analysis of p53 in vulval intraepithelial neoplasia and vulval squamous cell carcinoma. *Br. J. Cancer*, 2003 88, 251-256.

[297] Maclean, A. B., Jones, R. W., Scurry, J., Neill, S. Vulvar cancer and the need for awareness of precursor lesions. *J. Low Genit. Tract. Dis.*, 2009 13, 115-117.

[298] Goodman, A. Primary vaginal cancer. *Surg. Oncol. Clin. N. Am.*, 1998 7, 347-361.

[299] Verguts, J., Amant, F., Moerman, P., Vergote, I. HPV induced ovarian squamous cell carcinoma: case report and review of the literature. *Arch. Gynecol. Obstet.*, 2007 276, 285-289.

[300] Kaminski, P. F., Lyon, D. S., Sorosky, J. I., Wheelock, J. B., Podczaski, E. S. Significance of atypical cervical cytology in pregnancy. *Am. J. Perinatol.*, 1992 9, 340-343.

[301] Kosko, J. R., Derkay, C. S. Role of cesarean section in prevention of recurrent respiratory papillomatosis: is there one? *Int. J. Pediatr. Otorhinolaryngol.*, 1996 35, 31-38.
[302] Jayasinghe, Y., Garland, S. M. Genital warts in children: what do they mean? *Arch. Dis. Child*, 2006 91, 696-700.
[303] Bartholomew, D. A. Human papillomavirus infection in adolescents: a rational approach. *Adolesc. Med. Clin.*, 2004 15, 569-595.
[304] Campion, M. J. Clinical manifestations and natural history of genital human papillomavirus infection. *Obstet. Gynecol. Clin. North Am.*, 1987 14, 363-388.
[305] Campion, M. J. Clinical manifestations and natural history of genital human papillomavirus infection. *Dermatol. Clin.*, 1991 9, 235-249.
[306] Campion, M. J., Greenberg, M. D., Kazamel, T. I. Clinical manifestations and natural history of genital human papillomavirus infections. *Obstet. Gynecol. Clin. North Am.*, 1996 23, 783-809.
[307] Zanotti, K. M., Belinson, J. Update on the diagnosis and treatment of human papillomavirus infection. *Cleve. Clin. J. Med.,* 2002 69, 948.
[308] Sevin, B. U. Social implications of sexually transmitted cancer. *J. Womens Health Gend. Based Med.*, 1999 8, 759-766.
[309] Tristram, A. HPV information needs. *Best Pract. Res. Clin. Obstet. Gynaecol.*, 2006 20, 267-277.
[310] Herzog, T. J., Wright, J. D. The impact of cervical cancer on quality of life – The components and means for management. *Gynecol. Oncol.*, 2007 107, 572-527.
[311] Graziottin, A., Serafini, A. HPV infection in women: psychosexual impact of genital warts and intraepithelial lesions. *J. Sex. Med.*, 2009 6, 633-645.
[312] Bloch, B., Dehaeck, C. M. Human papillomavirus and the squamous epithelium of the female genital tract. *S. Afr. Med. J.*, 1987 72, 557-558.
[313] Fowler, J. Screening for cervical cancer. Current terminology, classification, and technique. *Postgrad. Med.*, 1993 93, 57-64.
[314] Schneider, A. Virologic screening. *Eur. J. Obstet. Gynecol. Reprod. Biol.*, 1996 65, 61-63.
[315] Ferenczy, A., Jenson, A. B. Tissue effects and host response. The key to the rational triage of cervical neoplasia. *Obstet. Gynecol. Clin. North Am.,* 1996 23, 759-782.
[316] Cox, J. T. Clinical role of HPV testing. *Obstet. Gynecol. Clin. North Am.,* 1996 23, 811-851.

[317] Cain, J. M., Howett, M. K. Preventing cervical cancer. *Science*, 2000 288, 1753-1755.

[318] Trofatter, K. F. Jr. Diagnosis of human papillomavirus genital tract infection. *Am. J. Med.*, 1997 102, 21-27.

[319] Spitzer, M. Cervical screening adjuncts: recent advances. *Am. J. Obstet. Gynecol.*, 1998 179, 544-556.

[320] Kaufman, R. H., Adam, E. Is human papillomavirus testing of value in clinical practice? *Am. J. Obstet. Gynecol.*, 1999 180, 1049-1053.

[321] Ledger, W. J., Jeremias, J., Witkin, S. S. Testing for high-risk human papillomavirus types will become a standard of clinical care. *Am. J. Obstet. Gynecol.*, 2000 182, 860-865.

[322] Bovicelli, A., Bristow, R. E., Montz, F. J. HPV testing: where are we now? *Anticancer Res.*, 2000 20, 4673-4680.

[323] Ball, C., Madden, J. E. Update on cervical cancer screening. Current diagnostic and evidence-based management protocols. *Postgrad. Med.*, 2003 113, 59-64.

[324] Van Hamont, D., Bekkers, R. L., Massuger, L. F., Melchers, W. J. Detection, management, and follow-up of pre-malignant cervical lesions and the role for human papillomavirus. *Rev. Med. Virol.*, 2008 18, 117-132.

[325] Cox, J. T., American Society for Colposcopy and Cervical Pathology. The clinician's view: role of human papillomavirus testing in the American Society for Colposcopy and Cervical Pathology Guidelines for the management of abnormal cervical cytology and cervical cancer precursors. *Arch. Pathol. Lab. Med.*, 2003 127, 950-958.

[326] Falkner, C. A., Walker, J. L. Management of atypical and low-grade cervical cytology. *Cancer J.*, 2003 9, 377-381.

[327] Spitzer, M., Apgar, B. S., Brotzman, G. L. Management of histologic abnormalities of the cervix. *Am. Fam. Physician*, 2006 73, 105-112.

[328] Moore, K. N., Walker, J. L. High risk human papillomavirus testing: guidelines for use in screening, triage, and follow-up for the prevention and early detection of cervical cancer. *J. Natl. Compr. Canc. Netw.*, 2004 2, 589-596.

[329] Crosbie, E. J., Kitchener, H. C. Human papillomavirus in cervical screening and vaccination. *Clin. Sci.* (Lond.), 2006 110, 543-552.

[330] Koliopoulos, G., Arbyn, M., Martin-Hirsch, P., Kyrgiou, M., Prendiville, W., Paraskevaidis, E. Diagnostic accuracy of human papillomavirus testing in primary cervical screening: a systematic review and meta-

analysis of non-randomized studies. *Gynecol. Oncol.*, 2007 104, 232-246.

[331] Spitzer, M. Screening and management of women and girls with human papillomavirus infection. *Gynecol. Oncol.*, 2007 107, S14-S18.

[332] Chelmow, D., Waxman, A., Cain, J. M., Lawrence, H. C. 3rd. The evolution of cervical screening and the specialty of obstetrics and gynecology. *Obstet. Gynecol.*, 2012 119, 695-699.

[333] Lui, R. Clinical utility of HPV testing. *Clin. Obstet. Gynecol.*, 2013 56, 17-24.

[334] Garrett, L. A., McCann, C. K. Abnormal cytology in 2012: management of atypical squamous cells, low-grade intraepithelial neoplasia, and high-grade intraepithelial neoplasia. *Clin. Obstet. Gynecol.*, 2013 56, 25-34.

[335] Cronjé, H. S. Screening for cervical cancer in developing countries. *Int. J. Gynaecol. Obstet.*, 2004 84, 101-108.

[336] Cronjé, H. S. Screening for cervical cancer in the developing world. *Best Pract. Res. Clin. Obstet. Gynaecol.*, 2005 19, 517-529.

[337] Hoppenot, C., Stampler, K., Dunton, C. Cervical cancer screening in high- and low-resource countries: implications and new developments. *Obstet. Gynecol. Surv.*, 2012 67, 658-667.

[338] Breitenecker, G., Gitsch, G. What's new in diagnosis and treatment of HPV-associated cervical lesions. *Pathol. Res. Pract.*, 1992 188, 242-247.

[339] Reid, R. Biology and colposcopic features of human papillomavirus-associated cervical disease. *Obstet. Gynecol. Clin. North Am.*, 1993 20, 123-151.

[340] Powell, J. L. Pitfalls in cervical colposcopy. *Obstet. Gynecol. Clin. North Am.*, 1993 20, 177-188.

[341] Prendiville, W. Recent innovations in colposcopy practice. *Best Pract. Res. Clin. Obstet. Gynaecol.*, 2005 19, 779-792.

[342] Gagné, H. M. Colposcopy of the vagina and vulva. *Obstet. Gynecol. Clin. North Am.*, 2008 35, 659-669.

[343] Tsoumpou, I., Arbyn, M., Kyrgiou, M., Wentzensen, N., Koliopoulos, G., Martin-Hirsch, P., Malamou-Mitsi, V., Paraskevaidis, E. p16(INK4a) immunostaining in cytological and histological specimens from the uterine cervix: a systematic review and meta-analysis. *Cancer Treat. Rev.*, 2009 35, 210-220.

[344] Tworek, J. A., Henry, M. R., Blond, B., Jones, B. A. College of American Pathologists Gynecologic Cytopathology Quality Consensus Conference on good laboratory practices in gynecologic cytology:

background, rationale, and organization. *Arch. Pathol. Lab. Med.*, 2013 137, 158-163.

[345] Brainard, J. A., Birdsong, G. G., Elsheikh, T. M., Hartley, D. A., Naik, K., Neal, M. H., Souers, R. J., Henry, M. R. Prospective and retrospective review of gynecologic cytopathology: findings from the College of American Pathologists Gynecologic Cytopathology Quality Consensus Conference working group 2. *Arch. Pathol. Lab. Med.*, 2013 137, 175-182.

[346] Booth, C. N., Bashleben, C., Filomena, C. A., Means, M. M., Wasserman, P. G., Souers, R. J., Henry, M. R. Monitoring and ordering practices for human papillomavirus in cervical cytology: findings from the College of American Pathologists Gynecologic Cytopathology Quality Consensus Conference working group 5. *Arch. Pathol. Lab. Med.*, 2013 137, 214-219.

[347] Ostör, A. G., Mulvany, N. The pathology of cervical neoplasia. *Curr. Opin. Obstet. Gynecol.*, 1996 8, 69-73.

[348] Cervical cancer. *NIH Consens Statement*, 1996 14, 1-38.

[349] Kitchener, H. Evidence-based medicine applied to cervical cancer. *Virus Res.*, 2002 89, 175-181.

[350] Cox, J. T. Management of precursor lesions of cervical carcinoma: history, host defense, and a survey of modalities. *Obstet. Gynecol. Clin. North Am.*, 2002 29, 751-785.

[351] Rieck, G. C., Fiander, A. N. Human papillomavirus, cervical carcinogenesis and chemoprevention with Indole derivates – A review of pathomechanisms. *Mol. Nutr. Food Res.*, 2008 52, 105-113.

[352] Gall, S. A. Female genital warts: global trends and treatments. *Infect. Dis. Obstet. Gynecol.*, 2001 9, 149-154.

[353] Baulon, E., Vautravers, A., Rodriguez, B., Nisand, I., Baldauf, J. J. Imiquimod and immune response modifiers in gynaecology. *Gynecol. Obstet. Fertil.*, 2007 35, 149-157.

[354] Pepas, L., Kaushik, S., Bryant, A., Nordin, A., Dickinson, H. O. Medical interventions for high grade vulval intraepithelial neoplasia. *Cochrane Database Syst. Rev.*, 2011 4, CD007924.

[355] Trofatter, K. F. Jr. Interferon. *Obstet. Gynecol. Clin. North Am.*, 1987 14, 569-579.

[356] Trofatter, K. F. Jr. Interferon treatment of anogenital human papillomavirus-related diseases. *Dermatol. Clin.*, 1991 9, 343-352.

[357] Gall, S. A. Human papillomavirus infection and therapy with interferon. *Am. J. Obstet. Gynecol.*, 1995 172, 1354-1359.

[358] Krebs, H. B. The use of topical 5-fluorouracil in the treatment of genital condylomas. *Obstet. Gynecol. Clin. North Am.*, 1987 14, 559-568.

[359] Lindeque, B. G. Management of cervical premalignant lesions. *Best Pract. Res. Clin. Obstet. Gynaecol.*, 2005 19, 545-561.

[360] Kyrgiou, M., Tsoumpou, I., Vrekoussis, T., Martin-Hirsch, P., Arbyn, M., Prendiville, W., Mitrou, S., Koliopoulos, G., Dalkalitsis, N., Stamatopoulos, P., Paraskevaidis, E. The up-to-date evidence on colposcopy practice and treatment of cervical intraepithelial neoplasia: the Cochrane colposcopy and cervical cytopathology collaborative group (C5 group) approach. *Cancer Treat. Rev.*, 2006 32, 516-523.

[361] Wright, V. C., Chapman, W. Intraepithelial neoplasia of the lower female genital tract: etiology, investigation, and management. *Semin. Surg. Oncol.*, 1992 8, 180-190.

[362] Reid, R. Physical and surgical principles governing expertise with the carbon dioxide laser. *Obstet. Gynecol. Clin. North Am.*, 1987 14, 513-535.

[363] Schwartz, D. B., Greenberg, M. D., Daoud, Y., Reid, R. The management of genital condylomas in pregnant women. *Obstet. Gynecol. Clin. North Am.*, 1987 14, 589-599.

[364] Hillard, P. A., Biro, F. M., Wildey, L. Complications of cervical cryotherapy in adolescents. *J. Reprod. Med.*, 1991 36, 711-716.

[365] Jordan, L. B., Monaghan, H. Pathology of the cervix: recent developments. *Clin. Oncol.* (R. Coll. Radiol.), 2004 16, 248-254.

[366] Dedes, K. J., Dedes, M., Varga, Z., Zimmermann, D. R., Fink, D., Fehr, M. K. Curative treatment of a pelvic side wall recurrence after conization for microinvasive cervical cancer stage IA1: a case report and review of the literature. *J. Low Genit. Tract. Dis.*, 2007 11, 177-181.

[367] Paraskevaidis, E., Arbyn, M., Sotiriadis, A., Diakomanolis, E., Martin-Hirsch, P., Koliopoulos, G., Makrydimas, G., Tofoski, J., Roukos, D. H. The role of HPV DNA testing in the follow-up period after treatment for CIN: a systematic review of the literature. *Cancer Treat. Rev.*, 2004 30, 205-211.

[368] Bornstein, J., Schwartz, J., Perri, A., Harroch, J., Zarfati, D. Tools for post LEEP surveillance. *Obstet. Gynecol. Surv.*, 2004 59, 663-668.

[369] Kyrgiou, M., Koliopoulos, G., Martin-Hirsch, P., Kehoe, S., Flannelly, G., Mitrou, S., Arbyn, M., Prendiville, W., Paraskevaidis, E. Management of minor cervical cytological abnormalities: a systematic review and a meta-analysis of the literature. *Cancer Treat. Rev.*, 2007 33, 514-520.

[370] Lonky, N. M. Reducing death from cervical cancer examining the prevention paradigms. *Obstet. Gynecol. Clin. North Am.*, 2002 29, 599-611.

[371] Diaz, M. L. Human papilloma virus: prevention and treatment. *Obstet. Gynecol. Clin. North Am.*, 2008 35, 199-217.

[372] Fiander, A. N. The prevention of cervical cancer in Africa. *Womens Health* (Lond. Engl.), 2011 7, 121-132.

[373] Denny, L. Cervical cancer: prevention and treatment. *Discov. Med.*, 2012 14, 125-131.

[374] Michelin, M. A., Murta, E. F. Potential therapeutic vaccine strategies and relevance of the immune system in uterine cervical cancer. *Eur. J. Gynaecol. Oncol.*, 2008 29, 10-18.

[375] Einstein, M. H. Acquired immune response to oncogenic human papillomavirus associated with prophylactic cervical cancer vaccines. *Cancer Immunol. Immunother.*, 2008 57, 443-51.

[376] Hines, J. F., Ghim, S., Schlegel, R., Jenson, A. B. Prospects for a vaccine against human papillomavirus. *Obstet. Gynecol.*, 1995 86, 860-866.

[377] Tjiong, M. Y., Out, T. A., Ter Schegget, J., Burger, M. P., Van Der Vange, N. Epidemiologic and mucosal immunologic aspects of HPV infection and HPV-related cervical neoplasia in the lower female genital tract: a review. *Int. J. Gynecol. Cancer*, 2001 11, 9-17.

[378] Lehtinen, M., Paavonen, J. Efficacy of preventive human papillomavirus vaccination. *Int. J. STD AIDS*, 2001 12, 771-776.

[379] Steller, M. A. Cervical cancer vaccines: progress and prospects. *J. Soc. Gynecol. Investig.*, 2002 9, 254-264.

[380] Lehtinen, M., Paavonen, J. Effectiveness of preventive human papillomavirus vaccination. *Int. J. STD AIDS*, 2003 14, 787-792.

[381] Tjalma, W. A., Arbyn, M., Paavonen, J., van Waes, T. R., Bogers, J. J. Prophylactic human papillomavirus vaccines: the beginning of the end of cervical cancer. *Int. J. Gynecol. Cancer,* 2004 14, 751-761.

[382] Ault, K. A. Vaccines for the prevention of human papillomavirus and associated gynaecologic diseases: a review. *Obstet. Gynecol. Surv.*, 2006 61, S26-S31.

[383] Paavonen, J., Lehtinen, M. Introducing human papillomavirus vaccines – Questions remain. *Ann. Med.,* 2008 40, 162-166.

[384] Frederick, P. J., Huh, W. K., PATRICIA Study Group. Evaluation of the interim analysis from the PATRICIA study group: efficacy of a vaccine against HPV 16 and 18. *Expert Rev. Anticancer Ther.*, 2008 8, 701-705.

[385] Bornstein, J. The HPV vaccines – Which to prefer? *Obstet. Gynecol. Surv.*, 2009 64, 345-350.

[386] Petry, K. U. What does HPV vaccination mean for gynecologic cancer screening? *Hautarzt*, 2007 58, 501-506.

[387] Chan, J. K., Berek, J. S. Impact of the human papilloma vaccine on cervical cancer. *J. Clin. Oncol.*, 2007 25, 2975-2982.

[388] Ault, K., Reisinger, K. Programmatic issues in the implementation of an HPV vaccination program to prevent cervical cancer. *Int. J. Infect. Dis.*, 2007 11 Suppl. 2, S26-S28.

[389] Ault, K. A. Long-term efficacy of human papillomavirus vaccination. *Gynecol. Oncol.*, 2007 107, S27-S30.

[390] Agorastos, T., Chatzigeorgiou, K., Brotherton, J. M., Garland, S. M. Safety of human papillomavirus (HPV) vaccines: a review of the international experience so far. *Vaccine*, 2009 27, 7270-7281.

[391] Herzog, T. J., Huh, W. K., Downs, L. S., Smith, J. S., Monk, B. J. Initial lessons learned in HPV vaccination. *Gynecol. Oncol.*, 2008 109, S4-S11.

[392] Harper, D. M., Paavonen, J. Age for HPV vaccination. *Vaccine*, 2008 26 Suppl. 1, A7-A11.

[393] Saleem, A., Tristram, A., Fiander, A., Hibbitts, S. Prophylactic HPV vaccination: a major breakthrough in the fight against cervical cancer? *Minerva Med.*, 2009 100, 503-523.

[394] Bello, F. A., Enabor, O. O., Adewole, I. F. Human papilloma virus vaccination for control of cervical cancer: a challenge for developing countries. *Afr. J. Reprod. Health*, 2011 15, 25-30.

[395] Tay, S. K. Cervical cancer in the human papillomavirus vaccination era. *Curr. Opin. Obstet. Gynecol.*, 2012 24, 3-7.

[396] Joura, E. A., Garland, S. M., Paavonen, J., Ferris, D. G., Perez, G., Ault, K. A., Huh, W. K., Sings, H. L., James, M. K., Haupt, R. M., FUTURE I and II Study Group. Effect of the human papillomavirus (HPV) quadrivalent vaccine in a subgroup of women with cervical and vulvar disease: retrospective pooled analysis of trial data. *BMJ*, 2012 344, e 1401.

[397] Crosbie, E. J., Kitchener, H. C. Human papillomavirus as a target for management, prevention and therapy. *Int. J. Hyperthermia*, 2012 28, 478-488.

[398] Santin, A. D., Bellone, S., Roman, J. J., Burnett, A., Cannon, M. J., Pecorelli, S. Therapeutic vaccines for cervical cancer: dendritic cell-based immunotherapy. *Curr. Pharm. Des.*, 2005 11, 3485-3500.

[399] Bellone, S., Pecorelli, S., Cannon, M. J., Santin, A. D. Advances in dendritic-cell-based therapeutic vaccines for cervical cancer. *Expert Rev. Anticancer Ther.*, 2007 7, 1473-1486.

[400] Lin, K., Roosinovich, E., Ma, B., Hung, C. F., Wu, T. C. Therapeutic HPV DNA vaccines. *Immunol. Res.*, 2010 47, 86-112.

[401] De Lorenzo, B. H., Ramos Mde, C., Michelin, M. A., Murta, E. F. Progress in the use of immunotherapy to treat uterine cervical cancer. *Tumori*, 2009 95, 1-7.

[402] Van Esch, E. M., Welters, M. J., Jordanova, E. S., Trimbos, J. B., van der Burg, S. H., van Poelgeest, M. I. Treatment failure in patients with HPV 16-induced vulvar intraepithelial neoplasia: understanding different clinical responses to immunotherapy. *Expert Rev. Vaccines*, 2012 11, 821-840.

[403] Brewster, W. R., Monk, B. J., Burger, R. A., Bergen, S., Wilczynski, S. P. Does human papillomavirus have a role in cancers of the uterine corpus? *Gynecol. Oncol.*, 1999 75, 51-54.

[404] Yamazawa, K., Matsui, H., Seki, K., Mitsuhashi, A., Kawamata, Y., Shirasawa, H., Sekiya, S. Human papillomavirus-positive well-differentiated villoglandular adenocarcinoma of the uterine cervix: A case report and review of the literature. *Gynecol. Oncol.*, 2000 77, 473-477.

[405] Chew, G. K., Cruickshank, M. E. Human papillomavirus as a form of risk assessment. *Best Pract. Res. Clin. Obstet. Gynaecol.*, 2001 15, 759-768.

[406] Cox, J. T. Management of atypical squamous cells of undetermined significance and low-grade squamous intra-epithelial lesion by human papillomavirus testing. *Best Pract. Res. Clin. Obstet. Gynaecol.*, 2001 15, 715-741.

[407] Bekkers, R. L., Massuger, L. F., Bulten, J., Melchers, W. J. Epidemiological and clinical aspects of human papillomavirus detection in the prevention of cervical cancer. *Rev. Med. Virol.*, 2004 14, 95-105.

[408] Simon, P., Roumeguere, T., Christophe Noël, J. Human papillomavirus infection in couples with female low-grade intraepithelial cervical lesion. *Eur. J. Obstet. Gynecol. Reprod. Biol.*, 2010 153, 8-11.

[409] Agorastos, T., Sotiriadis, A., Chatzigeorgiou, K. Can HPV testing replace the pap smear? *Ann. N. Y. Acad. Sci.*, 2010 1205, 51-56.

[410] Kyrgiou, M., Valasoulis, G., Founta, C., Koliopoulos, G., Karakitsos, P., Nasioutziki, M., Navrozoglou, I., Dalkalitsis, N., Paraskevaidis, E.

Clinical management of HPV-related disease of the lower genital tract. *Ann. N. Y. Acad. Sci.*, 2010 1205, 57-68.

[411] Herzog, T. J., Huh, W. K., Einstein, M. H. How does public policy impact cervical screening and vaccination strategies? *Gynecol. Oncol.*, 2010 119, 175-180.

[412] No, J. H., Kim, M. K., Jeon, Y. T., Kim, Y. B., Song, Y. S. Human papillomavirus vaccine: widening the scope for cancer prevention. *Mol. Carcinog.,* 2011 50, 244-253.

[413] Schmeink, C. E., Bekkers, R. L., Massuger, L. F., Melchers, W. J. The potential role of self-sampling for high-risk human papillomavirus detection in cervical cancer screening. *Rev. Med. Virol.*, 2011 21, 139-153.

[414] Cronjé, H. S. Cervical screening strategies in resourced and resource-constrained countries. *Best Pract. Res. Clin. Obstet. Gynaecol.*, 2011 25, 575-584.

[415] Lacour, D. E., Trimble, C. Human papillomavirus in infants: transmission, prevalence, and persistence. *J. Pediatr. Adolesc. Gynecol.*, 2012 25, 93-97.

[416] Seoud, M., Tjalma, W. A.,Ronsse, V. Cervical adenocarcinoma: moving towards better prevention. *Vaccine*, 2011 29, 9148-9158.

[417] Denny, L. Cytological screening for cervical cancer prevention. *Best Pract. Res. Clin. Obstet. Gynaecol.*, 2012 26, 189-196.

[418] Brown, A. J., Trimble, C. L. New technologies for cervical cancer screening. *Best Pract. Res. Clin. Obstet. Gynaecol.*, 2012 26, 233-242.

[419] Bhatla, N., Singla, S., Awasthi, D. Human papillomavirus deoxyribonucleic acid testing in developed countries. *Best Pract. Res. Clin. Obstet. Gynaecol.*, 2012 26, 209-220.

[420] Hinten, F., Meeuwis, K. A., van Rossum, M. M., de Hullu, J. A. HPV-related (pre)malignancies of the female anogenital tract in renal transplant recipients. *Crit. Rev. Oncol. Hematol.*, 2012 84, 161-180.

[421] Erickson, B. K., Alvarez, R. D., Huh, W. K. Human papillomavirus: what every provider should know. *Am. J. Obstet. Gynecol.,* 2013 208, 169-175.

[422] Del Pino, M., Rodriguez-Carunchio, L., Ordi, J. Pathways of vulvar intraepithelial neoplasia and squamous cell carcinoma. *Histopathology*, 2013 62, 161-175.

[423] Hagemann, A. R., Wilkinson-Ryan, I., Kuroki, L. M., Squires, K. Discussion: "Comparison of cervical cancer screening strategies", by Cox et al. *Am. J. Obstet. Gynecol.*, 2013 208, e1-4.

[424] De Vincenzo, R., Ricci, C., Conte, C., Scambia, G. HPV vaccine cross-protection: Highlights on additional clinical benefit. *Gynecol. Oncol.*, 2013 130, 642-651.

[425] Duff, P. Hepatitis in pregnancy. *Semin. Perinatol.*, 1998 22, 277-283.

[426] Han, G. R., Xu, C. L., Zhao, W., Yang, Y. F. Management of chronic hepatitis B in pregnancy. *World J. Gastroenterol.*, 2012 18, 4517-4521.

[427] Dinsmoor, M. J. Hepatitis in the obstetric patient. *Infect. Dis. Clin. North Am.,* 1997 11, 77-91.

[428] Shi, Z., Yang, Y., Wang, H., Ma, L., Schreiber, A., Li, X., Sun, W., Zhao, X., Yang, X., Zhang, L., Lu, W., Teng, J., An, Y. Breastfeeding of newborns by mothers carrying hepatitis B virus: a meta-analysis and systematic review. *Arch. Pediatr. Adolesc. Med.,* 2011 165, 837-846.

[429] Samuels, P., Cohen, A. W. Pregnancies complicated by liver disease and liver dysfunction. *Obstet. Gynecol. Clin. North Am.*, 1992 19, 745-763.

[430] Babb, R. R. Hepatitis B antigen: a review of its importance in the practice of obstetrics and gynecology. *Am. J. Obstet. Gynecol.*, 1976 126, 602-606.

[431] Greenspoon, J. S., Martin, J., Greenspoon, R. L., McNamara, B. T. Necessity for routine obstetric screening for hepatitis B surface antigen. *J. Reprod. Med.*, 1989 34, 655-658.

[432] Kitau, M. J., Grint, P. C., Heath, R. B., Chard, T. Serum alphafetoprotein levels in subjects infected with hepatitis B virus. *J. Med. Virol.*, 1988 26, 437-442.

[433] Sangkomkamhang, U. S., Lumbiganon, P., Laopaiboon, M. Hepatitis B vaccination during pregnancy for preventing infant infection. *Cochrane Database Syst. Rev.*, 2011 3, CD007879.

[434] Gall, S. A. Expanding the use of hepatitis vaccines in obstetrics and gynecology. *Am. J. Med.,* 2005 118 Suppl. 10A, 96S-99S.

[435] Gonik, B. The role of obstetrician/gynecologists in the management of hepatitis C virus infection. *Infect. Dis. Obstet. Gynecol.*, 2008 2008, 374517.

[436] Lynch-Salamon, D. I., Combs, C. A. Hepatitis C in obstetrics and gynecology. *Obstet. Gynecol.*, 1992 79, 621-629.

[437] Dinsmoor, M. J. Hepatitis C in pregnancy. *Curr. Womens Health Rep.*, 2001 1, 27-30.

[438] Madzime, S., William, M. A., Mohamed, K., October, T., Adem, M., Mudzamiri, S., Woelk, G. B. Seroprevalence of hepatitis C virus infection among indigent urban pregnant women in Zimbabwe. *Cent. Afr. J. Med.*, 2000 46, 1-4.

[439] Airoldi, J., Berghella, V. Hepatitis C and pregnancy. *Obstet. Gynecol. Surv.*, 2006 61, 666-672.
[440] Hiratsuka, M., Minakami, H., Koshizuka, S., Sato, I. Administration of interferon-alpha during pregnancy: effects on fetus. *J. Perinat. Med.*, 2000 28, 372-376.
[441] Prasad, M. R., Honegger, J. R. Hepatitis C virus in pregnancy. *Am. J. Perinatol.*, 2013 30, 149-159.
[442] Scott, L. L., Hollier, L. M., Dias, K. Perinatal herpesvirus infections. Herpes simplex, varicella, and cytomegalovirus. *Infect. Dis. Clin. North Am.*, 1997 11, 27-53.
[443] Hollier, L. M., Grissom, H. Human herpes viruses in pregnancy: cytomegalovirus, Epstein-Barr virus, and varicella zoster virus. *Clin. Perinatol.*, 2005 32, 671-696.
[444] Riley, L. E. Herpes simplex virus. *Semin. Perinatol.*, 1998 22, 284-292.
[445] Frederick, D. M., Bland, D., Gollin, Y. Fatal disseminated herpes simplex virus infection in a previously healthy pregnant woman. A case report. *J. Reprod. Med.*, 2002 47, 591-596.
[446] Greenspoon, J. S., Wilcox, J. G., McHutchison, L. B., Rosen, D. J. Acyclovir for disseminated herpes simplex virus in pregnancy. A case report. *J. Reprod. Med.*, 1994 39, 311-317.
[447] Kang, A. H., Graves, C. R. Herpes simplex hepatitis in pregnancy: a case report and review of the literature. *Obstet. Gynecol. Surv.*, 1999 54, 463-468.
[448] Johnson, L. G., Saldana, L. R. Herpes simplex virus hepatitis in pregnancy. A case report. *J. Reprod. Med.*, 1994 39, 544-546.
[449] Fagnant, R. J., Monif, G. R. How rare is congenital herpes simplex? A literature review. *J. Reprod. Med.*, 1989 34, 417-422.
[450] Petersen, E. E. Infections with herpes viruses in gynecology and obstetrics. *Fortschr. Med.*, 1989 107, 526-528.
[451] ACOG Committee on Practice Bulletins – Gynecology. ACOG practice bulletin: Clinical management guidelines for obstetrician-gynecologists, number 57, November 2004. Gynecologic herpes simplex virus infections. *Obstet. Gynecol.,* 2004 104, 1111-1118.
[452] Sperling, R. S., Berkowitz, R. L. Obstetric management of women with a history of recurrent genital herpes. *Am. J. Perinatol.*, 1989 6, 275-277.
[453] Landy, H. J., Grossman, J. H. 3rd. Herpes simplex virus. *Obstet. Gynecol. Clin. North Am.*, 1989 16, 495-515.

[454] Cleary, K. L., Paré, E., Stamilio, D., Macones, G. A. Type-specific screening for asymptomatic herpes infection in pregnancy: a decision analysis. *BJOG*, 2005 112, 731-736.

[455] Dupuis, O., Audibert, F., Fernandez, H., Frydman, R. Herpes simplex virus encephalitis in pregnancy. *Obstet. Gynecol.*, 1999 94, 810-812.

[456] Brown, Z. A., Gardella, C., Wald, A., Morrow, R. A., Corey, L. Genital herpes complicating pregnancy. *Obstet. Gynecol.*, 2005 106, 845-856.

[457] Baker, D. A. Herpes simplex virus infections. *Curr. Opin. Obstet. Gynecol.*, 1992 4, 676-681.

[458] Steben, M., Money, D., Wong, T., Gruslin, A., Yudin, M., Cohen, H., Boucher, M., Mackinnon, C., Paquet, C., van Schalkwyk, J., Infectious Disease Committe; Executive and Council of the Society of Obstetritians and Gynecologist of Canada. Genital herpes: gynaecological aspects. *J. Obstet. Gynaecol. Can.,* 2008 30, 347-361.

[459] Baker, D. A. Valacyclovir in the treatment of genital herpes and herpes zoster. *Expert Opin. Pharmacother.*, 2002 3, 51-58.

[460] Brown, Z. A., Baker, D. A. Acyclovir therapy during pregnancy. *Obstet. Gynecol.*, 1989 73, 526-531.

[461] Reichel, R. P. Management of recurrent genital herpes virus infections in gynecology and obstetrics. *Gynakol Geburtshilfliche Rundsch*, 1993 33, 17-21.

[462] Scott, L. L. Prevention of perinatal herpes: prophylactic antiviral therapy? *Clin. Obstet. Gynecol.*, 1999 42, 134-148.

[463] Faro, S. A review of famciclovir in the management of genital herpes. *Infect. Dis. Obstet. Gynecol.*, 1998 6, 38-43.

[464] Brown, Z. Preventing herpes simplex virus transmission to the neonate. *Herpes*, 2004 11 Suppl. 3, 175A-186A.

[465] Hollier, L. M., Wendel, G. D. Third trimester antiviral prophylaxis for preventing maternal genital herpes simplex virus (HSV) recurrences and neonatal infection. *Cochrane Database Syst. Rev.,* 2008 1, CD004946.

[466] Maccato, M. L., Kaufman, R. H. Herpes genitalis. *Dermatol. Clin.*, 1992 10, 415-422.

[467] Baker, D. A. Antiviral therapy for genital herpes infections in pregnancy. *Expert Rev. Anti Infect. Ther.*, 2005 3, 385-392.

[468] Prober, C. G. Herpetic vaginitis in 1993. *Clin. Obstet. Gynecol.*, 1993 36, 177-187.

[469] Jaiyeoba, O., Amaya, M. I., Soper, D. E., Kilby, J. M. Preventing neonatal transmission of herpes simplex virus. *Clin. Obstet. Gynecol.*, 2012 55, 510-520.

[470] Straface, G., Selmin, A., Zanardo, V., De Santis, M., Ercoli, A., Scambia, G. Herpes simplex virus infection in pregnancy. *Infect. Dis. Obstet. Gynecol.,* 2012 2012, 385697.

[471] Gardella, C., Brown, Z. Prevention of neonatal herpes. *BJOG*, 2011 118, 187-192.

[472] Westhoff, G. L., Little, S. E., Caughey, A. B. Herpes simplex virus and pregnancy: a review of the management of antenatal and peripartum herpes infections. *Obstet. Gynecol. Surv*., 2011 66, 629-638.

[473] Gardella, C., Brown, Z. A. Managing varicella zoster infection in pregnancy. *Cleve. Clin. J. Med*., 2007 74, 290-296.

[474] Goldberg, J. M., Ziel, H. K., Burchette, R. Evaluation of varicella immune status in an obstetric population in relation to place of birth. *Am. J. Perinatol*., 2002 19, 387-394.

[475] Hudson, L. B., Perlman, S. E. Necrotizing genital ulcerations in a premenarcheal female with mononucleosis. *Obstet. Gynecol*., 1998 92, 642-644.

[476] Barnes, M. N., Barrett, J. C., Kimberlin, D. F., Kilgore, L. C. Burkitt lymphoma in pregnancy. *Obstet. Gynecol*., 1998 92, 675-678.

[477] Gaytant, M. A., Rours, G. I., Steegers, E. A., Galama, J. M., Semmekrot, B. A. Congenital cytomegalovirus infection after recurrent infection: case reports and review of the literature. *Eur. J. Pediatr*., 2003 162, 248-253.

[478] Cheong, J. L., Cowan, F. M., Modi, N. Gastrointestinal manifestations of postnatal cytomegalovirus infection in infants admitted to a neonatal intensive care unit over a five year period. *Arch. Dis. Child Fetal Neonatal. Ed.,* 2004 89, F367-F369.

[479] Daniel, Y., Gull, I., Peyser, M. R., Lessing, J. B. Congenital cytomegalovirus infection. *Eur. J. Obstet. Gynecol. Reprod. Biol*., 1995 63, 7-16.

[480] McCarthy, F. P., Giles, M. L., Rowlands, S., Purcell, K. J., Jones, C. A. Antenatal interventions for preventing the transmission of cytomegalovirus (CMV) from the mother to fetus during pregnancy and adverse outcomes in the congenitally infected infant. *Cochrane Database Syst. Rev*., 2011 3, CD008371.

[481] Nigro, G., Adler, S. P. Cytomegalovirus infections during pregnancy. *Curr. Opin. Obstet. Gynecol*., 2011 23, 123-128.

[482] Johnson, J., Anderson, B., Pass, R. F. Prevention of maternal and congenital cytomegalovirus infection. *Clin. Obstet. Gynecol*., 2012 55, 521-530.

[483] Von Dadelszen, P., Magee, L. A. Could an infectious trigger explain the differential maternal response to the shared placental pathology of preeclampsia and normotensive intrauterine growth restriction? *Acta Obstet. Gynecol. Scand.*, 2002 81, 642-648.

[484] Xie, F., Hu, Y., Magee, L. A., Money, D. M., Patrick, D. M., Krajden, M., Thomas, E., von Dadelszen, P., Toxemia Study Group. An association between cytomegalovirus infection and pre-eclampsia: a case-control study and data synthesis. *Acta Obstet. Gynecol. Scand.*, 2010 89, 1162-1167.

[485] British Andrology Society. British Andrology Society guidelines for the screening of semen donors for donor insemination (1999). *Hum. Reprod.,* 1999 14, 1823-1826.

[486] Liesnard, C., Strebelle, E., Englert, Y. Screening standards in assisted reproductive technologies. Is the British Andrology Society recommendation to recruit cytomegalovirus negative semen donors only, a reasonable one? *Hum. Reprod.*, 2001 16, 1789-1791.

[487] Syggelou, A., Iacovidou, N., Kloudas, S., Christoni, Z., Papaevangelou, V. Congenital cytomegalovirus infection. *Ann. N. Y. Acad. Sci.*, 2010 1205, 144-147.

[488] Malinger, G., Lev, D., Lerman-Sagie, T. Imaging of fetal cytomegalovirus infection. *Fetal Diagn. Ther.*, 2011 29, 117-126.

[489] Yinon, Y., Farine, D., Yudin, M. H. Screening, diagnosis, and management of cytomegalovirus infection in pregnancy. *Obstet. Gynecol. Surv.*, 2010 65, 736-743.

[490] Dogan, Y., Yuksel, A., Kalelioglu, I. H., Has, R., Tatli, B., Yildirim, A. Intracranial ultrasound abnormalities and fetal cytomegalovirus infection: report of 8 cases and review of the literature. *Fetal Diagn. Ther.*, 2011 30, 141-149.

[491] Ramirez, M. M., Mastrobattista, J. M. Diagnosis and management of human parvovirus B19 infection. *Clin. Perinatol.*, 2005 32, 697-704.

[492] Rodis, J. F., Hovick, T. J. Jr; Quinn, D. L., Rosengren, S. S., Tattersall, P. Human parvovirus infection in pregnancy. *Obstet. Gynecol.*, 1988 72, 733-738.

[493] Kumar, M. L. Human parvovirus B19 and its associated diseases. *Clin. Perinatol.*, 1991 18, 209-225.

[494] Boley, T. J., Popek, E. J. Parvovirus infection in pregnancy. *Semin. Perinatol.,* 1993 17, 410-419.

[495] Levy, R., Weissman, A., Blomberg, G., Hagay, Z.J. Infection by parvovirus B 19 during pregnancy: a review. *Obstet. Gynecol. Surv.*, 1997 52, 254-259.
[496] Yaegashi, N., Niinuma, T., Chisaka, H., Watanabe, T., Uehara, S., Okamura, K., Moffatt, S., Sugamura, K., Yajima, A. The incidence of, and factors leading to, parvovirus B19-related hydrops fetalis following maternal infection; report of 10 cases and meta-analysis. *J. Infect.*, 1998 37, 28-35.
[497] Eis-Hübinger, A. M., Dieck, D., Schild, R., Hansmann, M., Schneweis, KE. Parvovirus B19 infection in pregnancy. *Intervirology*, 1998 41, 178-184.
[498] Von Kaisenberg, C. S., Jonat, W. Fetal parvovirus B19 infection. *Ultrasound Obstet. Gynecol.*, 2001 18, 280-288.
[499] Al-Khan, A., Caligiuri, A., Apuzzio, J. Parvovirus B-19 infection during pregnancy. *Infect. Dis. Obstet. Gynecol.*, 2003 11, 175-179.
[500] Von Kaisenberg, C. S., Grebe, S., Schleider, S., Kuhling-von Kaisenberg, H., Venhoff, L., Meinhold-Heerlein, I. Successful intrauterine intracardiac transfusion in monochorionic twins affected by parvovirus B19. *Fetal Diagn. Ther.*, 2007 22, 420-424.
[501] Bekhit, M. T., Greenwood, P. A., Warren, R., Aarons, E., Jauniaux, E. In utero treatment of severe fetal anaemia due to parvovirus B19 in one fetus in a twin pregnancy – A case report and literature review. *Fetal Diagn. Ther.*, 2009 25, 153-157.
[502] Rosa, C. Rubella and rubeola. *Semin. Perinatol.*, 1998 22, 318-322.
[503] De Santis, M., Cavaliere, A. F., Straface, G., Caruso, A. Rubella infection in pregnancy. *Reprod. Toxicol.*, 2006 21, 390-398.
[504] Schoenhoff, D. D., Lane, T. W., Hansen, C. J. Primary prevention and rubella immunity: overlooked issues in the outpatient obstetric setting. *Infect. Control Hosp. Epidemiol.*, 1997 18, 633-636.
[505] Mylonas, I., Brüning, A., Kainer, F., Friese, K. HTLV infection and its implication in gynaecology and obstetrics. *Arch. Gynecol. Obstet.*, 2010 282, 493-501.
[506] Lynch, M. P., Kaumaya, P. T. Advances in HTLV-1 peptide vaccines and therapeutics. *Curr. Protein Pept. Sci.*, 2006 7, 137-145.
[507] Theiler, R. N., Rasmussen, S. A., Treadwell, T. A., Jamieson, D. J. Emerging and zoonotic infections in women. *Infect. Dis. Clin. North Am.*, 2008 22, 755-772.
[508] Longman, R. E., Johnson, T. R. Viral respiratory disease in pregnancy. *Curr. Opin. Obstet. Gynecol.*, 2007 19, 120-125.

[509] Satpathy, H. K., Lindsay, M., Kawwass, J. F. Novel H1N1 virus infection and pregnancy. *Postgrad. Med.*, 2009 121, 106-112.
[510] Toal, M., Agyeman-Duah, K., Schwenk, A., Yoong, W. Swine flu and pregnancy. *J. Obstet. Gynaecol.*, 2010 30, 97-100.
[511] Alford, C. E., Chen, G. L., Armstrong, A. Y. 2009 H1N1 influenza prevention and treatment: counseling infertility patients. *Fertil. Steril.*, 2010 94, 1178-1180.
[512] Klatt, T. E., Hopp, E. Effect of a best-practice alert on the rate of influenza vaccination of pregnant women. *Obstet. Gynecol.*, 2012 119, 301-305.
[513] Fridman, D., Steinberg, E., Azhar, E., Weedon, J., Wilson, T. E., Minkoff, H. Predictors of H1N1 vaccination in pregnancy. *Am. J. Obstet. Gynecol.,* 2011 204, S124-S127.
[514] Myers, E. R., Misurski, D. A., Swamy, G. K. Influence of timing of seasonal influenza vaccination on effectiveness and cost-effectiveness in pregnancy. *Am. J. Obstet. Gynecol.*, 2011 204, S128-S140.
[515] Nakai, A., Saito, S., Unno, N., Kubo, T., Minakami, H. Review of the pandemic (H1N1) 2009 among pregnant Japanese women. *J. Obstet. Gynaecol. Res.,* 2012 38, 757-762.
[516] Shavell, V. I., Moniz, M. H., Gonik, B., Beigi, R. H. Influenza immunization in pregnancy: overcoming patient and health care provider barriers. *Am. J. Obstet. Gynecol.*, 2012 207, S67-S74.
[517] Ault, K. A., Heine, R. P., Riley, L. E. Programmatic and research priorities for improving influenza immunization of pregnant women. *Am. J. Obstet. Gynecol.*, 2012 207, S75-S77.
[518] Laibl, V. R., Sheffield, J. S. Influenza and pneumonia in pregnancy. *Clin. Perinatol.*, 2005 32, 727-738.
[519] Ramsey, P. S., Ramin, K. D. Pneumonia in pregnancy. *Obstet. Gynecol. Clin. North Am.*, 2001 28, 553-569.
[520] Jamieson, D. J., Ellis, J. E., Jernigan, D. B., Treadwell, T. A. Emerging infectious disease outbreaks: old lessons and new challenges for obstetrician-gynecologists. *Am. J. Obstet. Gynecol.*, 2006 194, 1546-1555.
[521] Bruno, J., Rabito, F. J. Jr; Dildy, G. A. 3rd. West nile virus meningoencephalitis during pregnancy. *J. La State Med. Soc.*, 2004 156, 204-205.
[522] Jamieson, D. J., Kourtis, A. P., Bell, M., Rasmussen, S. A. Lymphocytic choriomeningitis virus: an emerging obstetric pathogen? *Am. J. Obstet. Gynecol.,* 2006 194, 1532-1536.

[523] Suarez, V. R., Hankins, G. D. Smallpox and pregnancy: from eradicated disease to bioterrorist threat. *Obstet. Gynecol.*, 2002 100, 87-93.

[524] Jamieson, D. J., Cono, J., Richards, C. L., Treadwell, T. A. The role of the obstetrician-gynecologist in emerging infectious diseases: monkeypox and pregnancy. *Obstet. Gynecol.*, 2004 103, 754-756.

[525] Sharma, J. B., Gulati, N. Potential relationship between dengue fever and neural tube defects in a northern district of India. *Int. J. Gynaecol. Obstet.*, 1992 39, 291-295.

[526] Waduge, R., Malavige, G. N., Pradeepan, M., Wijeyaratne, C. N., Fernando, S., Seneviratne, S. L. Dengue infections during pregnancy: a case series from Sri Lanka and review of the literature. *J. Clin. Virol.*, 2006 37, 27-33.

[527] Lin, H. Y., Linn, G., Liu, C. B., Chen, C. J., Yu, K. J. An immune-compromised woman with severe molluscum contagiosum that responded well to topical imiquimod: a case report and literature review. *J. Low Genit. Tract Dis.*, 2010 14, 134-135.

[528] Creatsas, G. Improving reproductive sexual health: a primary goal at the beginning of the new millennium. *Eur. J. Contracept. Reprod. Health Care,* 1999 4, 185-186.

[529] Creatsas, G., Deligeoroglou, E. Microbial ecology of the lower genital tract in women with sexually transmitted diseases. *J. Med. Microbiol.*, 2012 61, 1347-1351.

[530] Minnis, A. M., Padian, N. S. Effectiveness of female controlled barrier methods in preventing sexually transmitted infections and HIV: current evidence and future research directions. *Sex. Transm. Infect.*, 2005 81, 193-200.

[531] Mbizvo, M. T. Condom acceptance and HIV prevention in reproductive health: the challenges. *Cent. Afr. J. Med.*, 1991 37, 419-427.

[532] Minkoff, H., Willoughby, A. The future of prenatal HIV testing. *Acta Paediatr.* Suppl., 1997 421, 72-77.

[533] Corusić, A., Skrgatić, L., Mahovlić, V., Mandić, V., Planinić, P., Karadza, M. Cervical cancer as a public health issue – What next? *Coll Antropol.*, 2010 34, 301-307.

[534] Myers, E., Huh, W. K., Wright, J. D., Smith, J. S. The current and future role of screening in the era of HPV vaccination. *Gynecol. Oncol.*, 2008 109, S31-S39.

[535] Kadish, A. S., Einstein, M. H. Vaccine strategies for human papillomavirus-associated cancers. *Curr. Opin. Oncol.*, 2005 17, 456-461.

[536] Fathalla, M. F. Reproductive health for all: a commitment towards the new millennium. *Eur. J. Contracept. Reprod. Health Care*, 1999 4, 212-216.

In: Viral Infections
Editor: Deborah Shinn

ISBN: 978-1-63117-221-2

Chapter 2

MANAGEMENT OF HIV INFECTION BY CHINESE MEDICINE

***Beuy Joob*[1] *and Viroj Wiwanitkit*[2]**
[1]Sanitation 1 Medical Academic Center, Bangkok, Tailand
[2]Visiting Professor, Hainan Medical University, China
Faculty of Medicine, University of Nis, Serbia

ABSTRACT

Human immunodeficiency virus (HIV) is a retrovirus that causes the immunodeficiency illness. HIV infection is an important infectious disease that can be seen around the world. This disease is still a problematic public health threat since there is still no successful therapeutic option for HIV. The management of HIV by alternative medicine is an interesting topic. Here, the authors will briefly review and discuss on the role of Chinese medicine for management of HIV infection.

INTRODUCTION

Immunodeficiency is a common problem in clinical medicine. There are several causes of immunodeficiency. Of several causes, infection is an important issued to be discussed. Human immunodeficiency virus (HIV) is a retrovirus that causes the immunodeficiency illness. HIV infection is an important infectious disease that can be seen around the world. The patients with HIV infection will have several clinical features including abnormal opportunistic infections (such as rare parasitic infestations, fungal infections and viral infections, etc.) and malignancies (such as lymphoma and leukemia). This HV disease is still a problematic public health threat since there is still no successful therapeutic option for HIV. Around the world, many million people carry HIV and can transmit it to others. The management of HIV by alternative medicine is an interesting topic. Here, the authors will briefly review and discuss on the role of Chinese medicine for management of HIV infection.

HIV in Chinese Medicine Concept

HIV infection is a new disease, therefore, it has not been documented in the ancient Chinese Medicine text.

In Chinese work, HIV infection is known as "Àizībìng, 艾滋病" which means the disease relating to "love". It is classified as a sexually transmitted disease.

The application of Chinese Medicine for HIV management is widely discussed at present. Wu et al. proposed that "Traditional Chinese Medicine shows good efficacy for intervention in HIV/AIDS and could become an effective treatment option [1]."

Liu et al. also noted that "high efficacy and low toxicity anti-HIV drug from traditional Chinese medicine is an important and prospective research direction in the future [2]."

At present, there are many advances in the study of anti-HIV natural compounds derived from traditional Chinese medicines [3]. In this short communication, the authors will review and discuss on two important aspects of Chinese Medicine for HIV management. As a concept, Lü said that "drugs strengthening the patients' resistance could enhance the efficacy of AIDS treatment [4]."

So, it is no doubt that there are many ongoing researches on Chinese herbs for management of HIV infection [5 - 6].

Virtual screening of Chinese herbs has been continuously done to find new drugs [7]. Cui et al. concluded that "core TCM treatment of AIDS is replenishing Qi and detoxification, by which AIDS patients' immune system may be enhanced [8]."

Chinese Herb and HIV Management

There are a lot of Chinese herbs that can be available as pharmaceuticals and neutraceuticals at present. The effect of many Chinese herbs on HIV is proposed.

Here, the authors will introduce researches on some important Chinese herbs for management of HIV infection

A. Ginseng

Ginseng is one of the most well-known Chinese herbs. In Chinese Medicine, Ginseng is an herb that has positive promoting effect to health status. There are many reports on effect of ginseng on HIV [9]. Cho et al. reported that long-term intake of red ginseng could delay development of resistance mutation to zidovudine in HIV infected patients [10]. Jeong et al. found that ginsenoside rh1 could eliminate the cytoprotective phenotype of human immunodeficiency virus type 1-transduced human macrophages by inhibiting the phosphorylation of pyruvate dehydrogenase lipoamide kinase isozyme 1 and this implies usefulness of ginseng for management of HIV infection [11]. Sung et al. concluded that ginseng intake had clinical utility for delay the occurrence of resistant mutation to standard anti-HIV therapy [12].

B. Lingzhi

Lingzhi or reishi is another well-known Chinese herb. The anti-HIV effect of this herb is confirmed [13]. Min et al. reported that ganoderic acid beta, (24S)-lanosta-7,9(11)-diene-3 beta,24,25-triol (called lucidumol B), ganodermanondiol, ganodermanontriol and ganolucidic acid A which could be isolated from Lingzhi had significant anti-HIV-1 protease activity [14]. For molecular mechanism, Akbar and Yam concluded that "HIV-1 protease in general is a suitable target for ganoderic acid B [15]."

C. Gingko

Gingko is another well-known Chinese herb. The anti-HIV effect of this herb is also mentioned. Lü et al. mentioned that "ginkgolic acid effectively inhibits HIV protease activity in a cell free system and HIV infection in PBMCs without significant cytotoxicity [16]." Long chain phenols from the sarcotestas of Ginkgo biloba is proposed as active ingredient with anti-HIV property [17].

Acupuncture and HVI Management

The usefulness of Chinese acupuncture for HIV management is also widely mentioned [18 – 20]. Most reports usually claim for the advantage of acupuncture for control of HIV symptoms. For example, Anastasi and McMahon reported that acupuncture helped manage chronic diarrhea in HIV infected patients [21]. Ursini et al. reported the successful use of acupuncture on healing of giant wart in HIV infected patients [22]. Louie concluded that acupuncture was useful for symptom relief and improved quality of life in HIV management [23].

References

[1] Wu XF, Wang J, Li Y, Tang YL, Zhao DD. Thoughts on intervention in HIV/AIDS with traditional Chinese medicine. *J. Tradit. Chin. Med.* 2011 Dec;31(4):265-8.

[2] Liu ZM, Yang YS, Wang XL, Wen RX. Recent progress on anti-HIV research of traditional Chinese medicine and components. *Zhongguo Zhong Yao Za Zhi*. 2006 Nov;31(21):1753-8.

[3] Zhang X, Huang N, Zheng YT. Advances in the study of anti-HIV natural compounds derived from traditional Chinese medicines. *Yao Xue Xue Bao*. 2010 Feb;45(2):141-53.

[4] Lü W. Prospect for study on treatment of AIDS with traditional Chinese medicine. *J. Tradit. Chin. Med.* 1995 Mar;15(1):3-9.

[5] Wu B. Recent development of studies on traditional Chinese medicine in prophylaxis and treatment of AIDS. *J. Tradit. Chin. Med.* 1992 Mar;12(1):10-20.

[6] Chinese herb trial. *GMHC Treat Issues*. 1995 Dec;9(12):9.

[7] Ehrman TM, Barlow DJ, Hylands PJ. Virtual screening of Chinese herbs with Random Forest. *J. Chem. Inf. Model*. 2007 Mar-Apr;47(2):264-78.

[8] Cui M, Li J, Li H, Song C. Herbal compatibility of traditional Chinese medical formulas for acquired immunodeficiency syndrome. *J. Tradit. Chin. Med.* 2012 Sep;32(3):329-34.

[9] Can ginseng help suppress HIV? TreatmentUpdate. 2001 Jul;13(3):2-4.

[10] Cho YK, Sung H, Lee HJ, Joo CH, Cho GJ. Long-term intake of Korean red ginseng in HIV-1-infected patients: development of resistance

mutation to zidovudine is delayed. *Int. Immunopharmacol.* 2001 Jul;1(7):1295-1305.

[11] Jeong JJ, Kim B, Kim DH. Ginsenoside rh1 eliminates the cytoprotective phenotype of human immunodeficiency virus type 1-transduced human macrophages by inhibiting the phosphorylation of pyruvate dehydrogenase lipoamide kinase isozyme 1. *Biol. Pharm. Bull.* 2013;36(7):1088-94.

[12] Sung H, Jung YS, Cho YK. Beneficial effects of a combination of Korean red ginseng and highly active antiretroviral therapy in human immunodeficiency virus type 1-infected patients. *Clin. Vaccine Immunol.* 2009 Aug;16(8):1127-31.

[13] Sanodiya BS, Thakur GS, Baghel RK, Prasad GB, Bisen PS. Ganoderma lucidum: a potent pharmacological macrofungus. *Curr. Pharm. Biotechnol.* 2009 Dec;10(8):717-42.

[14] Min BS, Nakamura N, Miyashiro H, Bae KW, Hattori M. Triterpenes from the spores of Ganoderma lucidum and their inhibitory activity against HIV-1 protease. *Chem. Pharm. Bull* (Tokyo). 1998 Oct;46(10):1607-12.

[15] Akbar R, Yam WK. Interaction of ganoderic acid on HIV related target: molecular docking studies. *Bioinformation.* 2011;7(8):413-7.

[16] Lü JM, Yan S, Jamaluddin S, Weakley SM, Liang Z, Siwak EB, Yao Q, Chen C. Ginkgolic acid inhibits HIV protease activity and HIV infection in vitro. *Med. Sci. Monit.* 2012 Aug;18(8):BR293-298.

[17] Lee JS, Hattori M, Kim J. Inhibition of HIV-1 protease and RNase H of HIV-1 reverse transcriptase activities by long chain phenols from the sarcotestas of Ginkgo biloba. *Planta Med.* 2008 Apr;74(5):532-4.

[18] Wang J, Zou W. Practices, challenges, and opportunities: HIV/AIDS treatment with traditional Chinese medicine in China. *Front Med.* 2011 Jun;5(2):123-6.

[19] Wang J, Zou W. Recent advances of HIV/AIDS treatment with traditional Chinese medicine in China. *J. Tradit. Chin. Med.* 2010 Dec;30(4):305-8.

[20] Huson C. Acupuncture and traditional Oriental medicine in the treatment of HIV and AIDS. *STEP Perspect.* 1996 Spring;8(1):2-3.

[21] Anastasi JK, McMahon DJ. Testing strategies to reduce diarrhea in persons with HIV using traditional Chinese medicine: acupuncture and moxibustion. *J. Assoc. Nurses AIDS Care.* 2003 May-Jun;14(3):28-40.

[22] Ursini T, Polilli E, Congedo G, Tontodonati M, Di Masi F, Mazzotta E, Parruti G, Pippa L. Complete Healing of a Giant Wart in a Severely Immune-Compromised Patient with HIV Infection Treated with Acupuncture. *Case Rep. Dermatol.* 2011 May;3(2):175-80.

[23] Louie L, Pathanapornpandh N, Pultajuk U, Kaplan R, Hodgson I, Maund L, Greenlee H. The Mae On Project: using acupuncture for symptom relief and improved quality of life for people living with HIV and AIDS in rural Thailand. *Acupunct. Med.* 2010 Mar;28(1):37-41.

In: Viral Infections
Editor: Deborah Shinn

ISBN: 978-1-63117-221-2

Chapter 3

ANTIVIRAL ACTIVITY OF LACTOFERRIN: FROM BASIC RESEARCH TO MEDICAL APPLICATIONS

Paula E. Florian, Catalin Lazar, Norica Nichita and Anca Roseanu*

Institute of Biochemistry of the Romanian Academy,
Bucharest, Romania

Lactoferrin (Lf) is a multifunctional iron-binding glycoprotein present in most biological fluids of mammals, being abundant in milk and colostrum. It was shown that Lf is a key player in the innate immune defense, as it is rapidly released from the neutrophils during an inflammatory response. Besides the immunomodulatory activity, Lf plays a plethora of biological functions, such as anti-tumoral, bactericidal and antiviral. Most of these activities are associated with the N-terminal region of the protein.

As for other functions, the antiviral mechanism of Lf is a multifaceted property and not yet fully defined. Lf was demonstrated to exert *in vitro* and *in vivo* anti-viral activity against a broad range of RNA and DNA viruses such as influenza viruses, human immunodeficiency virus (HIV), rotaviruses, Japanese encephalitis virus (JEV), hepatitis B and C viruses (HBV and HCV) or poliovirus. The antiviral mechanisms of action of Lf were suggested to involve prevention of viral infection of the target cell by direct binding to virus particle or by competition for /or

* Corresponding author e-mail address: Dr. Anca Roseanu email: roseanua@gmail.com

blocking the common receptors/co-receptors at the cell membrane. Since Lf binds to most cells and Lf receptors with either low or high affinity for the protein have been described, intracellular antiviral activities of Lf involving apoptosis or inflammatory pathways have been proposed. Intriguingly, several peptides derived from Lf were shown to preserve the beneficial antiviral activity of the parental protein. Moreover, synergistic effects of antiviral drugs in combination with Lf or Lf -derived peptides were reported. However, only a few antiviral studies using Lf have reached the level of clinical trials.

Despite continuous improvement of current therapies, many viruses develop resistance during treatment, therefore the search for alternative antiviral strategies remains a very hot topic. Owing to its remarkable antiviral properties and lack of cellular toxicity Lf has recently received increasing attention from virologists and clinicians, much effort being devoted in subscribing this interesting protein to a therapeutic platform.

The present work is a critical overview of the mechanisms proposed to explain the antiviral activity of Lf and Lf-derived peptides, and their use as a possible novel strategy in antiviral therapeutics.

INTRODUCTION

Lactoferrin (Lf) is a multifunctional iron-binding glycoprotein belonging to the transferrin family present in high concentration in colostrum, milk and in many exocrine secretions of mammals, such as tears, saliva or fluids of the digestive tract [1-3].

Lf is a key player of the innate immune system in the mammalian organisms, being a major component released from the secondary granules of neutrophils during an inflammatory response [4, 5]. It was reported that in some pathologies, Lf plasma level is greatly increased from 0.4 to 2 mg/L reaching 200mg/L in septicemia [6].

The protein is a single polypeptide chain of 691 amino acid residues, folded into two globular lobes, the N-terminal (N-t, 1-333 amino acid residues) and the C-terminal (C-t, 345-691 amino acid residues) linked by a short hinge region, in α-helix conformation [7]. The N- and C-t halves of the protein share ~ 40% sequence identity. The bovine (B) and human (H) Lf share about 69% identity at the level of amino acid sequence [8]. All Lfs characterized so far are glycosylated, but the number of sites actually occupied and their location depend on the origin of the protein. Besides conferring an increased resistance to proteolysis, other roles of the glycans in the biological functions of Lf are not well characterized.

Lf is a highly basic protein, with positive charges distributed at the N-t (1–7 amino acid residues), along the outside of the first helix (13–30 amino acid residues), as well as in the interlobe region [9]. Many active clusters, for which the biological role has been described, are located in this basic domain [10]: a) the N-t peptide (1–5 amino acid residues) is the sequence for nuclear targeting [11]; b) lactoferricin (Lfcin), a pepsin-cleaved fragment (1-47 amino acid residues in HLf, and residues 17-41 of BLf) is responsible for the antimicrobial and antitumor activities and proteoglycans binding [12]; within this domain a sequence comprising seven amino acids (28-34 amino acid residues) [13] was shown to bind the bacterial endotoxin lipopolysaccharide (LPS), a component of the outer membrane of Gram-negative bacteria involved in induction of inflammatory processes.

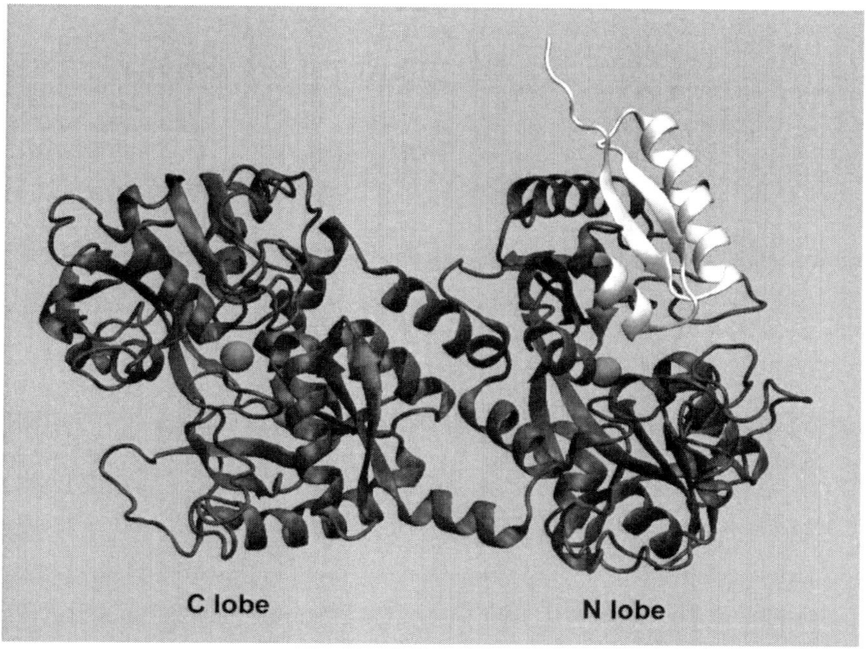

Figure 1. A ribbon diagram representation of the secondary structure of iron saturated human lactoferrin. The basic domain of N-t lobe (residues 1-50) is highlighted in white and the two iron atoms are shown in grey. (http://www.ks.uiuc.edu/Research/vmd/).

The biological functions of Lf range from iron metabolism regulation [14] and the well-established antimicrobial activity against various pathogens, including bacteria, viruses, fungi, and parasites, to immunomodulatory and anti-tumoral activities [10]. Some of these functions depend on the iron-saturation of the molecule (such as bacteriostatic, and immunomodulatory activities) while others rely on the interaction with the cell surface (antibacterial, antifungal and antiviral activities).

Regarding the antiviral property, Lf was demonstrated to inhibit the growth of a variety of both, naked and enveloped viruses, such as human immunodeficiency virus (HIV), Japanese encephalitis virus (JEV), rotaviruses, influenza viruses, hepatitis B and C viruses (HBV and HCV), poliovirus [15]. Similar to other functions played by this complex molecule, the antiviral activity of Lf is a multifaceted property, still incompletely defined. Possible mechanisms that could explain the Lf protection of host cells against viral infections involve a direct interaction with the viral particle, iron sequestration, or competitive binding to the cell membrane. Finally, an intracellular activity of Lf involving apoptosis or inflammatory pathways could account for antiviral effects in those cell lines permissive for Lf entry.

Several peptides derived from Lf were also shown to preserve the beneficial antiviral activity of the parental protein. Moreover, synergistic effects of antiviral drugs in combination with Lf or Lf-derived peptides were reported. Since many viruses develop resistance to current therapies it is hoped that the antiviral properties and the different mechanisms of Lf action may promote this protein as a clinically relevant, alternative therapeutic strategy.

The present work is a critical overview of the mechanisms proposed to explain the antiviral activity of Lf and Lf-derived peptides, and the feasibility of their use as potential antivirals.

Antiviral Mechanisms of Action

The antiviral mechanisms of Lf are complex and not yet fully understood. Based on the current data, two main modes of action were proposed: interaction with molecules of the host cell surface and direct interaction with virus particles.

INTERACTION WITH HOST CELLS

Many cells possess Lf specific and non-specific receptors, such as heparin sulphate (HS), glycosaminoglycans (GAG), low-density lipoprotein receptor (LDLR), nucleolin and asialoglycoprotein receptor (ASGPR). Interestingly, some of these molecules are also used by viruses to enter the target cells and initiate infection. Therefore, a direct competition between Lf and viral particles for binding the same sites on receptor molecules may occur, thus preventing viral infection.

HERPES SIMPLEX VIRUS (HSV)

Since 1994 it was shown that both BLf and HLf inhibit HSV infection and replication in human embryonic lung cells independently of iron-saturation status of the protein or the presence of sialic acid [16], despite the sensitivity to proteolysis acquired after sialic acid loss [9]. Later on BLf and HLf was reported to prevent the cytopathic effect and yield of both HSV-1 and HSV-2 in Vero cells [17, 18]. In order to detect the influence of iron saturation in the inhibition of viral infection, iron-free BLf (Apo-BLf), iron-saturated BLf (Holo-BLf) as well as Lf containing different metal ions such as Mn(II) or Zn(II) were tested for the activity against HSV infection. The results showed that all the metal-saturated forms of BLf acted at early steps of viral infection, more precisely during adsorption of the virus particles at the cell surface [18].

In an attempt to identify the mechanism of BLf action against HSV infection, one report has shown that BLf interfered with viral particle binding to GAG chains, HS or chondroitin sulphate (CS) [19]. This was in agreement with a previous study demonstrating that early steps of viral infection require HSV binding to GAGs, which can act as receptors for human herpetic viruses [20]. The viral glycoproteins gC or gB bind to HS or CS on the target cell surface, although HS is preferred. The BLf anti-viral activity proved to be efficient in cells expressing HS or CS or both and inefficient in mutant cells depleted of GAGs. The same results were obtained when cells were treated with GAG-degrading enzymes. Moreover, mutant gC-deficient viruses were less inhibited by BLf suggesting that Lf competes with viral gC for cell surface HS or CS binding [19]. Intriguingly, the same research group has published later the observation that BLf was able to inhibit plague-forming by HSV-2 in cells devoid of GAG expression, suggesting that unlike HSV-1, the mechanism of HSV-2 infection by BLf may imply the protein binding to a virus receptor of a non-GAG nature [21].

The inhibitory effect of peptides derived from Lf on HSV infection was also investigated and the effect was generally lower as compared with the parental protein. BLf tryptic digestion-derived peptides were assayed for antiviral activity and two high molecular weight peptides, one from C-lobe (345-689) and one from N-lobe (1-280), proved to be efficient. Two low molecular weight peptides (222-230 and 264-269) revealed antiviral effect only when added together in the antiviral assay. However, the effect was lower than that obtained when the larger fragments and the native molecule were used [22]. The experiments performed with BLf N-lobe and C-lobe demonstrated a 50- and 10-fold respectively, lower efficiency than that of the native protein [23]. Time of addition assays demonstrated an antiviral effect of two N-lobe derived peptides in the early steps of HSV infection. Introduction of negative charges by single amino acid substitutions did not influence the antiviral properties of these peptides. Based on these studies it was concluded that the anti-HSV mechanism of action of BLf should be more complicated than the simple competition between BLf and viral particle for target cell surface GAG binding.

Regarding potential mechanisms of action of Lfcin against HSV infection, the protein binding to HS was involved in Vero cells [24]. The authors also investigated a potential post-infection effect of both Lf and Lfcin, by studying the intracellular distribution of the immunogold-labeled protein and derived peptide using transmission electron microscope (TEM). A clear proof that Lf must be localized at the plasma membrane in order to inhibit HSV entry was obtained by detecting the labeled protein at the cell surface. On the contrary, Lfcin was detected randomly distributed in the cytoplasm of Vero cells and thus it was suggested an inhibitory effect on HSV at a later step of infection [24].

These results are in contradiction with previous report revealing a much lower efficiency of HLfcin in inhibiting clinical isolates of HSV-1 and HSV-2 infection as compared with BLfcin [25]. However, a synergistic effect between acyclovir (ACV) in combination with both Lf or Lfcin in inhibiting HSV infection was recorded [25].

Immunofluorescence studies on cellular uptake and intracellular trafficking of HSV-1 showed a significant reduction in HSV-1 cellular uptake in both, BLf- and BLfcin- treated cells [26]. Moreover, the few viral particles that were internalized revealed a delayed intracellular trafficking along microtubules, more precisely toward nucleus, thus affecting virus replication in Vero cells. The authors suggested that BLf and BLfcin exert also an intracellular antiviral effect, in addition to the inhibitory effect at entry of the virus.

The dependency of Lfcin inhibition of HSV infection on the presence of HS or CS on the target cell surface is not totally shared by cyclic and linear HLfcin and BLfcin derivatives [27, 28]. The study showed that affinity for HS does not predict the antiviral activity and that the native protein exhibits a much higher antiviral effect than the smaller peptides.

CYTOMEGALOVIRUS (CMV)

The inhibition of infection and replication of CMV *in vitro* by Lf was described initially in 1994 [16] and later confirmed by other research groups. The antiviral capacity was not associated with iron saturation or presence of sialic acid in the structure of the molecule, but rather with the protein moiety. The protein was found to be efficient at early steps of virus infection, preventing CMV adsorption and/or internalization in the target cells [16]. Later, in a study that has investigated native and chemically modified proteins from serum and milk for their antiviral activity on fibroblasts it was shown that only native BLf completely blocked CMV infection [29]. Moreover, it was shown that a conformational intact protein is required for antiviral effect to occur while addition of negatively charged groups by succinylation decreased the antiviral potency. In contrast, addition of positive charge by amination increased the anti-CMV activity of Lf [30]. N-t region seems to be important for anti-CMV activity of the protein, since N-t deletion variants were less efficient against CMV [30].

In another study investigating the antiviral potency of human milk against CMV *in vitro* it was observed that HLf inhibited the growth of the virus in cell culture [31]. It was suggested that the cationic feature of Lf was responsible for its anti-CMV activity at early steps of infection since cationic human serum albumin inhibited CMV replication in a similar way, when cells rather than virus particles were pre- incubated with the protein [32]. In a similar experimental setting, the Lfcin effect was seven-fold weaker as compared to the parental molecule [33].

HEPATITIS B VIRUS (HBV)

Inhibition of virus entry into target cells seems to be the antiviral mechanism of Lf action against HBV infection as well. Hara et al. have investigated the anti-HBV activity of Lf in human hepatocytes PH5CH8 cell line. Pre-treatment of cells with either BLf or HLf was required for inhibition of HBV infection, but pre-incubation of viral particles with the protein had no inhibitory effect. The authors hypothesized Lf prevented virus particle adsorption on cell surface by direct interaction with molecules from the plasma membrane [34]. In a more recent study, HepG2 cells were subjected to HBV infection in the presence or absence of iron- or zinc-saturated BLf or protein hydrolysate treatment. Using FQ-PCR, it was shown that BLf significantly decreased HBV DNA in a dose-dependent manner, while BLf hydrolysate was ineffective [35]. However, it is difficult to conclude the mechanism of anti-HBV activity of Lf since the authors employed cell lines with very poor HBV infectivity rate, although the use of human hepatocyte lines susceptible to HBV infection was claimed. In 2002, a French team established a cell line called HepaRG exhibiting hepatocyte-like morphology and expressing specific hepatocyte functions, which supports HBV infection at a rate comparable to primary cultures [36]. Evaluation of HBV infection in the presence of HLf in this new cellular infectivity model, by Southern blotting using encapsidated HBV DNA, revealed the potent activity of the protein in inhibiting HBV entry when added during infection [37].

We have also used the HepaRG cell line to study the anti-HBV activities of seven HLf-derived synthetic peptides (HLPs) belonging to the N-t domain [38]. Among the peptide investigated, HLP1-23 containing the GRRRR cationic cluster, proved most efficient in inhibiting HBV infection. Time of addition assays revealed that HLP1-23 was active only when it was pre-incubated for 1 h with viral inoculum. Surprisingly, while the parental protein exerts its antiviral effect at an early phase of viral infection, the derived peptide HLP1-23 was suggested to interact with the negatively charged residues on the viral particle [38].

Table 1. Effect of human lactoferrin-derived synthetic peptides (HLP) against HBV infection in HepaRG cells

Differentiated cells were infected with HBV inoculum. HLP were added together with the viral inoculum. The amount of HBV-specific RNA or encapsidated DNA in cells was quantified either by reverse transcription (RT) real time-PCR or real-time PCR [38].

	Peptide sequence	HBV inhibition (%)
1.	GRRRRSVQWCAVSQPEATKCFQW (HLP1-23)	82.8
2.	CFQWQRNMRKVRGPPVSCIKRDSPIQ (HLP20-45)	50
3.	TKCGQWQRN (HLP18-26F21G)	40
4.	TKCFGWGRN (HLP18-26Q22G/Q24G)	24
5.	TGCFQWQRN (HLP18-26K19G)	42
6.	TKCFQWQGN (HLP18-26R25G)	20
7.	FQWQRNMRKVR (HLP21-31)	16.5

The most common way of HBV infection and the main cause of chronicity is mother-to-child transmission. Researchers and clinicians have found viral markers in human milk and a correlation between colostral HBsAg and HBeAg titers and their corresponding levels in maternal blood [38, 40]. Since colostrum is enriched in Lf, breastfeeding was encouraged in many debates [41]. Moreover, the World Health Organization (WHO) postulates that chronic infection with HBV is not a reliable argument against breastfeeding. However, there are not sufficient studies in support of breastfeeding involving HBV-infected mothers and the ability of Lf to prevent potential mother-to-child transmission of the virus. It is worth mentioning that the American Academy of Pediatrics supports the notion that HBV infection is not a contraindication to breastfeeding of infants who received HBV vaccine and hepatitis B immune globulin treatment (HBIG).

Human Immunodeficiency Virus (HIV)

Both BLf and HLf in their native form efficiently prevent the cytopathic effect of HIV-1 *in vitro* on MT4 cells [29]. However, a 4-fold stronger anti-HIV-1 activity was recorded after addition of negatively charged groups to Lf by succinylation. In a study of antiviral capacity of plasma and milk proteins with modified charge it was shown that addition of positive charges through amination decreased anti-HIV effect [30]. Apo- and ferric, manganese or zinc-saturated forms of BLf were tested for their capacity to inhibit HIV-1 infection in C8166 T-cell line [42]. The study revealed that HIV-1 replication, as well as syncytium formation was inhibited in a dose-dependent manner when all Lf forms were added before viral inoculum or during the adsorption phase. A strong inhibitory effect of BLf on the viral reverse transcriptase but not on the protease and the integrase was observed in a study where different proteins isolated from bovine milk were assayed for inhibitory effects against HIV enzymes [43].

Dendritic cell-mediated HIV-1 transmission was efficiently inhibited by BLf by blocking the interaction established between the HIV receptor dendritic cell-specific intercellular adhesion molecule-3-grabbing non-integrin (DC-SIGN) and the viral gp120 on the surface of these cells [44]. Interestingly, BLf was more efficient in blocking HIV transmission from dendritic cells to CD4(+) T-cells than HLf. The efficacy of HLf in preventing HIV uptake by dendritic cells was confirmed by another group who also reported the capacity of HLf to limit specifically adsorption of R5- and X4-HIV-1-free particles on endometrial epithelial HEC-1A cells [45]. HLf inhibited virus adsorption on HS proteoglycans on epithelial cells, but not HIV transcytosis across monolayer of endometrial HEC-1A cells.

Interestingly, it was reported that Lf exhibits synergy with zidovudine in inhibition of HIV replication *in vitro* [46].

In an attempt to search for the domain of the native BLf that is responsible for its anti-HIV activity, an investigation of protein-derived peptides was performed. In this study BLfcin was found to exhibit a modest inhibition of HIV infection, while BLf inhibited HIV infection through a mechanism targeting the viral entry process. The results suggested that other regions than Lfcin within the parental molecule must be responsible for the anti-HIV activity of Lf [47, 48]. Recently, the same group has reported that HLf and a HLf-derived peptide Lf-33 peptide were able to modulate HIV binding to epithelial cells, but only the full length protein was able to inhibit by 40% the HIV mucosal transmission from dendritic cells to T-cells [49]. HLf inhibited the attachment of the virus to human endometrial HEC-1 cells and human colorectal HT-29 epithelial cells with a greater efficacy than the Lf-33 peptide.

ADENOVIRUS

Lf was able to inhibit adenovirus replication *in vitro* in a dose-dependent manner when added before viral adsorption, during virus infection or when present during the entire viral life cycle, including replication [50, 51]. Another report suggested that BLf inhibited adenovirus infection by a competition mechanism for the common receptor involving GAGs binding [52]. A role for positive charges- enriched N-t part of the protein in mediating antiviral mechanism was proposed since the C-t half rendered no inhibitory capacity on adenoviral infection of HEp-2 cells.

In contrast to the results shown above, other studies reported that HLf from tear fluid was able to promote adenoviral infection of corneal epithelial cells [53]. The infection with adenovirus in the presence of HLf was observed on polarized cells which do not express coxsackie- and adenovirus receptor (CAR) on the apical side and was considered an alternative mechanism for viral entry into the target cells. Lf in the tear fluid plays an important anti-microbial and anti-inflammatory role. The entry of the viral particles into the epithelial cells could be inhibited by Lf; however, a high concentration of Lf in tears could limit the opportunistic Lf mediated bridging of adenoviral particle and target cells, which occurs in other tissues [54].

Adams et al. reported that infection of human dendritic cells by adenovirus serotype 5 could be mediated by Lf and the proposed virus receptor DC-SIGN [55]. The viral-Lf complex entry required the high-mannose-type N-linked glycans present on the protein to interact with DC-SIGN. Recently, another study using clinical adenovirus 2C isolates showed that DC-SIGN mediates infection of monocyte-derived dendritic cells with the virus in the presence of BLf, but not HLf [56]. The difference in behavior of the two proteins could be explained by the difference in the high mannose carbohydrate content which is necessary for the interaction with DC-SIGN.

ALPHAVIRUS

HLf inhibited infection of BHK-21 by HS-adapted Sindbis virus or Semliki Forest virus by interfering with virus-receptor interaction. HLf failed to inhibit infection of the hamster kidney fibroblasts by HS non-adapted alphaviruses [57] Given the fact that charged-modified serum albumin had a similar effect on HS-adapted alphaviruses infection, this observation highlighted once again the important role of the positive charges of the HLf molecule.

Hantavirus

The effect of BLf and ribavirin on Seoul type hantavirus was investigated *in vitro* [58]. Pretreatment of Vero E6 cells with BLf proved to be highly efficient in inhibiting foci formation, but subsequent addition of ribavirin demonstrated a synergistic effect against hantavirus. It was suggested that Lf inhibited virus adsorption to target cells by interacting with cell surface, since washing the Lf-preincubated cells resulted in minimal focus reduction. Other reports showed that although saliva from healthy volunteers reduced only partially hantavirus infection, Lf was not able to inhibit Hantaan hantavirus in vitro [59].

Feline Calicivirus

It was shown that pre-incubation of BLf cells or addition of BLf together with feline calicivirus inoculum reduced infection of Crandel-Reese feline kidney (CRFK) [60]. A proof that Lf prevents virus attachment by interfering with virus binding to cellular membrane was detection of BLf on cell surface. BLfcin also proved to inhibit feline calicivirus infection in a similar manner as the parental protein. In a study comparing the effects of amination and acylation on the antiviral and antimicrobial capacity of Lf it was found that increasing the negative charges of Lf diminished substantially the anti-feline calicivirus activity of the protein [61].

Japanese Encephalitis Virus (JEV)

Using wild-type as well as laboratory-adapted strains of JEV it was shown that BLf was able to inhibit early events of JEV infection *in vitro*. The infectivity of HS-adapted viral strains was reduced to a greater extent compared to that of HS-non-adapted strains, supporting the hypothesis that BLf interaction with GAGs from the surface of the target cell is required for antiviral activity. Further experiments revealed that a HS-independent pathway involving cell surface-expressed LDLR may be used by BLf to inhibit JEV infection, since rLDLR and anti-LDLR antibodies decreased the antiviral capacity of BLf [62].

Influenza A Virus

It was shown that BLf interfere with caspase 3 function and thus inhibits influenza virus triggered apoptosis of infected cells [63]. Moreover, the same study demonstrated that BLf blocked viral particle assembly by inhibiting viral ribonucleoproteins nuclear transport.

In a study investigating the effect of esterified whey proteins on influenza A H5N1, both native Lf as well as its esterified form proved to be the most potent antiviral protein among the tested samples [64].

Pietrantoni et al. revealed that BLf was able to inhibit the influenza virus cytopathic effect regardless the ion saturation form or carbohydrate content [65]. The study investigated the antiviral activity of different forms of BLf when treatment was performed after the adsorption step on influenza virus or at early phases of infection. The authors concluded that the effect of Lf was exerted after the adsorption step, and was not influenced by the level of ion saturation of the protein or the carbohydrate content.

Recently, Ammendolia et al. demonstrated that the C-lobe of BLf is the active part in inhibiting influenza virus hemagglutination by binding to HA(2) region of the viral protein and diminishing infection of the cells by major virus subtypes [66]. Three peptides derived from the C-lobe of BLf exhibited antiviral activity at femtomolar concentrations by reducing viral hemagglutination and infection, as revealed by molecular docking studies.

Severe Acute Respiratory Syndrome (SARS)

It was reported recently that Lf was able to inhibit SARS pseudovirus infection in a dose-dependent manner by binding to cell surface HS and thus preventing viral spike protein attachment to Hek293E/ACE2-Myc host cells [67]. Co-localization studies revealed that Oregon Green-labeled Lf localize at the cell membrane and targets HS chains suggesting a protective role of the protein against viral insults. Moreover, heparinase treatment or exogenous heparin addition to Vero E6 or Caco-2 cells abolished SARS infection, confirming the essential role of HS proteoglycans for SARS entry into host cells. However, Lf failed to block the interaction between SARS and angiotensin-converting enzyme 2 (ACE2) which is a well-known receptor for SARS.

Human Papilloma Virus (HPV)

The anti-HPV activity of both, HLf and BLf was studied on HPV-16 virus-like particles labeled with carboxyfluorescein diacetate succinimidyl esther (CFDA-SE) that fluoresce only after virus internalization in human keratinocyte HaCaT cells, natural host for HPV. Flow cytometry analysis revealed a decrease in fluorescence, which is an indication that Lf was able to inhibit virus internalization. The mechanism was thought to be mediated by interaction of Lf with HS. Interestingly, BLf was shown to be more potent in inhibiting HPV entry as compared to human protein [68]. HLfcin and BLfcin were tested for their anti-HPV activity on HaCaT and C33A cell lines along with other HLfcin- and BLfcin-derived peptides adopting acyclic or linear conformation. The results revealed that a linear 15 amino acids residues peptide derived from BLfcin [17-31] was the most potent in inhibiting both HPV-5 and HPV-16 pseudovirus and both cell lines tested [69]. In contrast, only a modest antiviral activity was observed for HLfcin.

Picornavirus

In a study investigating the effect of Lf on enteric viruses it was shown that BLf was able to inhibit poliovirus infection in monkey embryo kidney cells when present throughout the infection period. Immunofluorescence experiments revealed the presence of BLf on the surface of the cells, indicating that BLf prevents virus attachment to susceptible cells. BLfcin, however, failed to inhibit poliovirus infection [60].

In conclusion, Lf was shown to bind to many common cell surface molecules such as HS, GAGs, nucleolin, ASGPR, LDLR, providing a rather non-specific shield against a variety of cell pathogens. It was therefore suggested that the antiviral activity of Lf involves inhibition of virus entry into host cells by a protection mechanism involving blocking of their access to cellular receptors.

Direct Interaction with Viral Particles

HSV

BLf was reported to inhibit HSV-1 infection of Green Monkey Kidney cells using a mechanism dependent on the specific interaction between Lf and viral structural proteins VP-16 (major capsid protein) and ICP-5 (viral tegument protein). Co-localization of HSV-1 and BLf at early stages of infection was observed, as well as an impaired transport of the viral protein VP-16 to the nucleus in the presence of BLf. Moreover, the immunofluorescence microscopy experiments revealed that BLf was able to inhibit cell-to-cell spread of the virus infection at 16h post infection [70]. Further, the same research group has published a paper addressing the antiviral activity of both, HLf and BLf against HSV-2 [21]. It was found that BLf does not interact with viral glycoprotein C (gC) since the antiviral effect of BLf against wild-type or gC-truncated derivative HSV-2 was similar. On the contrary, the HLf effect against HSV-2 infection was potentiated when the virus contained the defective glycoprotein, indicating that HLf may bind other viral proteins which are not available for interaction in the wild-type virus. Overall, the authors concluded that BLf was more effective in inhibiting HSV-2 infection as compared to the human protein [21].

In a study investigating the anti-HSV-1 activity of Lf and lysozyme, another highly cationic protein from the mucosal immune system, it was observed for the first time that only HLf in its apo-or iron-saturated form displayed HSV-1 virus neutralization properties when pre-incubated with the virus [71]. Cell-to-cell spreading of HSV-1 with mutated glycoprotein D (gD) remained unmodified, suggesting that the inhibition of virus propagation in culture is dependent at least in part by gD.

HCV

The anti-HCV activity of Lf was not addressed until 1997 when the group of Yi et al. has reported that HCV envelope proteins expressed in bacteria or mammalian cells-are able to bind HLf and BLf, regardless the presence of the N-t loop in the human or bovine protein [72]. Pre-incubation of the viral inoculum with BLf or HLf was required for the inhibition of HCV infection of human hepatocytes PH5CH8 [73]. The inhibition of HCV infection of

PH5CH8 hepatocytes and MT-2C T-cells was due to direct and very rapid interaction of BLf with the virus particles, but the anti-HCV effect was reversed by heating at 65 °C. Infection with hepatitis G virus, a virus distantly related to HCV, was inhibited by Lf in a manner similar to HCV infection [74].

BLf was reported to inhibit specifically the infection of the pseudotype vesicular stomatitis virus possessing HCV envelope proteins in HepG2 cells confirming the anti-HCV mechanism of Lf by direct interaction with viral proteins [75].

Interestingly, camel Lf pre-incubated with HCV but not with human leukocytes was shown to inhibit virus entry into the cells after seven days of incubation [76]. Recent studies have compared the anti-HCV activity of native and recombinant full-length camel Lf (ncLf and rcLf) with its N and C lobes on Huh-7 cells [77]. The results showed that rcLf as well as its N lobe inhibit HCV entry by direct interaction with the virus and exhibit a similar antiviral activity as compared to their native counterparts, thus underlining the efficiency of the recombinant protein for potential clinical applications. Pretreatment of PBMCs and Huh7.5 cells with different proteins from camel milk did not prevent HCV infection [78]. The study showed that only camel IgG and cLf were able to inhibit the HCV entry in the cell systems tested by direct interaction between the two milk proteins and the virus particle. The anti-HCV activity of the cLf was further compared with HLf, BLf and sheep Lf, however the cLf was demonstrated to possess the highest inhibitory effect against HCV infection and amplification in HepG2 cells [79].

It is worth mentioning that incubation of hepatic cell lines stably expressing viral nonstructural proteins NS3- NS5B with holo-Lf in order to increase the concentration of iron in cell culture, did not reduce HCV replication [80].

It was demonstrated that BLfcin had no anti-HCV effect, even at 300 μg/ml, confirming the experiments of Yi et al. using truncated-Lf [74].

In an attempt to clarify the antiviral mechanism of HLf involving direct binding to HCV particles, several bacterial expressed thioredoxin-fused regions from HLf were investigated. It was found that the 93 carboxyl amino acids of HLf bind to HCV E2 envelope protein in a specific manner; using deletions of this region it was further demonstrated that the binding property leading to HCV inhibition is restricted to the 33 amino acids residues termed C-s3-33 (aminoacids 600-632) or the Nozaki peptide [81]. The amino acids from the carboxyl region revealed partial homology with CD81, the co-receptor of HCV on the surface of target cell. Moreover, the 93 amino acids from Lfs derived from horse and bovine cells were found to bind to E2 viral protein, demonstrating that the fragment is a conserved region. Furthermore, the presence of Cys at aminoacid 628 is required for binding to the E2 viral protein, as shown by site-directed mutagenesis [81]. An increased activity against HCV (VSV pseudotype bearing the native forms of HCV E1 and E2 protein) in PH5CH8 cells was obtained when the 33 aminoacid peptide C-s3-33 was repeated in tandem two or three times (82). In another study, starting from the 33 amino acids fragment (the Nozaki peptide) of HLf, a number of 5 biotin-linked peptides were synthesized and two peptides with the highest helical content were found to bind E2 protein of the N strain of HCV in a concentration-dependent manner [83].

HIV

Peptide-scanning studies have shown that modifications of the native Lf charges by succinylation or aconitylation do not change the capacity of the protein to bind to the V3 loop of gp120 envelope protein [84]. It was proposed that shielding of this domain could impair virus-cell fusion and consequent entry of the viral particle into target cell.

Adenovirus

It was shown that pre-incubation of cells with BLf was not sufficient to totally abolish adenovirus infection, since there may be viral receptors on the plasma membrane other than GAGs [85]. However, pre-incubation of BLf for 1h with adenovirus led to 95% inhibition of viral antigen synthesis. Western blot analysis has demonstrated the specific binding of BLf to the virus penton base (polypeptide III); in addition, negative-stain electron microscopy revealed that biotinylated BLf interacts directly with external structures on adenovirus particle labeled with streptavidin-gold [85].

Rotavirus

Apo- and holo-Lf interfered with early stages of rotavirus infection of human enterocyte-like cells HT-29 by direct binding to the viral particle and inhibition of virus attachment to intestinal cells [86]. The competition for common binding sites on cell surface of HT-29 cells was ruled out, since SA-11 rotavirus is well known to bind to glucidic residues different from GAGs. The results obtained suggested that apo-Lf was the most potent in inhibiting rotavirus antigen synthesis and viral replication in a concentration-dependent manner in HT-29 cells, as well as rotavirus haemagglutination of human erythrocytes. Further, the research group investigated the effect of metal saturation on the anti-SA-11 rotavirus activity of BLf and the results revealed a decreased effect of the manganese- or zinc-saturated BLf as compared to apo- or holo-BLf [87]. Intriguingly, when sialic acid was removed from BLf molecule, the anti-rotavirus activity was increased. It was suggested that the removal of the sialic acid residues could unmask some secondary viruses binding sites on Lf molecule.

On the contrary to the results discussed above, a study performed on MA104 and Caco-2 cells using neuraminidase-resistant Wa rotavirus showed that milk-fat globule protein lactadherine was able to inhibit viral infectivity, whereas BLf failed to suppress the rotavirus strain tested [88].

Regarding the anti-rotavirus activity of Lf-derived peptides, it was shown that a large fragment from the N-lobe as well as a small fragment of only six amino acids residues from the N half (YLTTLK) were able to inhibit rotavirus infection; however the effect was lower than that obtained with the full length protein [87].

PICORNAVIRUS

Experiments on poliovirus infection in Vero cells revealed that viral cytopathic effect was prevented by apo-, iron, manganese-, and zinc- saturated BLf and HLf in a dose-dependent manner [89]. Interestingly, only zinc-saturated Lf was able to inhibit infection after poliovirus internalization into the Vero cells.

Both BLf and HLf were reported to be potent inhibitors of enterovirus 71 infection in human embryonic rhabdomyosarcoma cells [90]. Moreover, it was shown that BLf protected also neuroblastoma SK-N-SH cell line from enterovirus 71 infection when added at various times and is able to bind VP1 viral protein [91].

The activity of BLf against echovirus 6 was assessed in GMK cells and the results revealed that Lf was able to inhibit intranucleosomal breakdown of cellular DNA, an effect of viral-induced programmed cell death [92]. The results were confirmed by electron micrographs of thin sections of GMK cells infected with echovirus 6, which exhibited no injury in the presence of BLf. In contrast, in the absence of treatment morphological markers of apoptosis, such as formation of micronuclei, cytosol derangement and big paracrystalline inclusion were observed. The same authors have further demonstrated that the inhibitory effect of BLf on echovirus 6 infection is due to direct interaction with viral capsid proteins that led to incapacity of the virus to uncoat [70]. Tryptic fragments of BLf were tested for anti-echovirus 6 effects on GMK cells at various times of addition and the results showed that the N-t cationic peptide (Lfcin) is very potent in inhibiting early steps of viral infection [93].

BLf digested with different human gastrointestinal enzymes exhibited inhibitory effect against echovirus 5 in cell culture when added before virus infection or at the same time with the viral inoculum [94]. The results obtained highlighted the importance of peptides released during the digestion process in prevention of viral infection.

Respiratory Syncytial Virus (RSV)

HLf was able to inhibit the growth of RSV in cell culture at a concentration 10 times lower than that found in milk [95]. In another study it was demonstrated that Lf inhibited the adsorption and growth of RSV in cell culture, but the antiviral activity decreased dramatically from 85% to only 30% when the protein was added to an infant formula [96]. It was not until 2003 when an attempt to decipher the anti-RSV mechanism of Lf was made by the study of Sano and co-workers. This study showed that Lf binds the RSV F protein, the viral glycoprotein responsible for penetration, resulting in reduction of both, the viral titer and the FITC-labeled RSV uptake [97]. Lf was demonstrated to interact directly with the F(1) subunit, which contains the antigenic sites of viral F surface glycoprotein and with F(2) subunit after deglycosylation.

Polyomavirus

Lf was shown to inhibit early steps of BK polyomavirus infection in Vero cells through a potential mechanism involving interaction with capsidic structures as revealed by electron micrograph of negatively–stained BK polyomavirus particles [98]. The authors mentioned however that an alternative mechanism involving Lf binding to plasma membrane receptors could be used in interfering with viral infection.

In summary, in the case of some viral infections, full length Lf and Lf-derived peptides are able to interfere with the early phases of the viral life-cycle by directly interacting with components of the viral particles and neutralizing binding epitopes important for adsorption on the cell surface

The mechanism of action of Lf and Lf-derived peptides are summarized in Fig. 2.

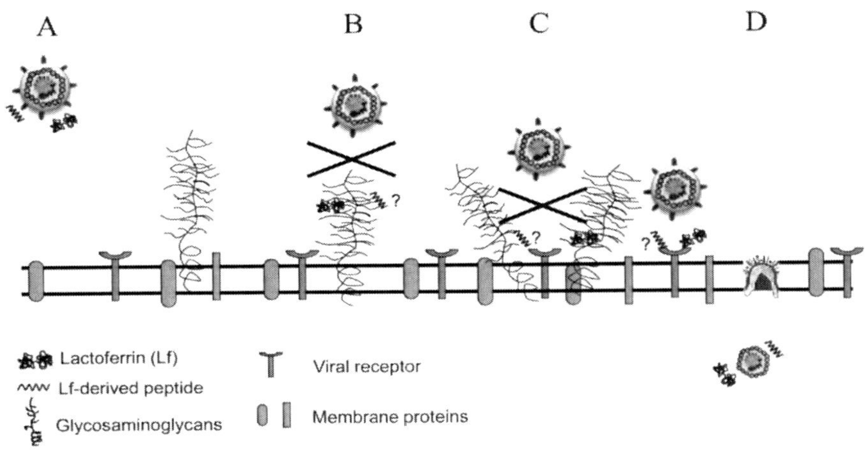

Figure 2. Schematic representation of the antiviral mechanisms of lactoferrin (Lf) and Lf-derived peptides. Lf inhibits viral infections by direct interaction with the virus (A), with specific and non-specific viral receptor molecules on the host cell surface (B,C), or by modulating intracellular pathways (D).

INDIRECT MECHANISMS OF ACTION-*IN VIVO* STUDIES ON ANIMALS

HSV

As early as 1995 it was reported that Lf was able to inhibit HSV-1 infection in mouse cornea by preventing plaque formation when administrated before viral inoculums [99]. However, Lf failed to inhibit virus propagation.

In another study, it was shown that BLf was able to inhibit the appearance of skin lesions when mice were fed with Lf ten days before HSV-1 cutaneous infection [100]. Although Lf did not abolish totally HSV-1 infection, it prevented body loss and the decrease of splenocytes. Moreover, it increases the level of anti-inflammatory cytokines IL-18 and IL-12 and the production of the antiviral molecule interferon (IFN)-γ.

Intriguingly, BLfcin but not BLf inhibited HSV-2 in a genital model of viral infection in mice when admixed with the virus inoculum prior to infection [101]. Although both BLf and BLfcin failed to stimulate chemokines production in splenocytes *in vitro*, they succeeded to induce CCL-5 vaginal production in C57/BL6 mice when inoculated intravaginally at 200 μg/mouse. There was no effect detected when the compounds were administrated 24h prior to HSV-2 infection. When BLfcin was given as a single dose 24h post-infection it was able to reduce viral load 15-fold and delay infection onset by 3 days, indicating the potential use of the peptide as a therapeutically approach at a post-infection stage.

Feline Immunodeficiency Virus (FIV)

Oral administration of BLf (40 mg/kg of body weight) improved intractable stomatitis in FIV-positive cats after 14 days of treatment [102]. It was suggested that phagocytic activity of neutrophils was improved after Lf administration, as showed using nonopsonized hydrophilic 2 microns polymer particles. The same group published later the results obtained in the study of anti-inflammatory effects of BLf on persistent immune activation status in FIV-infected cats [103]. Lf was shown to suppress FIV-induced apoptosis in feline PBMCs as well as concanavalin A-induced IL-2 production suggesting that Lf may improve the function of overactivated lymphocytes.

Friend Virus Complex (FVC)

Since 1987, *in vivo* studies on mice infected with FVC revealed the beneficial effects of intravenously administrated HLf (200 μg/mouse) on the development of erythroleukemia in the spleens [104]. The study reported that Lf administration prolonged survival and improved general architecture of the spleen, with the red pulp showing no modifications while the white pulp revealed no leukemic cells infiltrate as compared with controls. However, some mice did not respond to Lf treatment and exhibited splenomegaly. It is notable that the treatment applied 7 days before or after encountering viral infection did not have any beneficial effects. The conclusion of the study was that the time of treatment application is crucial for successful outcome and ideally it should be administered as early following FVC infection, as possible. In another study, the protective role of Lf was demonstrated on mice infected with polycythemia-inducing strain of FVC (FVC-P); the treatment prolonged the survival rates and decreased the titer of spleen focus-forming viruses [105]. Lf was administrated in a dosage of 200 μg and it exerted an antiviral effect when given 3 days before or after FVC-P infection. Since *in vitro* results showed that Lf did not interact directly with the virus particle, a protector role on cells was suggested. Later, a synergistic suppressive effect of recombinant murine IFN-γ and purified iron-saturated HLf was observed after treatment of mice which had been intravenously injected with FVC-P [106]. HLf was administrated sub-cutaneous in a dosage of 100 μg at day 7, whereas recombinant IFN-γ treatment started at day 6 and it lasted for 3 days. The decreased activity of natural killer (NK) cells recorded after FVC-P infection was restored after combined treatment.

CMV

Experiments in BALB/c mice demonstrated that the administration of 1 mg/g body weight of BLf before CMV infection resulted in an increased activation of NK cells induced by T lymphocytes [107]. In a study of pharmacokinetic behavior in rats, a high affinity of HLf for endothelial cells and leukocytes was observed as well as the ability to reach general circulation after intraperitoneal administration [108]. The authors underlined the importance of these findings as these type of cells are crucial for CMV replication and concluded that Lf could be a good candidate for antiviral therapeutic studies in the future since the human protein was able to reach blood circulation and showed increased bioavailability after multiple administrations (from 0.6 up to 3.6%). The same group also reported the beneficial effects of intravenous Lf administration at 6h after CMV infection, for three times a week. The treatment led to a 10-fold decrease in the virus titer after 4 weeks from initial infection in immunocompromised rats [32]. Notably, the anti-viral effect of Lf was successful when the rats received cell-free virus, instead of virus-infected leukocytes as a viral inoculum. The antiviral activity of Lf was suggested to involve inhibition of the initial stage of virus entry into the cell and not modulation of the immune system.

HANTAVIRUS

An interesting study reported that administration of 60 mg/kg of Lf prior to viral challenge to hantavirus-infected suckling mice increased survival rates to 70%, for single administration and up to 94% for double administration. The results obtained were comparable with those obtained after ribavirin treatment, which was shown to inhibit viral RNA synthesis [109].

INFLUENZA

The beneficial effects of BLf administration in H1N1 influenza virus-infected mice were evaluated by reduced lung consolidation score and decreased amount of leukocytes in bronchoalveolar lavage fluid [110]. BLf treatment by gavage administration started one day prior to influenza virus infections at a dosage of 62.5 mg/mouse. Notably, the virus yield in the bronchoalveolar fluid was not affected by Lf treatment. Consecutively, the group reported that the antiviral mechanism of action of BLf could involve modulation of host immunity by enhancing transcription of immune-related genes such as IL-12p40, IFN-β, and NOD2 [111].

ROTAVIRUS

A reduced incidence in diarrhoea episodes from 90% to 60% was observed in group A rotavirus-infected suckling rats which have previously received daily supplements of Lf combined with bovine whey protein concentrate from day 3 of life [112]. Moreover, serum level of anti-rotavirus antibodies, the proliferation of splenocytes as well as IFN-γ secretion were dramatically decreased in rats receiving combined treatment. Moreover, the supplementation received also succeeded to control the virus-induced increase in the proportion of mucosal T cells (IE-T CD8 alphaalpha+) in the intraepithelial intestinal compartment.

Enterovirus 71

It was reported that BLf was able to protect mice infected with enterovirus 71 [91] and recombinant porcine Lf was shown to increase survival rates in neonatal mice infected with a lethal dose of enterovirus type 71 [113].

RSV

Administration of BLf even at 10 mg/animal/day did not reveal any beneficial effects concerning lung inflammation, RSV replication and cytokines status to murine model of RSV [114].

In Human Experiments-Clinical Trials

HIV

A study on 22 children with a mean age of 9 years, infected vertically with HIV evaluated the effect of oral administration of BLf (1g every 8h, a total of 3g/day) for a period of 6 months [115]. No patient revealed any new symptoms related to HIV infection and no side effects were detected consecutive the BLf treatment. It was recorded that plasma viral load (log10) decreased from 4.54 (+/-0.65) to 4.28 (+/-0.6), but viral load did not differ significantly 2 months after the BLf treatment has stopped. However, immune parameters such as CD4+ cell number increased from 21.5% up to 24.5% and the percentage continued to remain higher than the baseline. Noticeably, combined antiretroviral and BLf therapy was shown to be more potent in enhancing CD4+ T cell subsets as compared to BLf treatment alone. These encouraging results recommend the natural protein in addition to conventional antiretroviral therapeutic program. More comprehensive studies on a larger number of subjects should be performed in order to establish the Lf dosage and administration program and evaluate the long term clinical effects.

An interesting study on children vertically infected with HIV performed over a 12 year period reported a high level of iron, Lf, transferrin and haptoglobin in urine. These findings revealed the potential use of Lf and other iron binding proteins as biomarkers for detection of HIV-associated nephropathy and hemolytic uremic syndrome [116].

HCV

The first pilot study which made use of beneficial attributes of BLf in chronic HCV infected patients was described by Tanaka and coworkers [117]. BLf (1.8 and 3.6 g/day) was given for 8 weeks to 11 patients and 3 out of 4 patients exhibited a decrease in the level of serum alanine aminotransaminase (ALT) and also lower viral RNA levels. It is worth mentioning that the 3 patients presented lower serum levels of HCV RNA before BLf treatment. No significant modifications were recorded in patients with high pretreatment levels of viral RNA.

In a further study conducted by the Japanese team BLf was administrates orally at a maximum of 7.2 g/day for a period of 8 weeks to 45 patients and after that biochemical and virological parameters levels were measured [118]. Only 4 patients have revealed a decrease in viral level by 50% or higher and 2 patients in ALT level, also by 50% or higher. No correlation between BLf dosage (1.8-7.2 g/day) and anti-HCV effect was detected. BLf treatment was tolerated very well, with no toxicity detected, suggesting the need for further trials including a higher number of patients.

A long-term follow-up of 63 chronic HCV patients treated orally with 600 mg/day BLf for 12 month revealed that after only 3 months of treatment, the serum levels of IL-18 was increased then decreased gradually throughout the investigation period [119]. IFN-γ+/ IL-4- (Th1) cell number were slightly, but not significantly enhanced, while serum levels of ALA, viral RNA and IL-10 were not modified in the BLf-treated group. The authors concluded that eradication of HCV in chronically infected patients by IFN treatment could be potentiated by concomitant administration of BLf, which provides a Th1-cytokine dominant environment.

Several other studies have investigated the role of BLf administration to a small number of HCV chronically infected patients receiving IFN therapy. In a study where 21 patients were assigned to either a consensus IFN monotherapy group or an IFN and BLf (3 g per day) group, no difference concerning virological response was recorded [120]. In another randomized controlled trial, 36 HCV patients were evaluated for their virological response after receiving IFN-α 2b, ribavirin and BLf (0.6g/day) combined therapy and compared to IFN-α 2b, ribavirin and placebo [121]. As with the previous clinical trial, no significant difference could be observe since 6 of 18 patients and 5 of 18 patients respectively, exhibited a complete virological response in either group.

It was shown that BLf may inhibit oxidative stress-induced lipid peroxidation in a study which enrolled 90 patients chronically infected with HCV in Japan [122]. The patients received a dose of 3.6 g/day BLf as monotherapy, but no modification in serum viral RNA level or iron metabolism markers were detected. However, some beneficial results following BLf treatment was observed, as the protein induced a decrease in lipid peroxidation marker 8-isoprostane in plasma from 8.6+/-3.7 down to 6.9+/-2.1 pg/ml, which correlated with an improvement in ALT level.

Unfortunately this promising result was not confirmed, in a randomized, double-blind phase III trial in patients chronically infected with HCV [123]. One hundred and ninety-eight patients with ages between 20 and 74 years were evaluated in this study and divided in 97 patients in BLf group who received tablets containing 1.8 g/day orally twice a day for 12 weeks and 101 patients in placebo group. Importantly, none of the patients enrolled received any IFN, corticosteroid, immunomodulatory or intravenously administrated glycirrhizin therapy. Regarding the serum HCV RNA level, as well as IL-18 levels and percentages of CD4+, CD8+, CD16+, and CD56+ lymphocytes investigated in the study, there was no significant difference between the two groups. Also, no decrease in biochemical parameter level, serum ALT, was observed in BLf group, indicating no efficacy of the bovine protein as a monotherapy in viral infection. However, a randomized study enrolling 111 Japanese patients with chronic HCV infection showed decrease reduction of the viral titer after Lf monotherapy [124]. Importantly the daily dose of Lf was doubled compared with the previous study by Ueno and coworkers leading to sustained virological response (55% as compared to 18% in control). These controversial results regarding Lf efficiency in treating HCV may arise from the heterogeneity of the patients and their genetic background and also, the incomplete characterization of the stage of the disease at the time of patients' enrollment in the clinical trials.

ROTAVIRUS AND EV71

In a prospective, randomized, single blind trial on healthy unvaccinated Taiwanese children the supplementation of infant formula with 70 mg/day BLf for 3 month did not revealed any beneficial effects in preventing enterovirus or rotavirus infection [125].

RSV

A potential protective effect of Lf on the immune regulation was investigated in a study on 18 infants with severe bronchiolitis [126]. Eleven infants enrolled in the study were formula fed, whereas seven were breastfed. IL-8, MCP-1 and cellular components from nasopharyngeal aspirates were quantified. The results revealed the presence of secondary granules of neutrophils in the nasal airways, which correlated with an increased Lf concentration. This increase of Lf concentration may be involved in the up-regulation of the innate immune response at the site of viral infection.

SARS

It was found that Lf gene, along with S100A9 and lipocalin2 genes, was highly up-regulated in PBMCs from patients infected with SARS, suggesting that an innate inflammatory response, rather than a specific cytokine response was triggered [127].

Lf as Biomarker

Development of early diagnostic biomarkers is very important for an efficient therapy, especially for pathogenesis lacking specific symptoms at the onset of the disease. Very relevant for biomarkers discovery are tissue proteins that can be released into the body fluids at early stages or during progression of the disease, since their levels can be easily monitored, avoiding invasive procedures. From this point of view, secreted Lf could make a good biomarker candidate; however, relevant studies in this area are scarce.

Data collected from 226 evaluations for 117 individuals revealed that fecal Lf could be a useful marker for prediction and monitoring inflammatory status in infectious diarrhea in children [128]. The level of fecal Lf was increased in *Salmonella* (11.17 μg/g ± 2.73 μg/g) or *Campylobacter* (10.32 μg/g ± 2.94 μg/g), but decreased in rotavirus (2.82 μg/g ± 1.27 μg/g) or norovirus (3.16 μg/g ± 1.18 μg/g) infected patients. Moreover, the level of fecal Lf correlated with severe and moderate disease. These are certainly promising results that deserve future investigation in a larger number of samples from patients for potential clinical validation.

All these clinical observations revealed that Lf may exert an indirect effect by activation and regulation of an innate or adaptive host immune response. It is conceivable to propose the protein as a natural adjuvant in the common antiviral therapy. Interestingly, Lf was demonstrated to be a potential useful biomarker for viral infection evaluation and detection of viral-associated inflammation.

Conclusion and Potential Medical Applications

The antiviral mechanism of action of Lf is complex and still not completely understood. Although the mechanism varies greatly from one cell model to another, major breakthroughs have been made in the last years indicating the potential use of this mucosal barrier protein as an adjuvant in common antiviral therapeutic scheme. This is of particular interest since there is a constant search for new drugs/nutraceuticals with less toxicity. Lf could meet all these requirements since it is a natural protein with proven antiviral activity. Moreover, Lf is a promising alternative to conventional therapies, which often induce side effects and selection of viral resistance.

For the majority of viral infections, both HLf and BLf have demonstrated a protective antiviral activity when present at an early stage of the viral life-cycle, which may be very relevant in preventive therapies.

The iron-binding capacity if Lf seems to have no relevance for the antiviral activity of the protein, on the contrary, it was shown that other metal ions are important for this property in the case of certain viruses.

As compared to the full-length protein, Lfcin and other Lf-derived peptides demonstrated only modest inhibition of viral infections. The differences observed between HLfcin and BLfcin could be explained by the different secondary structure adopted by the peptides. It was demonstrated that most antiviral peptides are generally highly cationic molecules [28]. In the case of Lf-derived peptides it was revealed that the spatial position of amino acids plays a more important role than the overall charge itself. Moreover, It was suggested that the peptide might exert an intracellular effect, rather than at the cell surface. [27].

In vivo studies on animal models have demonstrated the beneficial effects of LF in inhibiting viral infections. Consecutively, clinical trials on human subjects revealed the potential use of the protein as a natural adjuvant, in combination with current antiviral therapeutic approaches. Further clinical trials with larger patient cohorts are required to establish the potential use of Lf as *in vivo* treatment of viral infections.

REFERENCES

[1] Legrand, D., and J. Mazurier. (2010). A critical review of the roles of host lactoferrin in immunity. *Biometals : an international journal on the role of metal ions in biology, biochemistry, and medicine* 23:365-376.
[2] Teng, C. T. (2010). Lactoferrin: the path from protein to gene. *Biometals : an international journal on the role of metal ions in biology, biochemistry, and medicine* 23:359-364.
[3] Ward, P. P., S. Uribe-Luna, and O. M. Conneely. (2002). Lactoferrin and host defense. *Biochemistry and cell biology = Biochimie et biologie cellulaire* 80:95-102.
[4] Masson, P. L., J. F. Heremans, and E. Schonne. (1969). Lactoferrin, an iron-binding protein in neutrophilic leukocytes. *The Journal of experimental medicine* 130:643-658.
[5] Slater, K., and J. Fletcher. (1987). Lactoferrin derived from neutrophils inhibits the mixed lymphocyte reaction. *Blood* 69:1328-1333.
[6] Baynes, R. D., W. R. Bezwoda, Q. Khan, and N. Mansoor. (1986). Plasma lactoferrin content: differential effect of steroid administration and infective illnesses: lack of effect of ambient temperature at which specimens are collected. *Scandinavian journal of haematology* 37:353-359.
[7] Anderson, B. F., H. M. Baker, G. E. Norris, D. W. Rice, and E. N. Baker. (1989). Structure of human lactoferrin: crystallographic structure analysis and refinement at 2.8 A resolution. *Journal of molecular biology* 209:711-734.
[8] Pierce, A., D. Colavizza, M. Benaissa, P. Maes, A. Tartar, J. Montreuil, and G. Spik. (1991). Molecular cloning and sequence analysis of bovine lactotransferrin. European journal of biochemistry / *FEBS* 196:177-184.
[9] Baker, E. N., and H. M. Baker. (2005). Molecular structure, binding properties and dynamics of lactoferrin. *Cellular and molecular life sciences : CMLS* 62:2531-2539.
[10] Legrand, D., A. Pierce, E. Elass, M. Carpentier, C. Mariller, and J. Mazurier. (2008). Lactoferrin structure and functions. *Advances in experimental medicine and biology* 606:163-194.

[11] Penco, S., S. Scarfi, M. Giovine, G. Damonte, E. Millo, B. Villaggio, M. Passalacqua, M. Pozzolini, C. Garre, and U. Benatti. (2001). Identification of an import signal for, and the nuclear localization of, human lactoferrin. *Biotechnology and applied biochemistry* 34:151-159.

[12] Bellamy, W., M. Takase, K. Yamauchi, H. Wakabayashi, K. Kawase, and M. Tomita. (1992). Identification of the bactericidal domain of lactoferrin. *Biochimica et biophysica acta* 1121:130-136.

[13] Elass-Rochard, E., A. Roseanu, D. Legrand, M. Trif, V. Salmon, C. Motas, J. Montreuil, and G. Spik. (1995). Lactoferrin-lipopolysaccharide interaction: involvement of the 28-34 loop region of human lactoferrin in the high-affinity binding to Escherichia coli 055B5 lipopolysaccharide. *The Biochemical journal* 312 (Pt 3):839-845.

[14] Ando, K., K. Hasegawa, K. Shindo, T. Furusawa, T. Fujino, K. Kikugawa, H. Nakano, O. Takeuchi, S. Akira, T. Akiyama, J. Gohda, J. Inoue, and M. Hayakawa. (2010). Human lactoferrin activates NF-kappaB through the Toll-like receptor 4 pathway while it interferes with the lipopolysaccharide-stimulated TLR4 signaling. *The FEBS journal* 277:2051-2066.

[15] Berlutti, F., F. Pantanella, T. Natalizi, A. Frioni, R. Paesano, A. Polimeni, and P. Valenti. (2011). Antiviral properties of lactoferrin--a natural immunity molecule. *Molecules* 16:6992-7018.

[16] Hasegawa, K., W. Motsuchi, S. Tanaka, and S. Dosako. (1994). Inhibition with lactoferrin of in vitro infection with human herpes virus. *Japanese journal of medical science & biology* 47:73-85.

[17] Marchetti, M., C. Longhi, M. P. Conte, S. Pisani, P. Valenti, and L. Seganti. (1996). Lactoferrin inhibits herpes simplex virus type 1 adsorption to Vero cells. *Antiviral research* 29:221-231.

[18] Marchetti, M., S. Pisani, G. Antonini, P. Valenti, L. Seganti, and N. Orsi. (1998). Metal complexes of bovine lactoferrin inhibit in vitro replication of herpes simplex virus type 1 and 2. *Biometals : an international journal on the role of metal ions in biology, biochemistry, and medicine* 11:89-94.

[19] Marchetti, M., E. Trybala, F. Superti, M. Johansson, and T. Bergstrom. (2004). Inhibition of herpes simplex virus infection by lactoferrin is dependent on interference with the virus binding to glycosaminoglycans. *Virology* 318:405-413.

[20] Shukla, D., and P. G. Spear. (2001). Herpesviruses and heparan sulfate: an intimate relationship in aid of viral entry. *The Journal of clinical investigation* 108:503-510.

[21] Marchetti, M., M. G. Ammendolia, and F. Superti. (2009). Glycosaminoglycans are not indispensable for the anti-herpes simplex virus type 2 activity of lactoferrin. *Biochimie* 91:155-159.
[22] Siciliano, R., B. Rega, M. Marchetti, L. Seganti, G. Antonini, and P. Valenti. (1999). Bovine lactoferrin peptidic fragments involved in inhibition of herpes simplex virus type 1 infection. *Biochemical and biophysical research communications* 264:19-23.
[23] Seganti, L., A. M. Di Biase, B. Rega, B. De Giulio, M. Nicoletti, G. Antonini, and P. Valenti. (2001). Involvement of bovine lactoferrin moieties in the inhibition of herpes simplex virus type 1 infection. *International journal of immunopathology and pharmacology* 14:71-79.
[24] Andersen, J. H., H. Jenssen, K. Sandvik, and T. J. Gutteberg. (2004). Anti-HSV activity of lactoferrin and lactoferricin is dependent on the presence of heparan sulphate at the cell surface. *Journal of medical virology* 74:262-271.
[25] Andersen, J. H., H. Jenssen, and T. J. Gutteberg. (2003). Lactoferrin and lactoferricin inhibit Herpes simplex 1 and 2 infection and exhibit synergy when combined with acyclovir. *Antiviral research* 58:209-215.
[26] Marr, A. K., H. Jenssen, M. R. Moniri, R. E. Hancock, and N. Pante. (2009). Bovine lactoferrin and lactoferricin interfere with intracellular trafficking of Herpes simplex virus-1. *Biochimie* 91:160-164.
[27] Jenssen, H. (2005). Anti herpes simplex virus activity of lactoferrin/lactoferricin -- an example of antiviral activity of antimicrobial protein/peptide. *Cellular and molecular life sciences : CMLS* 62:3002-3013.
[28] Jenssen, H., J. H. Andersen, L. Uhlin-Hansen, T. J. Gutteberg, and O. Rekdal. (2004). Anti-HSV activity of lactoferricin analogues is only partly related to their affinity for heparan sulfate. *Antiviral research* 61:101-109.
[29] Harmsen, M. C., P. J. Swart, M. P. de Bethune, R. Pauwels, E. De Clercq, T. H. The, and D. K. Meijer. (1995). Antiviral effects of plasma and milk proteins: lactoferrin shows potent activity against both human immunodeficiency virus and human cytomegalovirus replication in vitro. *The Journal of infectious diseases* 172:380-388.
[30] Swart, P. J., M. C. Harmsen, M. E. Kuipers, A. A. Van Dijk, B. W. Van Der Strate, P. H. Van Berkel, J. H. Nuijens, C. Smit, M. Witvrouw, E. De Clercq, M. P. de Bethune, R. Pauwels, and D. K. Meijer. (1999). Charge modification of plasma and milk proteins results in antiviral

active compounds. *Journal of peptide science : an official publication of the European Peptide Society* 5:563-576.

[31] Clarke, N. M., and J. T. May. (2000). Effect of antimicrobial factors in human milk on rhinoviruses and milk-borne cytomegalovirus in vitro. *Journal of medical microbiology* 49:719-723.

[32] Beljaars, L., B. W. van der Strate, H. I. Bakker, C. Reker-Smit, A. M. van Loenen-Weemaes, F. C. Wiegmans, M. C. Harmsen, G. Molema, and D. K. Meijer. (2004). Inhibition of cytomegalovirus infection by lactoferrin in vitro and in vivo. *Antiviral research* 63:197-208.

[33] Andersen, J. H., S. A. Osbakk, L. H. Vorland, T. Traavik, and T. J. Gutteberg. (2001). Lactoferrin and cyclic lactoferricin inhibit the entry of human cytomegalovirus into human fibroblasts. *Antiviral research* 51:141-149.

[34] Hara, K., M. Ikeda, S. Saito, S. Matsumoto, K. Numata, N. Kato, K. Tanaka, and H. Sekihara. (2002). Lactoferrin inhibits hepatitis B virus infection in cultured human hepatocytes. *Hepatology research : the official journal of the Japan Society of Hepatology* 24:228.

[35] Li, S., H. Zhou, G. Huang, and N. Liu. (2009). Inhibition of HBV infection by bovine lactoferrin and iron-, zinc-saturated lactoferrin. *Medical microbiology and immunology* 198:19-25.

[36] Gripon, P., S. Rumin, S. Urban, J. Le Seyec, D. Glaise, I. Cannie, C. Guyomard, J. Lucas, C. Trepo, and C. Guguen-Guillouzo. (2002). Infection of a human hepatoma cell line by hepatitis B virus. *Proceedings of the National Academy of Sciences of the United States of America* 99:15655-15660.

[37] Lazar, C., D. Durantel, A. Macovei, N. Zitzmann, F. Zoulim, R. A. Dwek, and N. Branza-Nichita. (2007). Treatment of hepatitis B virus-infected cells with alpha-glucosidase inhibitors results in production of virions with altered molecular composition and infectivity. *Antiviral research* 76:30-37.

[38] Florian, P. E., A. Macovei, C. Lazar, A. L. Milac, I. Sokolowska, C. C. Darie, R. W. Evans, A. Roseanu, and N. Branza-Nichita. (2013). Characterization of the anti-HBV activity of HLP1-23, a human lactoferrin-derived peptide. *Journal of medical virology* 85:780-788.

[39] de Oliveira, P. R., A. Y. Yamamoto, C. B. de Souza, N. M. de Araujo, S. de Andrade Gomes, A. R. Heck, J. F. de Castro Figueiredo, and M. M. Mussi-Pinhata. (2009). Hepatitis B viral markers in banked human milk before and after Holder pasteurization. *Journal of clinical virology : the*

official publication of the Pan American Society for Clinical Virology 45:281-284.

[40] Lin, H. H., H. Y. Hsu, M. H. Chang, P. J. Chen, and D. S. Chen. (1993). Hepatitis B virus in the colostra of HBeAg-positive carrier mothers. *Journal of pediatric gastroenterology and nutrition* 17:207-210.

[41] Petrova, M., and V. Kamburov. (2010). Breastfeeding and chronic HBV infection: clinical and social implications. *World journal of gastroenterology : WJG* 16:5042-5046.

[42] Puddu, P., P. Borghi, S. Gessani, P. Valenti, F. Belardelli, and L. Seganti. (1998). Antiviral effect of bovine lactoferrin saturated with metal ions on early steps of human immunodeficiency virus type 1 infection. *The international journal of biochemistry & cell biology* 30:1055-1062.

[43] Ng, T. B., T. L. Lam, T. K. Au, X. Y. Ye, and C. C. Wan. (2001). Inhibition of human immunodeficiency virus type 1 reverse transcriptase, protease and integrase by bovine milk proteins. *Life sciences* 69:2217-2223.

[44] Groot, F., T. B. Geijtenbeek, R. W. Sanders, C. E. Baldwin, M. Sanchez-Hernandez, R. Floris, Y. van Kooyk, E. C. de Jong, and B. Berkhout. (2005). Lactoferrin prevents dendritic cell-mediated human immunodeficiency virus type 1 transmission by blocking the DC-SIGN--gp120 interaction. *Journal of virology* 79:3009-3015.

[45] Saidi, H., J. Eslahpazir, C. Carbonneil, L. Carthagena, M. Requena, N. Nassreddine, and L. Belec. (2006). Differential modulation of human lactoferrin activity against both R5 and X4-HIV-1 adsorption on epithelial cells and dendritic cells by natural antibodies. *Journal of immunology* 177:5540-5549.

[46] Viani, R. M., T. J. Gutteberg, J. L. Lathey, and S. A. Spector. (1999). Lactoferrin inhibits HIV-1 replication in vitro and exhibits synergy when combined with zidovudine. *Aids* 13:1273-1274.

[47] Berkhout, B., R. Floris, I. Recio, and S. Visser. (2004). The antiviral activity of the milk protein lactoferrin against the human immunodeficiency virus type 1. *Biometals : an international journal on the role of metal ions in biology, biochemistry, and medicine* 17:291-294.

[48] Berkhout, B., J. L. van Wamel, L. Beljaars, D. K. Meijer, S. Visser, and R. Floris. (2002). Characterization of the anti-HIV effects of native lactoferrin and other milk proteins and protein-derived peptides. Antiviral research 55:341-355.

[49] Carthagena, L., P. Becquart, H. Hocini, M. D. Kazatchkine, H. Bouhlal, and L. Belec. (2011). Modulation of HIV Binding to Epithelial Cells and HIV Transfer from Immature Dendritic Cells to CD4 T Lymphocytes by Human Lactoferrin and its Major Exposed LF-33 Peptide. *The open virology journal* 5:27-34.

[50] Arnold, D., A. M. Di Biase, M. Marchetti, A. Pietrantoni, P. Valenti, L. Seganti, and F. Superti. (2002). Antiadenovirus activity of milk proteins: lactoferrin prevents viral infection. *Antiviral research* 53:153-158.

[51] Seganti, L., A. M. Di Biase, M. Marchetti, A. Pietrantoni, A. Tinari, and F. Superti. (2004). Antiviral activity of lactoferrin towards naked viruses. *Biometals : an international journal on the role of metal ions in biology, biochemistry, and medicine* 17:295-299.

[52] Di Biase, A. M., A. Pietrantoni, A. Tinari, R. Siciliano, P. Valenti, G. Antonini, L. Seganti, and F. Superti. (2003). Heparin-interacting sites of bovine lactoferrin are involved in anti-adenovirus activity. *Journal of medical virology* 69:495-502.

[53] Johansson, C., M. Jonsson, M. Marttila, D. Persson, X. L. Fan, J. Skog, L. Frangsmyr, G. Wadell, and N. Arnberg. (2007). Adenoviruses use lactoferrin as a bridge for CAR-independent binding to and infection of epithelial cells. *Journal of virology* 81:954-963.

[54] Flanagan, J. L., and M. D. Willcox. (2009). Role of lactoferrin in the tear film. *Biochimie* 91:35-43.

[55] Adams, W. C., E. Bond, M. J. Havenga, L. Holterman, J. Goudsmit, G. B. Karlsson Hedestam, R. A. Koup, and K. Lore. (2009). Adenovirus serotype 5 infects human dendritic cells via a coxsackievirus-adenovirus receptor-independent receptor pathway mediated by lactoferrin and DC-SIGN. *The Journal of general virology* 90:1600-1610.

[56] Gunther, P. S., E. Mikeler, K. Hamprecht, J. Schneider-Schaulies, G. Jahn, and K. M. Dennehy. (2011). CD209/DC-SIGN mediates efficient infection of monocyte-derived dendritic cells by clinical adenovirus 2C isolates in the presence of bovine lactoferrin. *The Journal of general virology* 92:1754-1759.

[57] Waarts, B. L., O. J. Aneke, J. M. Smit, K. Kimata, R. Bittman, D. K. Meijer, and J. Wilschut. (2005). Antiviral activity of human lactoferrin: inhibition of alphavirus interaction with heparan sulfate. *Virology* 333:284-292.

[58] Murphy, M. E., H. Kariwa, T. Mizutani, K. Yoshimatsu, J. Arikawa, and I. Takashima. (2000). In vitro antiviral activity of lactoferrin and ribavirin upon hantavirus. *Archives of virology* 145:1571-1582.

[59] Hardestam, J., L. Petterson, C. Ahlm, M. Evander, A. Lundkvist, and J. Klingstrom. (2008). Antiviral effect of human saliva against hantavirus. *Journal of medical virology* 80:2122-2126.

[60] McCann, K. B., A. Lee, J. Wan, H. Roginski, and M. J. Coventry. (2003). The effect of bovine lactoferrin and lactoferricin B on the ability of feline calicivirus (a norovirus surrogate) and poliovirus to infect cell cultures. *Journal of applied microbiology* 95:1026-1033.

[61] Pan, Y., J. Wan, H. Roginski, A. Lee, B. Shiell, W. P. Michalski, and M. J. Coventry. (2007). Comparison of the effects of acylation and amidation on the antimicrobial and antiviral properties of lactoferrin. *Letters in applied microbiology* 44:229-234.

[62] Chien, Y. J., W. J. Chen, W. L. Hsu, and S. S. Chiou. (2008). Bovine lactoferrin inhibits Japanese encephalitis virus by binding to heparan sulfate and receptor for low density lipoprotein. *Virology* 379:143-151.

[63] Pietrantoni, A., E. Dofrelli, A. Tinari, M. G. Ammendolia, S. Puzelli, C. Fabiani, I. Donatelli, and F. Superti. (2010). Bovine lactoferrin inhibits influenza A virus induced programmed cell death in vitro. *Biometals : an international journal on the role of metal ions in biology, biochemistry, and medicine* 23:465-475.

[64] Taha, S. H., M. A. Mehrez, M. Z. Sitohy, A. G. Abou Dawood, M. M. Abd-El Hamid, and W. H. Kilany. (2010). Effectiveness of esterified whey proteins fractions against Egyptian Lethal Avian Influenza A (H5N1). *Virology journal* 7:330.

[65] Pietrantoni, A., M. G. Ammendolia, and F. Superti. (2012). Bovine lactoferrin: involvement of metal saturation and carbohydrates in the inhibition of influenza virus infection. *Biochemistry and cell biology = Biochimie et biologie cellulaire* 90:442-448.

[66] Ammendolia, M. G., M. Agamennone, A. Pietrantoni, F. Lannutti, R. A. Siciliano, B. De Giulio, C. Amici, and F. Superti. (2012). Bovine lactoferrin-derived peptides as novel broad-spectrum inhibitors of influenza virus. *Pathogens and global health 1*06:12-19.

[67] Lang, J., N. Yang, J. Deng, K. Liu, P. Yang, G. Zhang, and C. Jiang. (2011). Inhibition of SARS pseudovirus cell entry by lactoferrin binding to heparan sulfate proteoglycans. *PloS one* 6:e23710.

[68] Drobni, P., J. Naslund, and M. Evander. (2004). Lactoferrin inhibits human papillomavirus binding and uptake in vitro. *Antiviral research* 64:63-68.

[69] Mistry, N., P. Drobni, J. Naslund, V. G. Sunkari, H. Jenssen, and M. Evander. (2007). The anti-papillomavirus activity of human and bovine lactoferricin. *Antiviral research* 75:258-265.

[70] Ammendolia, M. G., M. Marchetti, and F. Superti. (2007). Bovine lactoferrin prevents the entry and intercellular spread of herpes simplex virus type 1 in Green Monkey Kidney cells. *Antiviral research* 76:252-262.

[71] Valimaa, H., J. Tenovuo, M. Waris, and V. Hukkanen. (2009). Human lactoferrin but not lysozyme neutralizes HSV-1 and inhibits HSV-1 replication and cell-to-cell spread. *Virology journal* 6:53.

[72] Yi, M., S. Kaneko, D. Y. Yu, and S. Murakami. (1997). Hepatitis C virus envelope proteins bind lactoferrin. *Journal of virology* 71:5997-6002.

[73] Ikeda, M., K. Sugiyama, T. Tanaka, K. Tanaka, H. Sekihara, K. Shimotohno, and N. Kato. (1998). Lactoferrin markedly inhibits hepatitis C virus infection in cultured human hepatocytes. *Biochemical and biophysical research communications* 245:549-553.

[74] Ikeda, M., A. Nozaki, K. Sugiyama, T. Tanaka, A. Naganuma, K. Tanaka, H. Sekihara, K. Shimotohno, M. Saito, and N. Kato. (2000). Characterization of antiviral activity of lactoferrin against hepatitis C virus infection in human cultured cells. *Virus research* 66:51-63.

[75] Matsuura, Y., H. Tani, K. Suzuki, T. Kimura-Someya, R. Suzuki, H. Aizaki, K. Ishii, K. Moriishi, C. S. Robison, M. A. Whitt, and T. Miyamura. (2001). Characterization of pseudotype VSV possessing HCV envelope proteins. *Virology* 286:263-275.

[76] Redwan el, R. M., and A. Tabll. (2007). Camel lactoferrin markedly inhibits hepatitis C virus genotype 4 infection of human peripheral blood leukocytes. *Journal of immunoassay & immunochemistry* 28:267-277.

[77] Liao, Y., E. El-Fakkarany, B. Lonnerdal, and E. M. Redwan. (2012). Inhibitory effects of native and recombinant full-length camel lactoferrin and its N and C lobes on hepatitis C virus infection of Huh7.5 cells. *Journal of medical microbiology* 61:375-383.

[78] El-Fakharany, E. M., N. Abedelbaky, B. M. Haroun, L. Sanchez, N. A. Redwan, and E. M. Redwan. (2012). Anti-infectivity of camel polyclonal antibodies against hepatitis C virus in Huh7.5 hepatoma. *Virology journal* 9:201.

[79] El-Fakharany, E. M., L. Sanchez, H. A. Al-Mehdar, and E. M. Redwan. (2013). Effectiveness of human, camel, bovine and sheep lactoferrin on

the hepatitis C virus cellular infectivity: comparison study. *Virology journal* 10:199.

[80] Lehmann, E., W. H. El-Tantawy, M. Ocker, R. Bartenschlager, V. Lohmann, S. Hashemolhosseini, G. Tiegs, and G. Sass. (2010). The heme oxygenase 1 product biliverdin interferes with hepatitis C virus replication by increasing antiviral interferon response. *Hepatology* 51:398-404.

[81] Nozaki, A., M. Ikeda, A. Naganuma, T. Nakamura, M. Inudoh, K. Tanaka, and N. Kato. (2003). Identification of a lactoferrin-derived peptide possessing binding activity to hepatitis C virus E2 envelope protein. *The Journal of biological chemistry* 278:10162-10173.

[82] Abe, K., A. Nozaki, K. Tamura, M. Ikeda, K. Naka, H. Dansako, H. O. Hoshino, K. Tanaka, and N. Kato. (2007). Tandem repeats of lactoferrin-derived anti-hepatitis C virus peptide enhance antiviral activity in cultured human hepatocytes. *Microbiology and immunology* 51:117-125.

[83] Beleid, R., D. Douglas, N. Kneteman, and K. Kaur. (2008). Helical peptides derived from lactoferrin bind hepatitis C virus envelope protein E2. *Chemical biology & drug design* 72:436-443.

[84] Swart, P. J., M. E. Kuipers, C. Smit, R. Pauwels, M. P. deBethune, E. de Clercq, D. K. Meijer, and J. G. Huisman. (1996). Antiviral effects of milk proteins: acylation results in polyanionic compounds with potent activity against human immunodeficiency virus types 1 and 2 in vitro. *AIDS research and human retroviruses* 12:769-775.

[85] Pietrantoni, A., A. M. Di Biase, A. Tinari, M. Marchetti, P. Valenti, L. Seganti, and F. Superti. (2003). Bovine lactoferrin inhibits adenovirus infection by interacting with viral structural polypeptides. *Antimicrobial agents and chemotherapy* 47:2688-2691.

[86] Superti, F., M. G. Ammendolia, P. Valenti, and L. Seganti. (1997). Antirotaviral activity of milk proteins: lactoferrin prevents rotavirus infection in the enterocyte-like cell line HT-29. *Medical microbiology and immunology* 186:83-91.

[87] Superti, F., R. Siciliano, B. Rega, F. Giansanti, P. Valenti, and G. Antonini. (2001). Involvement of bovine lactoferrin metal saturation, sialic acid and protein fragments in the inhibition of rotavirus infection. *Biochimica et biophysica acta* 1528:107-115.

[88] Kvistgaard, A. S., L. T. Pallesen, C. F. Arias, S. Lopez, T. E. Petersen, C. W. Heegaard, and J. T. Rasmussen. (2004). Inhibitory effects of human and bovine milk constituents on rotavirus infections. *Journal of dairy science* 87:4088-4096.

[89] Marchetti, M., F. Superti, M. G. Ammendolia, P. Rossi, P. Valenti, and L. Seganti. (1999). Inhibition of poliovirus type 1 infection by iron-, manganese- and zinc-saturated lactoferrin. *Medical microbiology and immunology* 187:199-204.

[90] Lin, T. Y., C. Chu, and C. H. Chiu. (2002). Lactoferrin inhibits enterovirus 71 infection of human embryonal rhabdomyosarcoma cells in vitro. *The Journal of infectious diseases* 186:1161-1164.

[91] Weng, T. Y., L. C. Chen, H. W. Shyu, S. H. Chen, J. R. Wang, C. K. Yu, H. Y. Lei, and T. M. Yeh. (2005). Lactoferrin inhibits enterovirus 71 infection by binding to VP1 protein and host cells. *Antiviral research* 67:31-37.

[92] Tinari, A., A. Pietrantoni, M. G. Ammendolia, P. Valenti, and F. Superti. (2005). Inhibitory activity of bovine lactoferrin against echovirus induced programmed cell death in vitro. *International journal of antimicrobial agents* 25:433-438.

[93] Pietrantoni, A., M. G. Ammendolia, A. Tinari, R. Siciliano, P. Valenti, and F. Superti. (2006). Bovine lactoferrin peptidic fragments involved in inhibition of Echovirus 6 in vitro infection. *Antiviral research* 69:98-106.

[94] Furlund, C. B., A. B. Kristoffersen, T. G. Devold, G. E. Vegarud, and C. M. Jonassen. (2012). Bovine lactoferrin digested with human gastrointestinal enzymes inhibits replication of human echovirus 5 in cell culture. *Nutrition research* 32:503-513.

[95] Grover, M., O. Giouzeppos, R. D. Schnagl, and J. T. May. (1997). Effect of human milk prostaglandins and lactoferrin on respiratory syncytial virus and rotavirus. *Acta paediatrica* 86:315-316.

[96] Portelli, J., A. Gordon, and J. T. May. (1998). Effect of compounds with antibacterial activities in human milk on respiratory syncytial virus and cytomegalovirus in vitro. *Journal of medical microbiology* 47:1015-1018.

[97] Sano, H., K. Nagai, H. Tsutsumi, and Y. Kuroki. (2003). Lactoferrin and surfactant protein A exhibit distinct binding specificity to F protein and differently modulate respiratory syncytial virus infection. *European journal of immunology* 33:2894-2902.

[98] Longhi, G., V. Pietropaolo, M. Mischitelli, C. Longhi, M. P. Conte, M. Marchetti, A. Tinari, P. Valenti, A. M. Degener, L. Seganti, and F. Superti. (2006). Lactoferrin inhibits early steps of human BK polyomavirus infection. *Antiviral research* 72:145-152.

[99] Fujihara, T., and K. Hayashi. (1995). Lactoferrin inhibits herpes simplex virus type-1 (HSV-1) infection to mouse cornea. *Archives of virology* 140:1469-1472.

[100] Wakabayashi, H., M. Kurokawa, K. Shin, S. Teraguchi, Y. Tamura, and K. Shiraki. (2004). Oral lactoferrin prevents body weight loss and increases cytokine responses during herpes simplex virus type 1 infection of mice. *Bioscience, biotechnology, and biochemistry* 68:537-544.

[101] Shestakov, A., H. Jenssen, I. Nordstrom, and K. Eriksson. (2012). Lactoferricin but not lactoferrin inhibit herpes simplex virus type 2 infection in mice. *Antiviral research* 93:340-345.

[102] Sato, R., O. Inanami, Y. Tanaka, M. Takase, and Y. Naito. (1996). Oral administration of bovine lactoferrin for treatment of intractable stomatitis in feline immunodeficiency virus (FIV)-positive and FIV-negative cats. *American journal of veterinary research* 57:1443-1446.

[103] Kobayashi, S., R. Sato, T. Aoki, K. Omoe, O. Inanami, C. Hankanga, Y. Yamada, N. Tomizawa, J. Yasuda, and J. Sasaki. (2008). Effect of bovine lactoferrin on functions of activated feline peripheral blood mononuclear cells during chronic feline immunodeficiency virus infection. *The Journal of veterinary medical science / the Japanese Society of Veterinary Science* 70:429-435.

[104] Chen, L. T., L. Lu, and H. E. Broxmeyer. (1987). Effects of purified iron-saturated human lactoferrin on spleen morphology in mice infected with Friend virus complex. *The American journal of pathology* 126:285-292.

[105] Lu, L., G. Hangoc, A. Oliff, L. T. Chen, R. N. Shen, and H. E. Broxmeyer. (1987). Protective influence of lactoferrin on mice infected with the polycythemia-inducing strain of Friend virus complex. *Cancer research* 47:4184-4188.

[106] Lu, L., R. N. Shen, S. Z. Zhou, C. Srivastava, M. Harrington, K. Miyazawa, B. Wu, Z. H. Lin, S. Ruscetti, and H. E. Broxmeyer. (1991). Synergistic effect of human lactoferrin and recombinant murine interferon-gamma on disease progression in mice infected with the polycythemia-inducing strain of the Friend virus complex. *International journal of hematology* 54:117-124.

[107] Shimizu, K., H. Matsuzawa, K. Okada, S. Tazume, S. Dosako, Y. Kawasaki, K. Hashimoto, and Y. Koga. (1996). Lactoferrin-mediated protection of the host from murine cytomegalovirus infection by a T-

cell-dependent augmentation of natural killer cell activity. *Archives of virology* 141:1875-1889.
[108] Beljaars, L., H. I. Bakker, B. W. van der Strate, C. Smit, A. M. Duijvestijn, D. K. Meijer, and G. Molema. (2002). The antiviral protein human lactoferrin is distributed in the body to cytomegalovirus (CMV) infection-prone cells and tissues. *Pharmaceutical research* 19:54-62.
[109] Murphy, M. E., H. Kariwa, T. Mizutani, H. Tanabe, K. Yoshimatsu, J. Arikawa, and I. Takashima. (2001). Characterization of in vitro and in vivo antiviral activity of lactoferrin and ribavirin upon hantavirus. *The Journal of veterinary medical science / the Japanese Society of Veterinary Science* 63:637-645.
[110] Shin, K., H. Wakabayashi, K. Yamauchi, S. Teraguchi, Y. Tamura, M. Kurokawa, and K. Shiraki. (2005). Effects of orally administered bovine lactoferrin and lactoperoxidase on influenza virus infection in mice. *Journal of medical microbiology* 54:717-723.
[111] Yamauchi, K., H. Wakabayashi, K. Shin, and M. Takase. (2006). Bovine lactoferrin: benefits and mechanism of action against infections. *Biochemistry and cell biology = Biochimie et biologie cellulaire* 84:291-296.
[112] Perez-Cano, F. J., S. Marin-Gallen, M. Castell, M. Rodriguez-Palmero, M. Rivero, C. Castellote, and A. Franch. (2008). Supplementing suckling rats with whey protein concentrate modulates the immune response and ameliorates rat rotavirus-induced diarrhea. *The Journal of nutrition* 138:2392-2398.
[113] Chen, H. L., L. C. Wang, C. H. Chang, C. C. Yen, W. T. Cheng, S. C. Wu, C. M. Hung, M. F. Kuo, and C. M. Chen. (2008). Recombinant porcine lactoferrin expressed in the milk of transgenic mice protects neonatal mice from a lethal challenge with enterovirus type 71. *Vaccine* 26:891-898.
[114] Gualdi, L., S. Mertz, A. M. Gomez, O. Ramilo, A. Wittke, and A. Mejias. (2013). Lack of effect of bovine lactoferrin in respiratory syncytial virus replication and clinical disease severity in the mouse model. *Antiviral research* 99:188-195.
[115] Zuccotti, G. V., F. Salvini, E. Riva, and C. Agostoni. (2006). Oral lactoferrin in HIV-1 vertically infected children: an observational follow-up of plasma viral load and immune parameters. *The Journal of international medical research* 34:88-94.
[116] Soler-Garcia, A. A., D. Johnson, Y. Hathout, and P. E. Ray. (2009). Iron-related proteins: candidate urine biomarkers in childhood HIV-

associated renal diseases. *Clinical journal of the American Society of Nephrology : CJASN* 4:763-771.

[117] Tanaka, K., M. Ikeda, A. Nozaki, N. Kato, H. Tsuda, S. Saito, and H. Sekihara. (1999). Lactoferrin inhibits hepatitis C virus viremia in patients with chronic hepatitis C: a pilot study. *Japanese journal of cancer research : Gann* 90:367-371.

[118] Okada, S., K. Tanaka, T. Sato, H. Ueno, S. Saito, T. Okusaka, K. Sato, S. Yamamoto, and T. Kakizoe. (2002). Dose-response trial of lactoferrin in patients with chronic hepatitis C. *Japanese journal of cancer research : Gann* 93:1063-1069.

[119] Ishii, K., N. Takamura, M. Shinohara, N. Wakui, H. Shin, Y. Sumino, Y. Ohmoto, S. Teraguchi, and K. Yamauchi. (2003). Long-term follow-up of chronic hepatitis C patients treated with oral lactoferrin for 12 months. *Hepatology research : the official journal of the Japan Society of Hepatology* 25:226-233.

[120] Hirashima, N., E. Orito, K. Ohba, H. Kondo, T. Sakamoto, S. Matsunaga, A. Kato, H. Nukaya, K. Sakakibara, T. Ohno, H. Kato, F. Sugauchi, T. Kato, Y. Tanaka, R. Ueda, and M. Mizokami. (2004). A randomized controlled trial of consensus interferon with or without lactoferrin for chronic hepatitis C patients with genotype 1b and high viral load. *Hepatology research : the official journal of the Japan Society of Hepatology* 29:9-12.

[121] Ishibashi, Y., K. Takeda, N. Tsukidate, H. Miyazaki, K. Ohira, H. Dosaka-Akita, and M. Nishimura. (2005). Randomized placebo-controlled trial of interferon alpha-2b plus ribavirin with and without lactoferrin for chronic hepatitis C. *Hepatology research : the official journal of the Japan Society of Hepatology* 32:218-223.

[122] Konishi, M., M. Iwasa, K. Yamauchi, R. Sugimoto, N. Fujita, Y. Kobayashi, S. Watanabe, S. Teraguchi, Y. Adachi, and M. Kaito. (2006). Lactoferrin inhibits lipid peroxidation in patients with chronic hepatitis C. *Hepatology research : the official journal of the Japan Society of Hepatology* 36:27-32.

[123] Ueno, H., T. Sato, S. Yamamoto, K. Tanaka, S. Ohkawa, H. Takagi, O. Yokosuka, J. Furuse, H. Saito, A. Sawaki, H. Kasugai, Y. Osaki, S. Fujiyama, K. Sato, K. Wakabayashi, and T. Okusaka. (2006). Randomized, double-blind, placebo-controlled trial of bovine lactoferrin in patients with chronic hepatitis C. *Cancer science* 97:1105-1110.

[124] Kaito, M., M. Iwasa, N. Fujita, Y. Kobayashi, Y. Kojima, J. Ikoma, I. Imoto, Y. Adachi, H. Hamano, and K. Yamauchi. (2007). Effect of

lactoferrin in patients with chronic hepatitis C: combination therapy with interferon and ribavirin. *Journal of gastroenterology and hepatology* 22:1894-1897.

[125] Yen, M. H., C. H. Chiu, Y. C. Huang, and T. Y. Lin. (2011). Effects of lactoferrin-containing formula in the prevention of enterovirus and rotavirus infection and impact on serum cytokine levels: a randomized trial. *Chang Gung medical journal* 34:395-402.

[126] Dixon, D. L., K. M. Griggs, K. D. Forsyth, and A. D. Bersten. (2010). Lower interleukin-8 levels in airway aspirates from breastfed infants with acute bronchiolitis. *Pediatric allergy and immunology : official publication of the European Society of Pediatric Allergy and Immunology* 21:e691-696.

[127] Reghunathan, R., M. Jayapal, L. Y. Hsu, H. H. Chng, D. Tai, B. P. Leung, and A. J. Melendez. (2005). Expression profile of immune response genes in patients with Severe Acute Respiratory Syndrome. *BMC immunology* 6:2.

[128] Chen, C. C., C. J. Chang, T. Y. Lin, M. W. Lai, H. C. Chao, and M. S. Kong. (2011). Usefulness of fecal lactoferrin in predicting and monitoring the clinical severity of infectious diarrhea. *World journal of gastroenterology : WJG* 17:4218-4224.

In: Viral Infections
Editor: Deborah Shinn

ISBN: 978-1-63117-221-2

Chapter 4

ANTIVIRAL EFFECT OF PHYTOCHEMICALS OF THE MEDITERRANEAN MEDICINAL PLANTS

Ludmila Yarmolinsky[1,2], Jonathan Gorelick[1] and Shimon Ben-Shabat[2,*]

[1]Judea Regional Research and Development Center, Carmel, Israel
[2]Department of Clinical Biochemistry and Pharmacology, Faculty of Health Sciences, Ben-Gurion University of the Negev, Beer-Sheva, Israel

ABSTRACT

Viral infection is an important health problem worldwide due to the rapid development of resistant mutants against current therapeutic agents. There are only a few antiviral drugs available for the treatment of viral diseases and they have generally inadequate efficacy and a number of serious adverse effects. Medicinal plants may be an alternative strategy for treatment of viral diseases. Although many herbs have a very good folkloric reputation, their antiviral properties have not yet been investigated. Medicinal plants from the Mediterranean region have been used in medicine since ancient times and are well known for their successful therapeutic activity. Many phytochemicals including

* Corresponding author: Dr. Shimon Ben-Shabat. Tel: +972-8- 6479354, Fax: +972-8-6472984, E-mail: sbs@ bgu.ac.il.

glycosides, flavonoids, terpenoids, polyphenolics, coumarins, saponins, furil compounds, alkaloids, different sugars, proteins and peptides isolated from these plants demonstrated antiviral properties.

The purpose of this review is to provide the verified data on the antiviral activities of the herb extracts and pure compounds isolated from the medicinal plants of the Mediterranean flora and to discuss the various mechanisms of their actions.

1. INTRODUCTION

Viral infections remain one of the most important public health problems worldwide. Unfortunately blood transfusion, organ transplantation and the use of hypodermic syringes create new opportunities for viral infections. Many serious viral diseases such as Ebola, AIDS (acquired immunodeficiency syndrome), influenza, SARS (Severe acute respiratory syndrome) and others are a leading cause of morbidity and mortality globally. For example, influenza viruses are responsible for up to 250,000–500,000 human deaths annually worldwide [1]. Although some viral infections cause relatively mild diseases, an economic burden of these diseases is significant, particularly in loss of working hours and missed school days.

Some antiviral drugs are known for specific viruses such as HIV (Human immunodeficiency virus), herpes viruses, influenza A and B viruses and the hepatitis B and C viruses, which can cause liver cancer (Figure 1).

Anti-HIV drugs may transform HIV-1 disease into a treatable and somewhat chronic infection [2]. These drugs are classified into different groups (nucleoside or nucleotide reverse transcriptase inhibitors; non-nucleoside-reverse transcriptase inhibitors; HIV protease inhibitors; fusion, entry inhibitors and HIV integrase strand transfer inhibitors) according to their activity on the replicative cycle of HIV, which can be divided into different steps: virus-cell adsorption, virus-cell fusion, uncoating, reverse transcription, integration, DNA replication, transcription, translation, budding (assembly/ release)and maturation [3]. Acyclovir (ACV) and other nucleoside analogues are the most prescribed anti-herpetic drugs (Figure 1). Phosphorylation of this drug by the viral thymidine kinase and cellular enzymes activates the drug as a substrate for the viral DNA polymerase. The drug is then incorporated into the synthesized viral genomic DNA and prevents its elongation [4]. However, none of the available drugs can clear the hepatitis viruses. They can stop the virus from replicating, thus minimizing liver damage [5].

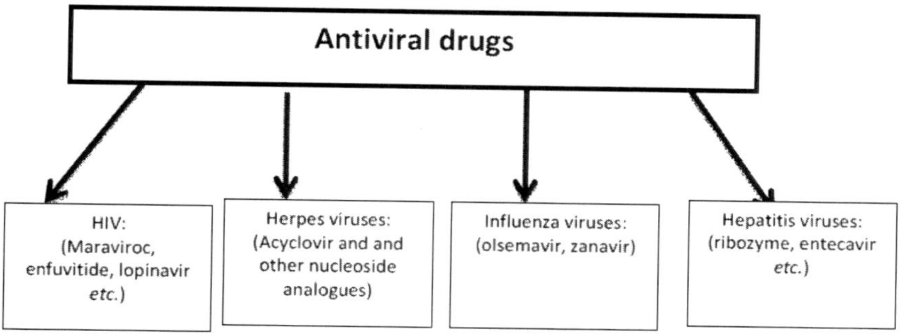

Figure 1. Antiviral drugs. The antiviral drugs are known for HIV (Human immune-deficiency virus), herpes viruses, influenza A and B viruses and the hepatitis B and C viruses. Some examples of the most prescribed drugs are shown in brackets.

The influenza drugs olseltamivir and zanavir are sialic acid-mimicking inhibitors of neuraminidase [6].

The development of antiviral agents is needed urgently to overcome the drawbacks of the above-mentioned antiviral drugs such as the expense, side effects and their limitations in activity due to viral resistance. In addition, there are no prescribed drugs for many other kinds of viruses.

The present review focuses on the antiviral activities of herb extracts and pure compounds isolated from the medicinal plants of the Mediterranean flora and the various mechanisms of their actions.

2. Antiviral Plants of the Mediterranean Region

Admittedly, medicinal plants from the Mediterranean region have been used in medicine since ancient times and are well known for their successful therapeutic activity.

Some studies have already been undertaken for estimation of the antiviral potential of various plants of the Mediterranean region against viruses. The majority of these plants are used in traditional medicine for treatment of diseases of possible viral origin.

Different kinds of extracts (aqueous, ethanolic, methanolic, hexane and so on) from various plant organs (roots, stems, leaves, buds, flowers, fruits and so on) were examined. The main findings related to antiviral plant extracts are summarized in table 1. The active compounds have not been isolated, purified and identified from the crude extracts which are mentioned in the table 1.

Table 1. Antiviral properties of plant extracts

Plant	Kind of extract	Virus	References
Achillea fragrantissima	Hydro-alcoholic extracts	Poliomyelitis-1 virus (POLIO)	[7]
Balanites aegyptica	n-Hexane leaf extract	VSV T2 (Vesicular Stomatitis Virus T2)	[8]
Capparis spinosa	Methanolic extract of buds	HSV-2	[9]
Cistus incanus	Polyphenol rich extract (CYSTUS052)	Avian and human influenza strains of different subtypes	[10, 11]
Cyperus rotundus	Hydro-alcoholic extracts	HSV-1	[7]
Dittrichia viscosa	Aqueous extracts	Vesicular stomatitis virus (VSV), HSV-1, poliovirus type 1	[18]
Euphorbia hirta	Aqueous extracts, methanol extracts	HIV-1, HIV-2, SIV (Simian immunodeficiency virus) mac 251	[21]
Ficus carica	The water extract from the leaves The hexanic and hexane-ethyl acetate from latex of fig fruit	HSV-1 HSV-1, echovirus type 11 (ECV-11) and adenovirus (ADV)	[12] [13]
Globularia arabica	Hydro-alcoholic extracts	Poliomyelitis-1 virus (POLIO)	[7]
Lilium candidum	Ethanol leaf extract	HSV-1, HSV-2	[14]
Melissa officinalis	Aqueous extracts	HSV-1 HSV-1, HSV-2 HIV	[15] [16] [17]
Moringa peregrina	Hydro-alcoholic extracts	HSV-1	[7]
Sanguisorba minor	Aqueous extracts	Vesicular stomatitis virus (VSV), HSV-1 HIV	[18] [19]
Solanum nigrum	Methanol and chloroform extracts of seeds	Hepatitis C Virus (HCV)	[20]
Tamarix nilotica	Hydro-alcoholic extracts	HSV-1	[7]
Tuberaria lignosa	An aqueous extract	HIV	[19]

All these extracts were tested in cell culture [7-21] but in vivo studies are still scarce [10, 17]. Majority of the publications were devoted to Herpes Simplex Virus 1 (HSV-1) [7, 8, 12-16, 18] and Herpes Simplex Virus 2 (HSV-2) [9, 16].

Mechanisms of the antiviral actions are considered in a few cases. *Cistusin canus* extract was able to interfere with the influenza virus surface and inhibit binding of the virus particles to cellular receptors [11]. Ethanol leaf extract of *Lilium candidum* inhibited HSV-1 and HSV-2 infections through direct inactivation of the virus infectivity [14].

Therefore, effective antiviral plant extracts are an important source for discovery of new antiviral drugs. Without doubt, the efficiency of these extracts encourages further exploration of the antiviral compounds occurring in plants.

3. Antiviral Compounds Isolated from Mediterranean Medicinal Plants

3.1. Alkaloids

Alkaloids are nitrogen-containing phytochemicals isolated and identified from plants that are very active against many kinds of viruses.

Lycorine is an alkaloid, found in a variety of Mediterranean plants of the family Amaryllidaceae (Figure 2). It has a wide range of antiviral effects including avian influenza virus H5N1 [22], flaviviruses [23], human immune-deficiency virus (HIV-1) [24, 25], severe acute respiratory syndrome-associated coronavirus (SARS-CoV) [26], poliovirus [27, 28], human enterovirus [29], HSV-1 [30], coxsackie virus [31] and measles virus [30].

Although it was shown that lycorine was able to inhibit protein synthesis [31-33], mechanisms of its antiviral actions are still not fully understood in many cases. It was shown that lycorine affected the proteins of poliovirus which were responsible for RNA replication and virus propagation. [27]. The antiviral effect of lycorine against West Nile virus was associated with a suppression of viral RNA synthesis [23]. Its anti-herpetic activity is connected with the blocking of viral DNA polymerase activity [30].

Some other alkaloids with a hexahydroindole ring with two functional hydroxyl groups from plants of the *Amaryllidaceae* family were active against HSV-1 [30].

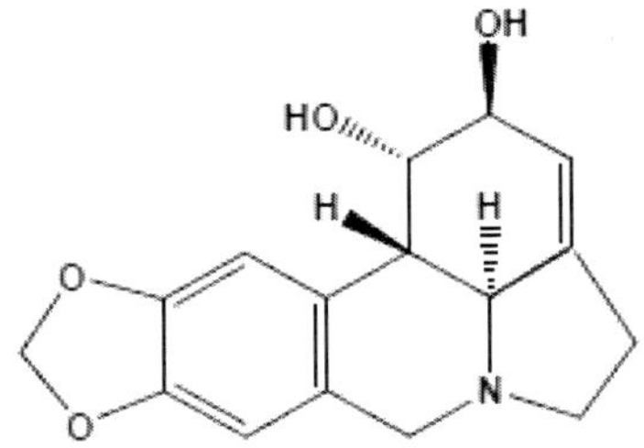

Figure 2. Lycorine is alkaloid, was isolated from many Mediterranean plants of the family *Amaryllidaceae*.

The mechanism of their antiviral action was similar to that of lycorine [30]. It was shown that bulbs of *Leucojumvernum (Amaryllidaceae)* also contain lycorine and other alkaloids: homolycorine and 2- O-acetyllycorine. These compounds were studied in vitro for HIV-1 replication inhibitory activity on MT4 cells, and their high antiretroviral activities (IC (50) = 0.4 - 7.3 micro g/mL) was marked [25]. Two alkaloids (5 Hydroxynoracronycine and acrimarine-F) from Citrus plants demonstrated inhibitory effects on an Epstein-Barr virus in vitro assay [34].

3.2. Glycosides

Glycosides are conjugates of sugars with small organic molecules. The sugar moiety likely plays an important role in their antiviral activity. This is evident from examples when glycosides have stronger antiviral activity compared to their aglycones [35, 36], (Figure 3). Another example is the inhibitory effect flavonoid rhamnoglycosides exhibit an on rotavirus infection, whereas their aglycones have no inhibitory activity [37].

Many antiviral glycosides were isolated and identified from plants of the Mediterranean flora (table 2). One of them is rutin which was active against Avian influenza virus [38], HSV-1, HSV-2 [36] and Parainfluenza-3 virus [39]. This flavonolglucoside is so widespread in the plant kingdom that it was isolated not only from Mediterranean plants and was active against Entero-virusA71 (EV-A71) [40] and HIV [41]. Rutin was modified to sodium rutinsulphate which showed a broad anti-HIV activity against R5 and X4 viruses with a selectivity index ranging from 197 to 575 and anti-herpetic activity [42].

Kaempferol ; R = H

kaempferol 3-O-rutinoside ; R = Glu-Rha

kaempferol 3-O-robinobioside ; R = Gala-Rha

Quercetin ; R = H

quercetin 3-O-rutinoside; R = Glu-Rha

Glu- glucose ; Gala-galactose ; Rha-Rhamnose

Figure 3. Chemical Structures of Three flavone glycosides; (1) quercetin 3-O-rutinoside, (2) kaempferol 3-O-rutinoside and (3) kaempferol 3-O-robinobioside of Ficus benjamina and their aglycons, quercetine and kaempferol. These three flavones were highly effective against HSV-1 reaching a selectivity index (SI) of 266, 100 and 666 for compound 1, 2 and3, respectively, while the SI of their aglycons, quercetin and kaempferol amounted only in 7.1 and 3.2, respectively.

Table 2. Antiviral properties of glycosides

Name of glycoside	Plant	Virus	References
Rutin, isoquercetin	*Capparis sinaica* Veill	Avian influenza strain H5N1	[38]
Rutin, kaempferol 3-O-rutinoside and kaempferol 3-O-robinobioside	*Ficus benjamina*	HSV-1, HSV-2	[36]
Flavonol glycosides, isorhamnetin 3-O-β-glucopyranoside-4'-O-β-xylopyranoside andkaempferol 3-O-β-glucopyranoside -4'-O-β-xylopyranoside .	*Diplotaxis harra*	Foot-and-mouth disease virus types A and O	[43]
quercetin-3-O-[beta-xylosyl-(1-2)-alpha-rhamnoside] 4'-O-alpha- rhamnoside	*Zizyphus spina-christi* L	HSV-1	[44]

Table 2. (Continued)

Name of glycoside	Plant	Virus	References
Rutin, 5,7-dimethoxyflavanone-4'-O-beta-D-glucopyranoside and 5,7,3'-trihydroxy-flavanone-4'-O-beta-D-glucopyranoside	*Galium fissurence, Viscum album, Cirsium hypoleucum*	Parainfluenza-3 virus	[39]
Skyrin-8-O-beta-D-glucopyranoside	*Hypericum triquetrifolium*	HSV-1	[45]
5,7-dimethoxyflavanone-4'-O-[2''-O-(5'''-O-trans-cinnamoyl)-beta-D-apiofuranosyl]-beta-D-glucopyranoside	*Galium fissurence, Viscum album, Cirsiumhy poleucum*	HSV-1	[39]
5,7,3',5'-tetrahydroxyflavanone 7-O-glucoside	*Hypericum hircinum* L.	HIV	[46]
Glycyrrhizin or glycyrrhizic acid	*Gkycyrthiza glabra*	Epstein-Barr virus (EBV), HSV-1 Varicella Zoster Virus (VZV) Hepatitis A virus Hepatitis B virus Hepatitis C virus HIV SARS-coronavirus Human cytomegalovirus Influenza virus	[47] [48] [49] [50] [51] [52, 53] [54, 55] [56] [57] [58]

Antiviral mechanisms were investigated in a few studies. The glycoside from *Hypericum hircitum* L. can affect DNA polymerase and Ribonuclease H which are both essential for HIV replication [46].

Although table 2 demonstrates many antiviral effects of glycyrrhizin [47-58], (Figure 4) the antiviral action of this glycoside is still poorly understood. Nevertheless, it was investigated for EBV.

Time of addition experiments suggested that glycyrrhizin interferes with an early step of the EBV replication cycle (possibly penetration) but does not influence viral adsorption [47]. It inhibits HCV full length viral particle and HCV core gene expression both at the RNA and protein level [52].

In addition, glycyrrhizin is able to inhibit phospholipase A2 (PLA2) of HCV [53]. It was also found that glycyrrhizin could influence HIV replication through interfering in virus–cell binding [54] and by inducing the production of beta-chemokines [55].

3.3. Flavonoids

Flavonoids are oxygen-containing aromatic compounds whose antiviral properties are well-known. Quercetin, found in a variety of Mediterranean plants, reduces the infectivity or replication of many viruses: rhinovirus in vivo and in vitro [59], highly pathogenic avian influenza strain H5N1 [38], dengue virus type-2 [60], HSV-1 [61], poliovirus type [62], adenovirus [61], respiratory syncytial virus [63], HCV [64] in vitro.

Mechanisms of its antiviral actions were considered in several cases. Quercetin inhibits rhinoviral infection at multiple stages, including endocytosis, transcription of the viral genome and viral protein synthesis [59]. It was also investigated that quercetin affected intracellular dengue virus type-2 replication but not the virus attachment and entry processes [60].

It was found that quercetin was able to inhibit HCV by attenuating the activity of some heat shock proteins (HSPs) which were involved in NS5A-mediated viral IRES translation [64]. The additional mechanisms of influence of quercetin on HCV were connected with its ability to inhibit HCV NS3 protease and HCV replication in a subgenomic HCV RNA replicon cell system [65].

Kaempferol, a polyhydric flavonol, was isolated from various plant sources including medicinal herbs of the Mediterranean region. Kaempferol exhibited activity against HSV-1 [66], and Japanese encephalitis virus (JEV), suppressing JEV replication and viral protein expression in BHK21 cells [67].

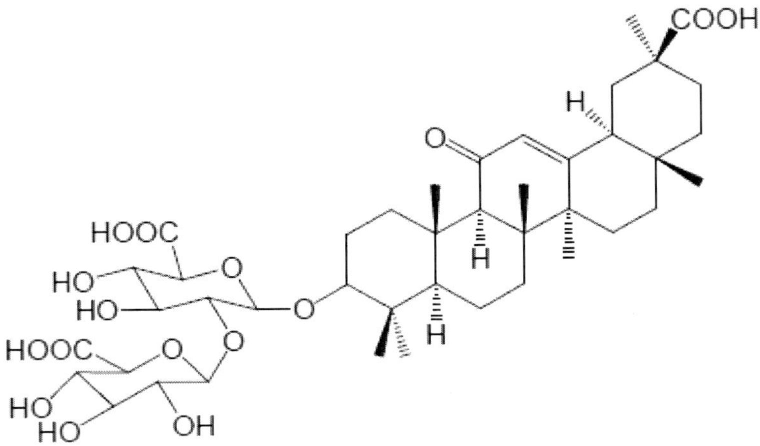

Figure 4. Glycyrrhizin or glycyrrhizic acid was isolated from extracts of *Gkycyrthiza glabra.*

Hypericin and pseudohypericin were isolated and identified from *Hypericum* species (Figure 5). Plants of this genus, for example *H. hircinum* L., *H. humifusum, H. languinosumare, H. maculatum* Crantz, *H. perfoliatum* L., *H. perforatum* L., *H. triquetrifolium* Turra and other species are widely distributed in the Mediterranean region [68].

These compounds inhibited HIV and HCV replication in cell cultures,and their antiviral activity was influenced by the presence of light and oxygen [69]. However, administration of hypericin on HIV-1 and hepatitis C virus patients gave disappointing results as no antiviral effect was observed [70].

In addition, hypericin inhibited human cytomegalovirus in vitro [69]. Xanthohumol, a constituent of *Humulus lupulis,* (Figure 6), was tested for antiviral activity against bovine viral diarrhea virus (BVDV) as a surrogate model of hepatitis C virus (HCV), human immunodeficiency virus (HIV), influenza A virus (FLU-A), influenza B virus (FLU-B), rhinovirus (Rhino), respiratory syncytial virus (RSV), yellow fever virus (YFV), cytomegalovirus (CMV), hepatitis B virus (HBV), and herpes simplex virus type 1 (HSV-1) and type 2 (HSV-2) and a low-to-moderate antiviral activity against these viruses was observed [71].

The mechanism of its anti-HIV-1 effect was investigated, and the inhibition of production of viral p24 antigen and reverse transcriptase in C8166 lymphocytes at non-cytotoxic concentration were demonstrated [72].

Silibinin was isolated from *Silybum marianum.*

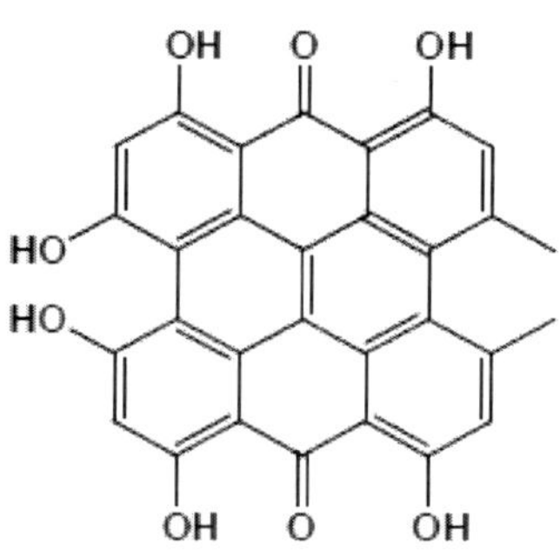

hypericin

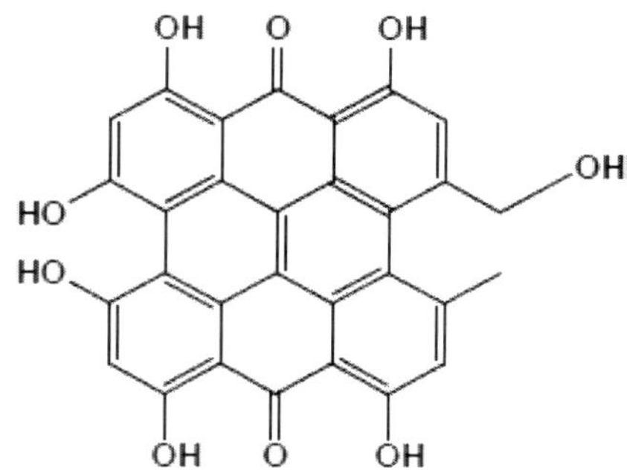

pseudohypericin

Figure 5. Hypericin and pseudohypericin were isolated from Hypericum species.

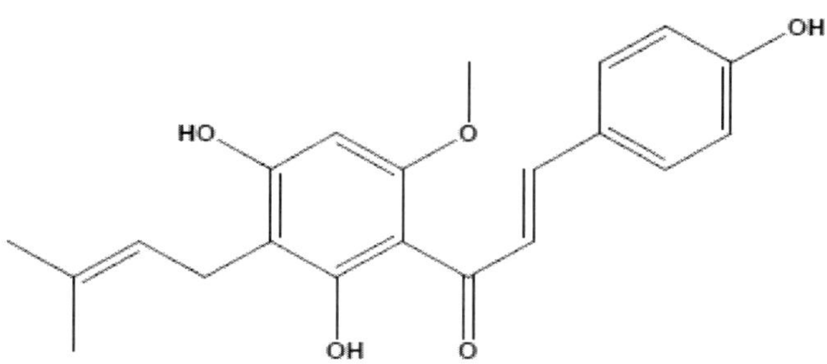

Figure 6. Xanthohumol was isolated from Humulus lupulis.

Investigations into this flavonoid for antiviral activities revealed its efficiency against Hepatitis C virus, reovirus, vesicular stomatitis and influenza viruses [73, 74]. Antiviral activity of silibinin against HCV is explained by inhibition of HCV RNA-dependent RNA polymerase activity [75] and early steps of infection by affecting endosomal trafficking of virions [74].

An analysis of the influence of silibinin on replication of subgenomic replicons from different HCV genotypes in vitro demonstrated a strong inhibition of RNA replication for genotype 1a, genotype 1b and a weak inhibition for genotype 2a. Further investigation of HCV resistance to silibin in in vitro and in vivo pointed to a novel mechanism involving nonstructural protein 4B [76].

Myricetin, a flavonoid found in many grapes, berries, fruits, vegetables, herbs of the Mediterranean region, possesses in vitro activity against HSV-1 [66] and SARS coronavirus [77]; in vitro and in vivo efficacy against different subtypes of influenza viruses including an oseltamivir-resistant strain [78]. Myrecetin inhibited the SARS-CoV helicase protein in vitro by affecting the ATPase activity [77].

Fisetin is a colouring agent of many Mediterranean plants. It inhibited HSV-1 [66], hematopoietic necrosis virus (IHNV), viral hemorrhagic septicemia virus (VHSV) [79] and Enterovirus A71 (EV-A71) [40].

3.4. Terpenes

Limonoids are an important group of triterpenes, isolated from various Mediterranean plants. Two of them, limonin and nomilin were found to inhibit the replication of the human retroviruses: HIV-1 [80] and HTLV-1 [81].

Olean-18-ene triterpenoids from *Cassine xylocarpa* and *Maytenus jelskii* inhibited HIV replication [82].

Carnosic acid (Figure 7) is a natural benzenediol abietane diterpene found in rosemary (*Rosmarinus officinalis*) and common sage (*Salvia officinalis*). The above-mentioned plants have been used in traditional medicine for treatment of diseases of possible viral origin since ancient times.

A replication of human respiratory syncytial virus (hRSV) was suppressed by carnosic acid, with the possible mechanism of its antiviral action due to the influence on the viral proteins and on the viral RNA synthesis [83]. In addition, carnosic acid inhibited HIV-1 protease [84] and HSV-1, HSV-2 [85].

Oleanolic acid and ursolic acid (Figure 7) are also found in rosemary.

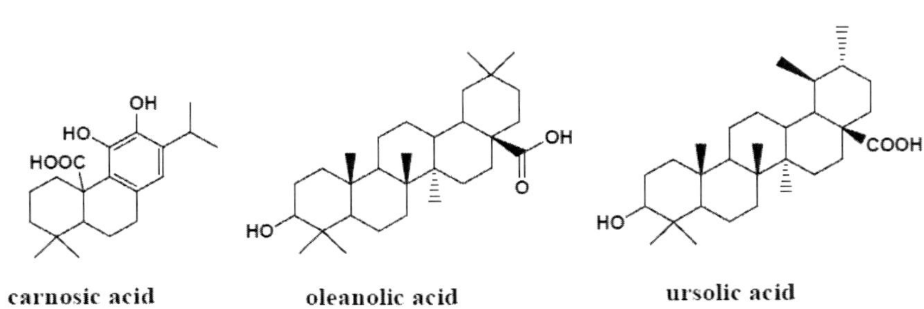

Figure 7. Antiviral constituents of rosemary (Rosmarinus officinalis): carnosic acid, oleanolic acid and ursolic acid.

They exhibited anti-HCV activity, one of the possible mechanisms was the suppression of HCV NS5B RNA-dependent RNA polymerase (RdRp) activity [86]. Ursolic acid but not oleanolic acid was effective against the Semliki Forest virus [87].

4. Mechanisms of Antiviral Agents of Plant Origin

Phytochemicals found in the Mediterranean plants exert their high level of antiviral activities through various complementary mechanisms of action, either inhibiting viral replication, or viral genome synthesis, as shown in Table 3.

Table 3. Antiviral mechanisms of plant phytochemicals

Compound	Virus	Suggested mode of action	References
Lycorine	Poliovirus	Influence on protein synthesis and genome replication of poliovirus	[27]
	West Nile virus	Suppression of viral RNA synthesis	[23]
	HSV-1	Blocking of viral DNA polymerase activity	[30]
5,7,3',5'-tetrahydroxyflavanone 7-O-glucoside	HIV	Blocking of viral DNA polymerase and Ribonuclease H	[46]
Glycyrrhizin	HCV	Influence on viral protein and RNA	[52, 53]
	HIV	Interfering in virus–cell binding	[54]
Quercetin	Rhinovirus	Inhibition of endocytosis, transcription of the viral genome and viral protein synthesis	[59]
	HCV	Influence on viral proteins	[64, 65]
Silibinin	HCV	Inhibition of RNA replication	[75, 76]
Carnosic acid	hRCV	Influence on the viral proteins and RNA synthesis	[83]

Four daphnanedeterpenes, HIV-inhibitors, (daphnetoxin, gnidicin, gniditrin and excoecariatoxin) were isolated and identified from the aerial parts of *Daphne gnidium* L, a small evergreen shrub that is widely distributed in the Mediterranean region [88]. It was shown that daphnetoxin abrogated the surface expression of two main HIV receptors: CXCR4 and CCR5 [88].

A review of the current literature has indicated that plant phytochemicals may affect virus binding to cell membranes, entry into the cell, replication, viral protein translation within the host cell, and formation of certain glycoprotein complexes of the virus envelope. All of these elements are present in antiviral activity of the compounds found in the plants of the Mediterranean region (Table 3).

Conclusion

With its cultural heritage and rich biodiversity, the Mediterranean region has promising therapeutic potentials, especially in the case of antiviral compounds. Further research priorities should include in vivo studies and a better understanding of the mechanisms of plant phytochemicals.

References

[1] Gasparini, R., Amicizia, D., Lai, P. L., Panatto, D. Clinical and socioeconomic impact of seasonal and pandemic influenza in adults and the elderly. *Human vaccines and immunotherapeutics*, 2011 July 18, volume 8, 21-28.

[2] Montagnier, L. 25 years after HIV discovery: prospects for cure and vaccine. *Virology*, 2010 February 20, volume 397, 248-254.

[3] Flexner, C. HIV drug development: the next 25 years. *Nature Reviews Drug Discovery,* 2007 December 3, volume 6, 959-966.

[4] Vere Hodge, R. A., Field, H. J. Antiviral agents for herpes simplex virus. *Advances in Pharmacology*, 2013, volume 68, 1-38.

[5] Neukam, K., Macías, J., Mira, J. A., Pineda, J. A. A review of current anti-HCV treatment regimens and possible future strategies. *Expert opinion on pharmacotherapy,* 2009 February, volume 10, 417-433.

[6] Das, K., Aramini, J. M., Ma, L. C., Krug, R. M., Amold, E. Structures of influenza A proteins and insights into antiviral drug targets. *Nature Structural and Molecular Biology*, 2010 April 11, volume 17, 530-538.

[7] Soltan, M. M., Zaki, A. K. Antiviral screening of forty-two Egyptian medicinal plants. *Journal of Ethnopharmacology*, 2009 October 29, volume 126, 102-107.

[8] Maregesi, S. M., Piebers, L., Ngassapa, O. D., Apers, S., Vingerhoets, R., Cos, P., Vanden Berghe, D. A., Vlientink, A. J. Screening of some Tanzanian medicinal plants from Bunda district for antibacterial antifungal and antiviral activities. *Journal of Ethnopharmacology*, 2008 September 2, volume 119, 58-66.

[9] Arena, A., Bisignano, G., Pavone, B., Tomaino, A., Bonina, F. P., Saija, A., Cristani, M., D'Arrigo, M., Trombetta, D. Antiviral and immune-modulatory effect of a lyophilized extract of Capparis spinosa L. buds. *Phytotherapy Research*, 2007 December 4, volume 22, 313-317.

[10] Droebner, K., Ehrhardt, C., Poetter, A., Ludwig, S., Planz, O. CYSTUS0 52, a polyphenol-rich plant extract, exerts anti-influenza virus activity in mice. *Antiviral Research*, 2007 May 15, volume 76, 1-10.

[11] Ehrhardt, C., Hrincius, E. R., Korte, V., Mazur, I., Droebner, K., Poetter, A., Dreschers, S., Schmolke, M., Planz, O., Ludwig, S. A polyphenol rich plant extract, CYSTUS052, exerts anti influenza virus activity in cell culture without toxic side effects or the tendency to induce viral resistance. *Antiviral Research*, 2007 June 4, volume 76, 38-47.

[12] Wang, G., Wang, H., Song, Y., Jia, C., Wang, Z., Xu, H. Studies on anti-HSV effect of Ficus carica leaves. *Zhong Yao Cai*, 2004 October 27, volume 10, 754-756.

[13] Lazreg Aref, H., Gaaliche, B., Fekih, A., Mars, M., Aouni, M., Pierre Chaumon, J., Said, K. In vitro cytotoxic and antiviral activities of Ficus carica latex extracts. *Natural Product Research*, 2011 February 25, volume 25, 310-319.

[14] Yarmolinsky, L., Zaccai, M., Ben-Shabat, S., Mills, D., Huleihel, M. Antiviral activity of ethanol extracts of Ficus binjamina and Lilium candidum in vitro. *New Biotechnology*, 2009 August 22, volume 26, 307-313.

[15] Astani, A., Reichling, J., Schnitzler, P. Melissa officinalis extract inhibits attachment of herpes simplex virus in vitro. *Chemotherapy*, 2012 February 23, volume 58, 70-77.

[16] Nolkemper, S., Reichling, J., Stintzing, F. C., Carle, R., Schnitzler, P. Antiviral effect of aqueous extracts from species of the Lamiaceae

family against Herpes simplex virus type 1 and type 2 in vitro. *Planta Medica*, 2006 November 7, volume 72, 1378-1382.

[17] Geuenich, S., Goffinet, C., Venzke, S., Nolkemper, S., Baumann, I., Plinkert, P., Reichling, J., Keppler, O. T. Aqueous extracts from peppermint, sage and lemon balm leaves display potent anti-HIV-1 activity by increasing the virion density. *Retrovirology*, 2008 March 20, volume 5, 5-27.

[18] Abad, M. J., Guerra, J. A., Bermejo, P., Irurzun, A., Carrasco, L. Search for antiviral activity in higher plant extracts. *Phytotherapy Research*, 2000 November 29, volume 14, 604-607.

[19] Bedoya, L. M., Sanchez-Palomino, S., Abad, M. J., Bermejo, P., Alcami, J. Anti-HIV activity of medicinal plant extracts. *Journal of Ethnopharmacology*, 2001 September 29, volume 77, 113-116.

[20] Javed, T., Ashfaq, U. A., Riaz, S., Rehman, S., Riazuddin, S. In-vitro antiviral activity of Solanum nigrum against Hepatitis C Virus. *Virology Journal*. 2011 January 19, volume 8, 8-26.

[21] Gyuris, A., Szlávik, L., Minárovits, J., Vasas, A., Molnár, J., Hohmann, J. Antiviral activities of Euphorbia hirta L. against HIV-1, HIV-2 and SIV mac 251. *In vivo*, 2009 March 31, volume 23, 429-432.

[22] He, J., Qi, W. B., Wang, L., Tian, J., Jiao, P. R., Liu, G. Q., Ye, W. C., Liao, M. Amaryllidaceae alkaloids inhibit nuclear-to-cytoplasmic export of ribonucleoprotein (RNP) complex of highly pathogenic avian influenza virus H5N1. *Influenza and other respiratory viruses*. 2012 November 8, in Press.

[23] Zou, G., Puig-Basagoiti, F., Zhang, B., Qing, M., Chen, L., Pankiewicz, K. W., Felczak, K., Yuan, Z., Shi, P. Y. A single-amino acid substitution in West Nile virus 2K peptide between NS4A and NS4B confers resistance to lycorine, a flavivirus inhibitor. *Virology*. 2009 February 5, volume 384, 242-252.

[24] Leven, M., Vanden Berghe, D. A., Vlietinck, A. J. Plant antiviral agents IV. Influence of lycorine on growth pattern of three animal viruses. *Planta Medica*. 1983 October 11, volume 49, 109–114.

[25] Szlávik, L., Gyuris, A., Minárovits, J., Forgo, P., Molnár, J., Hohmann Alkaloids from Leucojum vernum and antiretroviral activity of Amaryllidaceae alkaloids. *Planta Medica*. 2004 September 2, volume 70, 871-873.

[26] Li, S. Y., Chen, C., Zhang, H. Q., Guo, H. Y., Wang, H., Wang, L., Zhang, X., Hua, S. N., Yu, J., Xiao, P. G., Li, R. S., Tan, X. Identification of natural compounds with antiviral activities against

SARS-associated coronavirus. *Antiviral Research*, 2005 July 8, volume 67, 18-23.
[27] Schmid, M., Wimmer, E. IRES-controlled protein synthesis and genome replication of poliovirus. *Archives of virology*. Supplementum, 1994, volume 9, 279-289.
[28] Hwang, Y. C., Chu, J. J., Yang, P. L., Chen, W., Yates, M. V. Rapid identification of inhibitors that interfere with polovirus replication using a cell-based assay. *Antiviral Research*, 2008 January 16, volume 77, 232-236.
[29] Liu, J., Yang, Y., Xu, Y., Ma, C., Qin, C., Zhang, L. Lycorine reduces mortality of human enterovirus 71-infected mice by inhibiting virus replication. *Virology Journal*, 2011 October 27, volume 8, 483–489.
[30] Renard –Nozaki, J., Kim, T., Imakura, Y., Kihara, M., Kobayashi, S. Effect of alkaloids isolated from Amaryllidaceae on herpes simplex virus. *Research in Virology*, 1989 March-April, volume 140, 115-128.
[31] Ghosal, S., Saini, K. S., Razdan, S. Crinum Alkaloids: Their Chemistry and Biology. *Phytochemistry*. 1985, volume 24, 2141-2156.
[32] Jimenez, A., Santos, A., Alonso, G., Vazquez, D. Inhibitors of protein synthesis in eukarytic cells. Comparative effects of some amaryllidaceae alkaloids. *Biochimica et biophysica acta*, 1976 March 17, volume 425, 342-348.
[33] Kukhanova, M., Victorova, L., Krayevsky, A. Peptidyltransferase center of ribosomes. On the mechanism of action of alkaloid lycorine. *Federation of European Biochemical Societies Letters*, 1983 August 22, volume 160, 129-133.
[34] Takemura, Y., Ju-ichi, M., Ito, C., Furukawa, H., Tokuda, H. Studies on the inhibitory effects of some acridone alkaloids on Epstein-Barr virus activation. *Planta Medica*, 1995 August 15, volume 61, 366-368.
[35] Choi, H. G., Kim, J. H., Lee, C. H., Ahn, Y. J., Song, J. H., Back,S. H., Kwon, D. H. Antiviral activity of quercetin 7-rhamnoside against porcine epidemic diarrhea virus. *Antiviral Research*, 2009 January 6, volume 81, 77-81.
[36] Yarmolinsky, L., Huleihel, M., Zaccai, M., Ben-Shabat, S. Potent antiviral flavone glycosides from Ficus benjamina leaves. *Fitoterapia*, 2011 December 3, volume 83, 362-367.
[37] Bae, E. A., Han, M., Lee, M., Kim, D. H. In vitro inhibitory effect of some flavonoids on rotavirus infectivity. *Biological and pharmaceutical bulletin*, 2000 September 4, volume 23, 122-124.

[38] Ibrahim, A. K., Youssef, A. I., Arafa, A. S., Ahmed, S. A. Anti-H5N1 virus flavonoids from Capparis sinaica Veill. *Natural product research*, 2013 May 7, in Press.

[39] Orhan, D. D., Ozçelik, B., Ozgen, S., Ergun, F. Antibacterial, antifungal, and antiviral activities of some flavonoids. *Microbiological Research*, 2010 August 20, volume 165, 496-504.

[40] Lin, Y. J., Chang, Y. C., Hsiao, N. W., Hsieh, J. L., Wang, C. Y., Kung, S. H., Tsai, F. J., Lan, Y. C., Lin, C. W. Fisetin and rutin as 3C protease inhibitors of enterovirus A71. *Journal of Virological Methods*, 2012 June 15, volume 182, 93-98.

[41] Goo, H. R., Choi, J. S., Na, D. H. Simultaneous determination of quercetin and its glycosides from the leaves of Nelumbo nucifera by reversed-phase high-performance liquid-chromatography. *Archives of Pharmacological Research*, 2009 February 6, volume 32, 201-206.

[42] Tao, J., Qinxue, H., Yang, J., Li, R., Li, X., Lu, C., Chen, C, Wang, L., Shattock, R., Ben, K. In vitro anti-HIV and –HSV activity and safety of sodium rutin sulfate as a microbicide candidate. *Antiviral Research*, 2007 September 16, volume 75, 227-233.

[43] Kassem, M. E., Afifi, M. S., Marzouk, M. M., Mostafa, M. A. Two new flavonol glycosides and biological activities of Diplotaxis harra (Forssk.) Boiss. *Natural product research*, 2013 August 20, 7-14.

[44] Shahat, A. A., Pieters, L., Apers, S., Nazeif, N. M., Abdel-Azim, N. S., Berghe, D. V., Vlietinck, A. J. Chemical and biological investigations on Zizyphus spina-christi L. *Phytotherapy research*, 2000 September 29, volume 15, 593-597.

[45] Naithani, R., Huma, L. C., Holland, L. E., Shukla, D., McCormick, D. L., Mehta, R. G., Moriarty, R. M. Antiviral activity of phytochemicals: a comprehensive review. *Mini-Reviews in Medicinal Chemistry*, 2008 October 7, volume 8, 1106-1133.

[46] Esposito, F., Sanna, C., Del Vecchio, C., Cannas, V., Venditti, A., Corona, A., Bianco, A., Serrilli, A. M., Guarcini, L., Parolin, C., Ballero, M., Tramontano, E. Hypericum hircinum L. components as new single-molecule inhibitors of both HIV-1 reverse transcriptase-associated DNA polymerase and ribonuclease H activities. *Pathogens and disease*, 2013 July 2, volume 68, 116-124.

[47] Lin, J. C. Mechanism of action of glycyrrhizic acid in inhibition of Epstein-Barr virus replication in vitro. *Antiviral Research,* 2003 June 24, volume 59, 41-47.

[48] Ikeda, T., Yokomizo, K., Okawa, M., Tsuchihashi, R., Kinjo, J., Nohara, T., Uyeda, M. Anti-herpes virus type 1 activity of oleanane-type triterpenoids. *Biological and pharmaceutical bulletin*, 2005 September 2, volume 28, 1779-1781.
[49] Baba, M., Shigeta, S. Antiviral activity of glycyrrhizin against varicella-zoster virus in vitro. *Antiviral Research*, 1987 February 4, volume 7, 99-107.
[50] Crance, J. M., Biziagos, E., Passagot, J., Van cuyck-Gandre, H., Deloince, R. Inhibition of hepatitis A virus replication in vitro by antiviral compounds. *Journal of Medical Virology*, 1990 June 10, volume 31, 155-160.
[51] Sato, H., Goto, W., Yamamura, J., Kurokawa, M., Kageyama, S., Takahara, T., Watanabe, Ashiraki, K. Therapeutic basis of glycyrrhizin on chronic hepatitis B. *Antiviral Research*, 1996 May 5, volume 30, 171-177.
[52] Ashfaq, U. A., Masoud, M. S., Nawaz, Z., Riazuddin, S. Glycyrrhizin as antiviral agent against Hepatitis C Virus. *Journal of translational medicine*, 2011 July 18, volume 9, 112-116.
[53] Matsumoto, Y., Matsuura, T., Aoyagi, H., Matsuda, M., Hmwe, S. S., Date, T., Watanabe, N., Watashi, K., Suzuki, R., Ichinose, S., Wake, K., Suzuki, T., Miyamura, T., Wakita, T., Aizaki, H. Antiviral activity of glycyrrhizin against hepatitis C virus in vitro. *PLoS one*, 2013 July 18, volume 8, doi: 10.1371/journal.pone.0068992.
[54] Ito, M., Sato, A., Hirabayashi, K., Tanabe, F., Shigeta, S., Baba, M., De Clerq, E. (1988). Mechanism of inhibitory effect of glycyrrhizin on replication of human immunodeficiency virus (HIV). *Antiviral Research*, 1988 December 11, volume 10, 289-298.
[55] Sasaki, H., Takei, M., Kobayashi, M., Pollard, R. B., Suzuki, F. (2002). Effect of glycyrrhizin, an active component of licorice roots, on HIV replication in cultures of peripheral blood mononuclear cells from HIV-seropositive patients. *Pathobiology*, 2003 April 5, volume 70,:229-236.
[56] Hoever, G., Baltina, L., Michaelis, M., Kondratenko, R., Baltina, L., Tolstikov, G. A., Doerr, H. W., Cinatl, J. J. Antiviral activity of glycyrrhizic acid derivatives against SARS-coronavirus. *Journal of Medicinal Chemistry*, 2005 February 24, volume 48, 1256-1259.
[57] Harada, H., Suzu, S., Ito, T., Okada, S. Selective expansion and engraftment of human CD16+ NK cells in NOD/SCID mice. *European Journal of Immunology*, 2005 December 6, volume 35, 3599-3605.

[58] Utsunomiya, T., Kobayashi, M., Pollard, R. B., Suzuki, F. Glycyrrhizin, an active component of licorise roots reduces morbidity and mortality of mice infected with lethal doses of influenza virus. *Antimicrobal Agents and Chemotherapy,* 1997 March, volume 41, 551-556.

[59] Ganesan, S., Faris, A. N., Comstock, A T., Wang, Q., Nanua, S., Hershenson, M. B., Sajjan, U. S. Quercetin inhibits rhinovirus replication in vitro and in vivo. *Antiviral Research*, 2012 March 23, volume 94, 258-271.

[60] Zandi, K., Teoh, B. T., Sam, S. S., Wong, P. F., Mustafa, M. R., Abubakar, S. Antiviral activity of four types of bioflavonoid against dengue virus type-2. *Virology Journal*, 2011 December 28, volume 8,: 560-566.

[61] Chiang, L. C., Chiang, W., Liu, M. C., Liu, C. C. In vitro antiviral activities of Caesalpinia pulcherrima and its related flavonoids. *The Journal of Antimicrobial Chemotherapy*, 2003 July 1, volume 52, 194-198.

[62] Neznanov, N., Kondratova, A., Chumakov, K. M., Neznanova, L., Kondratov, R., Banerjee, A. K., Gudkov, A. V. Quercetinase pirin makes poliovirus replication resistant to flavonoid quercetin. *DNA and Cell Biology*, 2008 April 13, volume 27, 191-198.

[63] Li, Y. L., Li, K. M., Su, M. X., Leung, K. T., Chen, Y. W., Zhang, Y. W. Studies on antiviral constituents in stems and leaves of Pithecellibium clypearia. *Zhongguo Zhong Yao Za Zhi*, 2006 March 5, volume 31, 397-400.

[64] Gonzalez, O., Fontanes, V., Raychaudhuri, S., Loo, R., Loo, J., Arumugaswami, V., Sun, R., Dasgupta, A., French, S. W. The heat shock protein inhibitor Quercetin attenuates hepatitis C virus production. *Hepatology*, 2009 August 10, volume 50, 1656-1764.

[65] Bachmetov, L., Gal-Tanamy, M., Shapira, A., Vorobeychik, M., Giterman-Galam, T., Sathiyamoorthy, P., Golan-Goldhirsh, A., Benhar, I., Tur-Kaspa, R., Zemel, R. Suppression of hepatitis C virus by flavonoid quercetin is mediated by inhibition of NS3 protease activity. *Journal of Viral Hepatitis*, 2011 May 16, volume 19, 81-88.

[66] Lyu, S. Y., Rhim, J. Y., Park, W. B. Antiherpetic activities of flavonoids against Herpes Simplex Virus Type 1 (HSV-1) and Type 2 (HSV-2) in Vitro. *Archives of Pharmacal Research*, 2005 June 21, volume, 28, 1293-1301.

[67] Zhang, T., Wu, Z., Du, J., Hu, Y., Liu, L., Yang, F., Jin, Q. Anti-Japanese-encephalitis-viral effects of kaempferol and daidzin and their RNA-binding characteristics. *PLoS one*, 2011 December 12, volume 7.

[68] Gonzales-Tejero, M. R., Casares-Porcel, M., Sanches-Rojas, C. P., Ramiro-Gutierrez, J. M., Molero-Mesa, J., Pieroni, A., Giusti, H. E., Censorii, E., de Pasquale, C., Della, A., Paraskeva-Hadijchambi, D., Hadjichambis, A., Houmani, Z., El- Demerdash, M., El-Zayat, M., Hmamouchi, M., Eljohrig, S. (2008). Medicinal plants in the Mediterranean area: Synthesis of the results of the project Rubia. *Journal of Ethnopharmacology,* 2007 December 14, volume 116, 341-357.

[69] Karioti, A., Bilia, A. R. Hypericins as potential leads for new therapeutics. *International Journal of Molecular Sciences*, 2010 February 4, volume 11, 562-594.

[70] Kubin, A., Wierrani, F., Burner, U., Alth, G., Grünberger, W. Hypericin--the facts about a controversial agent. *Current pharmaceutical design*, 2005 March 8, volume 11, 233-253.

[71] Buckwold, V. E., Wilson, R. J., Nalca, A., Beer, B. B., Voss, T. G., Turpin, J. A., Buckheit, R. W., Wei, J., Wenzel-Mathers, M., Walton, E. M., Smith, R. J., Pallansch, M., Ward, P., Wells, J., Chuvala, L., Sloane, S., Paulman, R., Russell, J., Hartman, T., Ptak, R. Antiviral activity of hop constituents against a series of DNA and RNA viruses. *Antiviral Research*, 2004 January 5, volume 61, 57-62.

[72] Wang, Q., Ding, Z. H., Liu, J. K., Zheng, Y. T. Xanthohumol, a novel anti-HIV-1 agent purified from Hops Humulus lupulus. *Antiviral Research*, 2004 December 8, volume 64, 189-194.

[73] Dai, J. P., Wu, L. Q., Li, R., Zhao, X. F., Wan, Q. Y., Chen, X. X., Li, W. Z., Wang, G. F., Li, K. S. Identification of 23-(s)-2-amino-3-phenylpropanoyl-silybin as an antiviral agent for influenza a virus infection in vitro and in vivo. *Antimicrobial agents and chemotherapy*, 2013 July 8, volume 57, 4433-4443.

[74] Blaising, J., Lévy, P. L., Gondeau, C., Phelip, C., Varbanov, M., Teissier, E., Ruggiero, F., Polyak, S J., Oberlies, N. H., Ivanovic, T., Boulant, S., Pécheur, E. I. Silibinin inhibits hepatitis C virus entry into hepatocytes by hindering clathrin-dependent trafficking. *Cellular microbiology*, 2013 June 13, volume 15, 1866-1882.

[75] Ahmed-Belkacem, A., Ahnou, N., Barbotte, L., Wychowski, C., Pallier, C., Brillet, R., Pohl, R. T., Pawlotsky, J. M. Silibinin and related compounds are direct inhibitors of hepatitis C virus RNA-dependent

RNA polymerase. *Gastroenterology*, 2009 November 30, volume 38, 1112-1122.

[76] Esser-Nobis, K., Romero-Brey, I., Ganten, T. M., Gouttenoire, J., Harak, C., Klein, R., Schemmer, P., Binder, M., Schnitzler, P., Moradpour, D., Bartenschlager, R., Polyak, S. J., Stremmel, W., Penin, F., Eisenbach, C., Lohmann, V. Analysis of hepatitis C virus resistance to silibinin in vitro and in vivo points to a novel mechanism involving nonstructural protein 4B. *Hepatology*, 2013 February 7, volume 57, 953-963.

[77] Yu, M. S., Lee, J., Lee, J. M., Kim, Y., Chin, Y. W., Jee, J. G., Keum, Y. S., Jeong, Y. J. Identification of myricetin and scutellarein as novel chemical inhibitors of the SARS coronavirus helicase, nsP13. *Bioorganic and medicinal chemistry letters*, 2012 June 15, volume 22, 49-54.

[78] Park, S., Kim, J. I., Lee, I., Lee, S., Hwang, M. W., Bae, J. Y., Heo, J., Kim, D., Han, S. Z., Park, M. S. Aronia melanocarpa and its components demonstrate antiviral activity against influenza viruses. *Molecular Cell Biology Research Communication,* 2013 October 11, volume 440, 14-19.

[79] Kang, S. Y., Kang, J. Y., Oh, M. J. Antiviral activities of flavonoids isolated from the bark of Rhus verniciflua stokes against fish pathogenic viruses In Vitro. *Journal of Microbiology*, 2012 April 2, volume 50, 293-300.

[80] Rukachaisirikul, V., Pailee, P., Hiranrat, A., Tuchinda, P., Yoosook, C., Kasisit, J., Taylor, W. C., Reutrakul, V. Anti-HIV-1 protostane triterpenes and digeranylbenzophenone from trunk bark and stems of Garcinia speciosa. *Planta medica*, 2003 September 29, volume 69, 1141-1146.

[81] Balestrieri, E., Pizzimenti, F., Ferlazzo, A., Giofrè, S. V., Iannazzo, D., Piperno, A., Romeo, R., Chiacchio, M. A., Mastino, A., Macchi, B. Antiviral activity of seed extract from Citrus bergamia towards human retroviruses. *Bioorganic and medicinal chemistry*, 2011 March 15, volume 19, 2084-2089.

[82] Osorio, A. A., Muñóz, A., Torres-Romero, D., Bedoya, L. M., Perestelo, N. R., Jiménez, I. A., Alcamí, J., Bazzocchi, I. L. Olean-18-ene triterpenoids from Celastraceae species inhibit HIV replication targeting NF-kB and Sp1 dependent transcription. *European journal of medicinal chemistry*, 2012 June 12, volume 52, 295-303.

[83] Shin, H. B., Choi, M. S., Ryu, B., Lee, N. R., Kim, H. I., Choi, H. E., Chang, J., Lee, K. T., Jang, D. S., Inn, K. S. Antiviral activity of

carnosic acid against respiratory syncytial virus. *Virology Journal*, 2013 October 8, volume 10, 303-309.

[84] Paris, A., Strukelj, B., Renko, M., Turk, V., Pukl, M., Umek, A., Korant, B. D. Inhibitory effect of carnosic acid on HIV-1 protease in cell-free assays [corrected]. *Journal of Natural Products*, 1993 August 22, volume 56, 1426-1430.

[85] Gigante, B., Santos, C., Silva, A. M., Curto, M. J., Nascimento, M. S., Pinto, E., Pedro, M., Cerqueira, F., Pinto, M. M., Duarte, M. P., Laires, A., Rueff, J., Gonçalves, J., Pegado, M. I., Valdeira, M. L. Catechols from abietic acid synthesis and evaluation as bioactive compounds. *Bioorganic and medicinal chemistry*, 2003 April 17, volume 11, 1631-1638.

[86] Kong, L., Li, S., Liao, Q., Zhang, Y., Sun, R., Zhu, X., Zhang, Q., Wang, J., Wu, X., Fang, X., Zhu, Y. Oleanolic acid and ursolic acid: novel hepatitis C virus antivirals that inhibit NS5B activity. *Antiviral Research*, 2013 April 23, volume 98, 44-53.

[87] Mulholland, D. A., Mohammed, A. M., Coombes, P. H., Haque, S., Pohjala, L. L., Tammela, P. S., Crouch, N. R. Triterpenoid acids and lactones from the leaves of Fadogia tetraquetra var. tetraquetra (Rubiaceae). *Natural product communication*, 2011 November 6, volume 6, 1573-1576.

[88] Vidal, V., Potterat, O., Louvel, S., Hamy, F., Mojarrab, M., Sanglier, J. J., Klimkait, T., Hamburger, M. Library-based discovery and characterization of daphnane diterpenes as potent and selective HIV inhibitors in Daphne gnidium. *Journal of Natural Products*, 2011 December 8, volume 75, 414-419.

INDEX

A

B

C

D

E

F

G

H

J

K

L

M

N

O

P

Q

R

S

T

U

V

W

Y

Z